THE CASE REVIEWS YOU TRUST,

in a format you've been waiting for.

The most trusted radiology review book series is now online! With the new **Case Reviews Online**, you can review your way, with interactive features and customizable study tools that are accessible online, anytime.

Case Reviews Online allows you to:

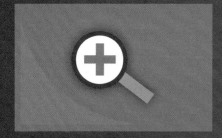

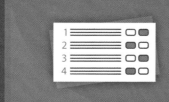

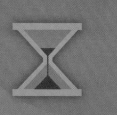

Accurately assess your board readiness with customizable tests that mimic the format of official exams.

Test your understanding of each case with the four multiple-choice questions that accompany them.

Spend more time reviewing and less time searching because cases are organized by radiologic subspecialty.

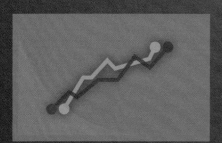

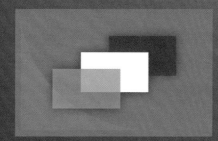

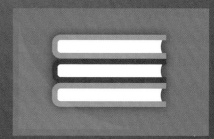

Confirm or challenge your diagnostic interpretations by selecting the label on/label off option.

Track your progress by comparing your previous test results with your latest scores.

Review cases from a variety of subspecialties including Musculoskeletal, Thoracic, Interventional, Spine, Pediatrics, Brain, Head and Neck, and Emergency Medicine.

SEE WHAT **CASE REVIEWS ONLINE** CAN DO FOR YOU.

To learn more, visit **casereviewsonline.com**

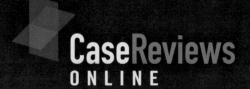

SEE WHAT **CASE REVIEWS ONLINE** CAN DO FOR YOU.

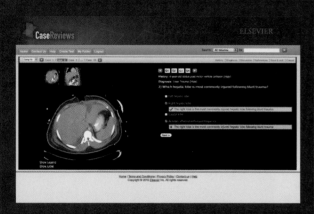

Practice Test questions on Case Reviews Online allow you to see rationale for both correct and incorrect questions as you take the test.

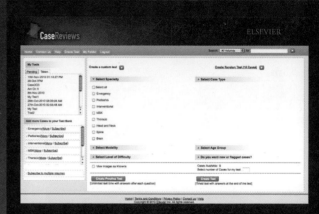

With Case Reviews Online, users can create a Practice Test with unlimited test time, or a "Real" Test that is timed and simulates the board-testing experience.

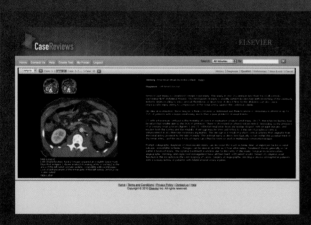

You can choose to take tests with or without help, with the ability to show or hide legends, labels, history, diagnosis, questions, discussion and review.

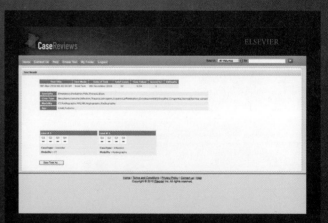

Results include full details on the test you took, along with test title, test mode, date and time, number of cases, score and difficulty.

To learn more, visit **casereviewsonline.com**

To inquire about Institutional Access contact
h.licensing@elsevier.com

CASE REVIEW
Gastrointestinal Imaging

Third Edition

Series Editor
David M. Yousem, MD, MBA
Professor of Radiology
Director of Neuroradiology
Russell H. Morgan Department of Radiology
and Radiological Science
The Johns Hopkins Medical Institutions
Baltimore, Maryland

Other Volumes in the CASE REVIEW Series
Brain Imaging, Second Edition
Breast Imaging
Cardiac Imaging
Duke Review of MRI Principles
Emergency Radiology
General and Vascular Ultrasound, Second Edition
Genitourinary Imaging, Second Edition
Musculoskeletal Imaging, Second Edition
Nuclear Medicine, Second Edition
Obstetric and Gynecologic Ultrasound, Second Edition
Pediatric Imaging, Second Edition
Spine Imaging, Second Edition
Thoracic Imaging, Second Edition
Vascular and Interventional Imaging

ELSEVIER
SAUNDERS

Vincent H.S. Low, MBBS, FRANZCR
Associate Professor
Department of Medicine and Pharmacology
University of Western Australia
Crawley, Western Australia

Consultant Radiologist
InSight Clinical Imaging
Joondalup, Western Australia

CASE REVIEW

Gastrointestinal Imaging

THIRD EDITION

CASE REVIEW SERIES

ELSEVIER
SAUNDERS

1600 John F. Kennedy Blvd.
Ste 1800
Philadelphia, PA 19103-2899

Notices

Knowledge and best practice in this field are constantly changing. As new research and experience broaden our understanding, changes in research methods, professional practices, or medical treatment may become necessary.

Practitioners and researchers must always rely on their own experience and knowledge in evaluating and using any information, methods, compounds, or experiments described herein. In using such information or methods they should be mindful of their own safety and the safety of others, including parties for whom they have a professional responsibility.

With respect to any drug or pharmaceutical products identified, readers are advised to check the most current information provided (i) on procedures featured or (ii) by the manufacturer of each product to be administered, to verify the recommended dose or formula, the method and duration of administration, and contraindications. It is the responsibility of practitioners, relying on their own experience and knowledge of their patients, to make diagnoses, to determine dosages and the best treatment for each individual patient, and to take all appropriate safety precautions.

To the fullest extent of the law, neither the Publisher nor the authors, contributors, or editors, assume any liability for any injury and/or damage to persons or property as a matter of products liability, negligence or otherwise, or from any use or operation of any methods, products, instructions, or ideas contained in the material herein.

ISBN: 978-0-323-08721-6

Content Strategist: Don Scholz
Content Development Specialist: Gina Donato
Publishing Services Manager: Patricia Tannian
Project Manager: Carrie Stetz
Design Direction: Steven Stave

Printed in the United States of America

Last digit is the print number: 9 8 7 6 5 4 3 2 1

Working together to grow libraries in developing countries

www.elsevier.com | www.bookaid.org | www.sabre.org

ELSEVIER | BOOK AID International | Sabre Foundation

To my dear and loving wife, Rena. Everything that I am, I am because of you. You have been by my side with unconditional love. You have been behind me with your loyalty, patience, and support. Thank you for being my sweetheart and my best friend.

I have been very gratified by the popularity and positive feedback that the authors of the *Case Review* series have received on the publication of the first and second editions of their volumes. Reviews in journals and word-of-mouth comments have been uniformly favorable. The authors have done an outstanding job filling the niche of an affordable, easy-to-read, case-based learning tool that supplements the material in *The Requisites* series. I have been told by residents, fellows, and practicing radiologists that the *Case Review* series is the ideal means for studying for oral board examinations and subspecialty certification tests.

Although some students learn best in a noninteractive study book mode, others need the anxiety or excitement of being quizzed. The selected format for the *Case Review* series (which consists of showing a few images needed to construct a differential diagnosis and then asking a few clinical and imaging questions) was designed to simulate the board examination experience. The only difference is that the *Case Review* texts provide the correct answer and immediate feedback. The limits and range of the reader's knowledge are tested through scaled cases ranging from relatively easy to very hard. The *Case Review* series also offers a brief discussion of each case, a link back to the pertinent *The Requisites* volume, and up-to-date references from the literature.

Because of the popularity of this series, we have been rolling out the second and third editions of the *Case Review* volumes. The expectation is that these editions will bring the content up to the current knowledge limits of the field, introduce new modalities and new techniques, and provide new and even more graphic examples of pathology. To adjust to the upcoming change from an oral board examination to a computer-based one, the *Case Review* series has changed. We have moved to an even more engaging live platform through the use of the Internet. The questions have been reframed into multiple-choice format, the links are dynamic to online references, and feedback is interactive with correct and incorrect answers. Please see the website www.casereviewsonline.com to see how the *Case Review* series has evolved to prepare trainees for the board examinations and practitioners for reading specialty cases. Personally, I am very excited about the future. Join us.

David M. Yousem, MD, MBA

When Drs. Halpert and Fescko declined the invitation to create the online version of the second edition of the *Gastrointestinal Imaging Case Review Series,* I asked around who was "the man" in gastrointestinal radiology these days. There was a consensus that the person with the most amazing material and the best talent for creating an online product was Vincent H.S. Low in Western Australia. Vincent accepted the offer eagerly and was immediately productive in creating a whole new feel and attraction to the cases and rewrote the material in expert fashion. The interactive format came alive in his hands, and the result is a vast improvement in the quality of the *Elsevier Case Review* product, in part because it is now online, with all the functionality that medium allows.

However, Dr. Low did not skimp on the hard copy version. This book will no doubt guide many residents through the boards and many radiologists through days in fluoroscopy and cross-sectional abdominal imaging.

My thanks and warm regards go out to Vincent Low, a new author and the latest contributor to the Elsevier *Case Review Series.*

David M. Yousem, MD, MBA

I was delighted to receive the call from Elsevier to serve as author of the third edition of *Gastrointestinal Imaging Case Review*. I was pleased to carry forward from the work of Dr. Peter Feczko in the first edition and Dr. Robert Halpert in the second edition.

Gastrointestinal imaging is considered by many, especially those of us in the specialty, to be the oldest of the specialities within radiology. Roentgen made his great discovery in 1895. Within a few months, pioneers began using the technology to observe gastrointestinal motility using ingested opaque materials such as liquid bismuth and beads of various materials. A lot has changed since then.

Almost all the cases in this book have been updated to reflect the changing trends in gastrointestinal imaging. A shift has occurred with a decline in the indications for barium studies and increasing reliance on cross-sectional techniques for making diagnoses. Cases have been updated to reflect this change in practice. However, modern radiologists need to maintain the skills to interpret basic radiology signs; this is also reflected in the cases presented in this edition. Fluoroscopy also remains a valuable diagnostic tool. There are conditions unique to gastrointestinal imaging in which fluoroscopy can most effectively and efficiently assist in making the diagnosis.

I have approached this book with the realization that it will be in the hands of trainees as they prepare for their oral board examinations. I have recalled all the lessons gifted to me by my teachers, and I have reflected on the feedback from all my trainees. The teaching of radiology has relied in large part on discussion around cases. This is reflected in teaching rounds and in the final hurdle for the trainee, the oral board or viva examination. The cases and their discussions in this book guide the reader through the thought process and steps that lead to the correct diagnosis. The student must realize that a good understanding of anatomy and physiology and a knowledge of pathology lead to a recognition of the radiologic signs. Knowing what to exclude from a differential diagnosis is as important as knowing what to include. As a teacher, it is important to me that my students learn the journey through the diagnostic process. This, I hope, will prepare them for their professional life as diagnosticians for decades to come.

Vincent H.S. Low, MBBS, FRANZCR

Opening Round

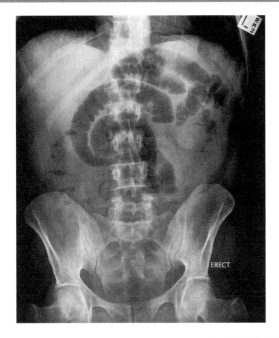

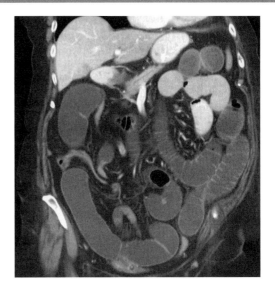

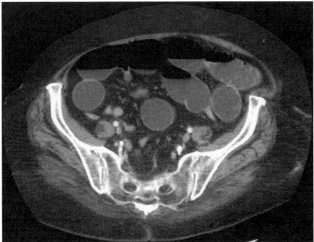

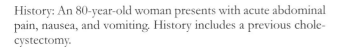

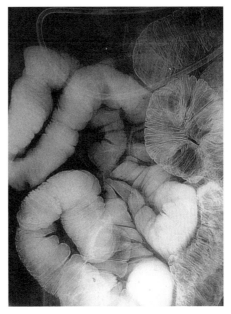

History: An 80-year-old woman presents with acute abdominal pain, nausea, and vomiting. History includes a previous cholecystectomy.

1. Which is the *best* diagnosis based on the location of the abnormality for this patient?
   A. Jejunum
   B. Ileum
   C. Right colon
   D. Diffuse

2. Which choice *best* describes the pathological process visible on CT for this patient?
   A. Hernia
   B. Tumor mass
   C. Inflammatory disease
   D. No etiology is demonstrated

3. The patient undergoes an enteroclysis 2 weeks later. Which choice *best* describes the findings?
   A. Adhesions
   B. Tumor
   C. Crohn's disease
   D. Hernia

4. At laparotomy, small bowel obstruction (SBO) was confirmed as imaged with dense adhesions the culprit. Which of the following regarding imaging of SBO is true?
   A. Plain film is diagnostic in 90% of cases.
   B. In ischemia, bowel wall may be hyperdense on noncontrast CT.
   C. Simple obstructed versus strangulated bowel can be differentiated based on clinical information and lab values.
   D. The small bowel feces sign is seen only in the setting of Crohn's.

Small Bowel Obstruction

1. B

2. D

3. A

4. B

References

Maglinte DD, Kelvin FM, Rowe MG, et al: Small bowel obstruction: optimizing radiologic investigation and nonsurgical management. *Radiology* 2001;218:39-46.

Silva AC, Pimenta M, Guimaraes LS: Small bowel obstruction: what to look for. *Radiographics* 2009;29:423-439.

Cross-Reference

Gastrointestinal Imaging: THE REQUISITES, 3rd ed, p 107.

Comment

Plain films of the abdomen should be the first step if bowel obstruction is suspected. The routine plain films of the abdomen are supine and upright images when possible. The classic differential air-fluid levels seen in the first 48 to 72 hours of a small bowel obstruction are almost pathognomonic of a mechanical small bowel obstruction. It is important to clearly understand what constitutes a differential air-fluid level. It represents two different air-fluid levels in the *same* loop of bowel. Air-fluid levels, in themselves, are nonspecific and can be seen in any number of conditions apart from mechanical obstruction. However, in mechanical obstruction, the motility of the bowel is exaggerated as it forcefully tries to push intestinal content past the narrowed segment, resulting in a to-and-fro movement of fluid. As a result there is an uneven distribution of fluid when the patient is raised to the upright position. Hence, differential air-fluid levels are seen in the same loop of bowel. With a paralytic ileus, on the other hand, the bowel movement is diminished or absent, and water distribution is equalized throughout the bowel; as a result, differential air-fluid levels are not seen.

Increasingly, CT of the abdomen is being done for an abdominal complaint, especially in the acute setting. CT is able to establish the diagnosis: The findings are dilated loops of small bowel and a transition zone from dilated to collapsed loops. Occasionally the cause is demonstrated. CT is of particular value in detecting closed-loop obstruction or strangulation. CT can also identify other causes of acute abdominal pain. If the diagnosis remains unclear, barium studies (enteroclysis) may be of value to delineate the level, cause, and severity of the obstruction.

Notes

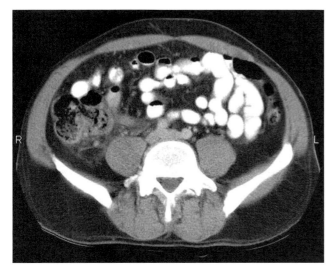

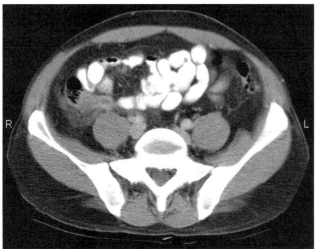

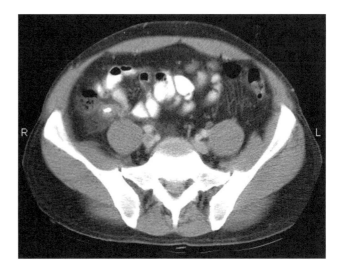

History: A 42-year-old man presents with acute abdomen and right lower quadrant pain and tenderness.

1. What is the *best* diagnosis for this patient based on the imaging?
   A. Appendicitis
   B. Ileitis
   C. Ureteric colic
   D. Right colitis

2. Which choice *best* characterizes the calcific density?
   A. Appendicolith
   B. Ureteric calculus
   C. Phlebolith
   D. Diverticulith

3. Which of the following statements about imaging of acute appendicitis is true?
   A. Plain abdominal radiography usually reveals nonspecific localized right lower quadrant paralytic ileus.
   B. An appendicolith is visible on plain radiography in 20% to 25% of cases.

C. Ultrasound is the modality of choice for children and young women.
D. Radionuclide scanning with ^{99m}Tc pertechnetate is highly sensitive and specific for the diagnosis of appendicitis.

4. Which of the following regarding CT imaging of the differential diagnosis of right lower quadrant pain is true?
   A. Angiodysplasia is suggested by right lower quadrant pain with rectal passage of altered blood and focal colonic wall enhancement.
   B. Pseudomembranous colitis is diagnosed by the presence of haustral thickening with submucosal edema (lucent stripe), described as the accordion sign.
   C. Crohn's disease is suggested by small bowel feces in the terminal ileum.
   D. Right colonic diverticulitis is suggested by pericolonic soft tissue stranding sparing the cecal pole.

C A S E   2

Acute Appendicitis

1. A

2. A

3. C

4. D

Reference

Duran JC, Beidle TR, Perret R, et al: CT imaging of acute right lower quadrant disease. *Am J Roentgenol* 1997;168:411-416.

Cross-Reference

Gastrointestinal Imaging: *THE REQUISITES,* 3rd ed, p 317.

Comment

Acute appendicitis is a common abdominal emergency condition. Indeed, it is the most common acute abdominal emergency in industrialized countries. Its incidence is approximately 10 to 11 per 10,000, but it has been slowly declining. The surface anatomy of the appendix was first described by McBurney in the 19th century, giving rise to the well-known McBurney's point in the right lower quadrant.

Although there has been much discussion about the merits of various modalities in the diagnosis, it is now clear that multidetector computed tomography (MDCT) is the imaging tool of choice. It is able to see the appendix easier than other methods, and it can also provide other crucial information, for example, regarding complications. Findings on MDCT include, in simple uncomplicated appendicitis, thickening of the appendix beyond 6 mm, appendiceal enhancement (vascular congestion), periappendiceal stranding, and occasionally small amounts of fluid around the appendix or in the cul-de-sac (see figures).

Plain film evaluation of appendicitis is usually not helpful. If a calcified appendicolith is seen in a patient with appropriate clinical symptoms, it is diagnostic (see figures). However, this is unusual. Occasionally one might see a focal ileus effect in the right lower quadrant, but by far the most common plain film finding is normal. Medical students and residents should discipline themselves to find the appendix on every abdominal CT case they encounter. Sometimes finding an unusually located appendix can be a chore. The more you do, the better you get at it.

Notes

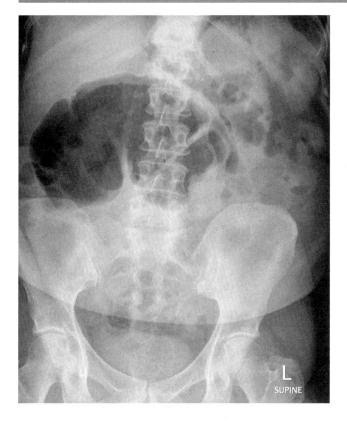

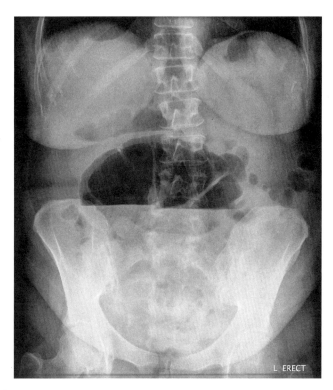

History: A 68-year-old woman presents with sudden onset of severe colicky abdominal pain and vomiting.

1. Which choice is the most likely diagnosis for this patient?
   A. Normal variant
   B. Cecal bascule
   C. Cecal volvulus
   D. Colonic ileus (Ogilvie's syndrome)

2. Which of the following regarding cecal volvulus is true?
   A. There is a mobile cecum due to a mobilization of the bowel at previous surgery.
   B. The cecum is a rare site of volvulus, accounting for 5% of colonic volvulus cases.
   C. The plain abdominal radiograph will allow a diagnosis of cecal volvulus in the majority of the cases.
   D. A contrast enema can demonstrate the classic bird-beak appearance of the twisted descending colon.

3. CT is a problem-solving tool suitable to aid in the diagnosis of cecal volvulus. Which of these choices is a sign of a cecal volvulus?
   A. Pneumatosis
   B. Bird beak sign
   C. "Swirl" sign at the root of the mesentery
   D. Displacement of the cecum adjacent to the liver

4. Which of the following regarding treatment of cecal volvulus is true?
   A. Colonoscopic reduction has the same long-term results as for sigmoid volvulus.
   B. Surgical reduction is a very risky option and is a management choice of last resort.
   C. The surgical treatment of choice is cecal resection with loop ileostomy.
   D. CT influences treatment by detecting complications of volvulus.

Cecal Bascule

1. B

2. C

3. B

4. D

References

Bobroff LM, Messinger NH, Subbarao K, et al: The cecal bascule. *Am J Roentgenol* 1972;115:249-252.

Moore CJ, Corl FM, Fishman EK: CT of cecal volvulus: unraveling the image. *Am J Roentgenol* 2001;177:95-98.

Cross-Reference

Gastrointestinal Imaging: *THE REQUISITES,* 3rd ed, p 310.

Comment

A volvulus is the twisting or torsion of a segment of bowel. The degree of severity and possibility of complications depend on the tightness of the twist and lack of spontaneous untwisting of the bowel. The number of volvuli that occur and spontaneously resolve is probably much higher than most radiologists appreciate.

The most common volvulus occurs in the sigmoid colon (50%-75% of cases). The cecum is the next most common site, seen in 20% to 40% of cases. Much less common are volvuli of the transverse colon and, rarely, the splenic flexure.

There are two types of cecal volvulus: the common torsion type and the much less common cecal bascule (about 10% of all cecal volvuli are bascules, as shown in this case). The more common cecal volvulus twists around its lumen axis. The torsion acts as an obstruction of the ascending colon. If the ileocecal valve is competent (allows only unidirectional flow) the luminal axis of the air-distended cecum is directed across the abdomen toward the spleen. Obviously, at a certain point, a greatly dilated thin-walled cecum will burst, resulting in perforation, spillage of colon contents, and peritonitis. If the ileocecal valve is not competent, the findings can be less clear.

In the case of a bascule, the cecum does not twist about its luminal axis but instead flips up and over an adhesion across the ascending colon, and the dilated cecum is seen clearly as a right-sided or midline subhepatic air-filled structure (see figures). The cause of the adhesion or band over which the cecum flips is unknown. It may be congenital.

Notes

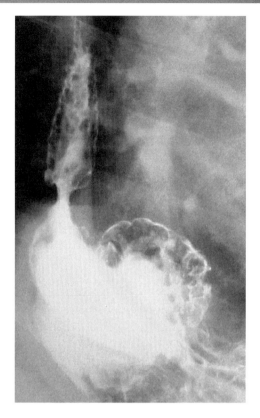
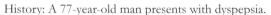
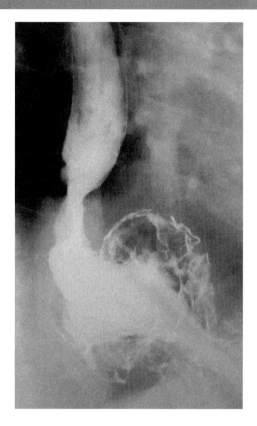

History: A 77-year-old man presents with dyspepsia.

1. Which of the following is the *best* diagnosis for the narrowing at the gastroesophageal junction?
   A. Normal physiologic
   B. Stricture, probably benign
   C. Stricture, probably malignant
   D. Extrinsic mass effect

2. What kind of diaphragmatic hernia is most associated with gastro-esophageal reflux disease (GERD)?
   A. Bochdalek
   B. Sliding
   C. Para-esophageal
   D. Rolling

3. Which of the following represent risk of GERD?
   A. Emphysema
   B. Bulimia
   C. Carcinoma
   D. Diabetes

4. Which of the following statements about GERD is true?
   A. There is almost a 2% prevalence of GERD in the population.
   B. Most patients with untreated chronic severe GERD will go on to develop Barrett's metaplasia.
   C. A manifestation of chronic GERD is episodic insomnia.
   D. The proximal esophagus is usually not spared in GERD.

Reflux Esophagitis

1. B

2. B

3. C

4. C

References

Eisenberg RL: Esophageal ulceration. In *Gastrointestinal Radiology: A Pattern Approach*, 4th ed. Baltimore, 2003, Lippincott Williams & Wilkins, pp 43-51.
Levine MS, Rubesin SE: Diseases of the esophagus: diagnosis with esophagography. *Radiology* 2001;237:414-427.

Cross-Reference

Gastrointestinal Imaging: *THE REQUISITES,* 3rd ed, p 16.

Comment

Radiologically, the findings of gastroesophageal reflux disease (GERD) are seen in the chronic phase. Radiographs are not yet able to identify the red mucosal coloring of early or acute disease. When seen in chronic disease, findings include fold thickening, granular appearance of the mucosa, superficial ulcerations, and developing luminal narrowing (see figures). Occasionally one encounters a "feline" esophagus in which fine transverse striations are seen transiently in the esophagus owing to brief contractions of the longitudinally orientated muscularis mucosae. This represents esophageal irritability in response to gastric acid on the mucosa. A similar finding characterized by fixed transverse folds, producing a "step-ladder" appearance, is believed to be due to scarring. This is similar to a finding in young patients with eosinophilic esophagitis. The presence of spontaneous gastroesophageal reflux and the way the esophagus handles it are most important. Is the gastric content cleared quickly from the esophagus by secondary wave activity? CT evaluation is less specific and might disclose some mild uniform thickening of the distal esophageal wall, a patulous esophagus, or fluid in the esophagus. The presence of a hiatal hernia, although not definitive, is associated with an increased incidence of reflux.

The complications of chronic GERD are Barrett's metaplasia (a condition in which the esophageal squamous mucosa begins to take on a somewhat disordered appearance of gastric or intestinal mucosa). Barrett's metaplasia is a precursor of adenocarcinoma in the distal esophagus and gastroesophageal junction. The other important complication is ulceration and strictures seen almost exclusively in the distal esophagus.

It is probably correct to assume that everyone, at some time or another, refluxes acid from the stomach up into the esophagus. However, the natural protective mechanisms—the lower esophageal sphincter (LES) and the secondary esophageal clearing wave that strips the acid back into the stomach—are usually sufficient to protect us from damage. Why this protective mechanism fails in some patients is not fully understood at this time. However, the incidence of GERD is increasing. Some have attributed the rise to increasing obesity in the general population and others have questioned the untoward side effect of many of the newer hypertensive and cardiac medications of lowering the pressure of the LES.

Notes

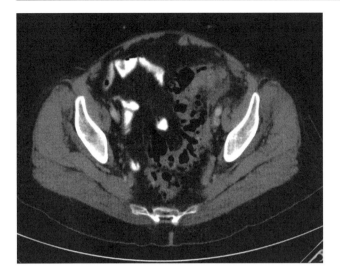

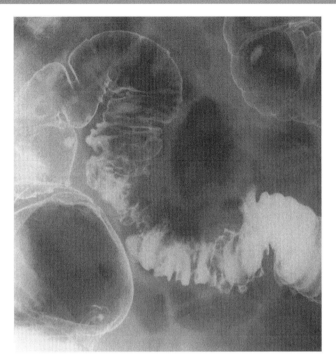

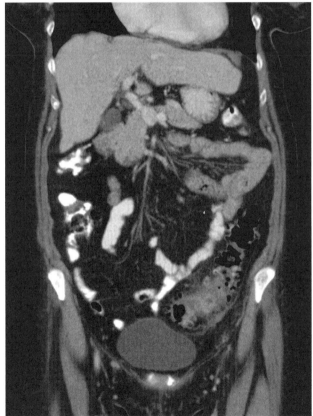

2. The referring clinician requests further imaging to assist with preoperative planning. Which study is most appropriate?
   A. Abdominal and pelvic ultrasound
   B. Contrast enema
   C. CT colonography
   D. Drainage: CT guided aspiration

3. Which of the following regarding colonic diverticular disease is true?
   A. Colonic diverticula are true diverticula.
   B. Diverticulitis is the most common cause of colovesical fistula.
   C. Diverticular hemorrhage usually ensues if diverticulitis is left untreated.
   D. Diverticulitis of the right colon is more likely to progress rapidly to complications.

4. Which of the following regarding the imaging of diverticular disease is true?
   A. On plain radiography, the most common appearance is a large bowel obstruction.
   B. On barium enema, the appearance of an intramural tract indicates diverticulitis.
   C. On CT, the appearance of the inflammatory mass simulates cancer in most cases.
   D. Percutaneous abscess drainage is contraindicated if there is large bowel obstruction.

History: A 74-year-old woman presents with left lower quadrant abdominal pain for several days.

1. Which of the following should be included in the differential diagnosis for this patient? (Choose all that apply.)
   A. Iliopsoas abscess
   B. Pneumatosis coli
   C. Colon cancer
   D. Diverticular disease

Sigmoid Diverticulitis

1. C and D

2. B

3. B

4. B

References

Cho KC, Morehouse HT, Alterman DD, Thornhill BA: Sigmoid diverticulitis: diagnostic role of CT comparison with barium enema studies. *Radiology* 1990;176:111-115.

Dahnert W: *Radiology Review Manual*, 6th ed. Philadelphia, 2007, Lippincott Williams & Wilkins, pp 821–823.

Cross-Reference

Gastrointestinal Imaging: *THE REQUISITES,* 3rd ed, p 302.

Comment

Diverticular disease of the colon is a very common condition. More than 60% of patients older than 60 years have colonic diverticula, 80% of which occur in the sigmoid segment. Most of these are asymptomatic. Some patients experience recurrent vague abdominal discomfort (spastic bowel), which might represent mild inflammatory changes (preceding frank diverticulitis) around the diverticula.

About 5% of the population has diverticulitis. This occurs with perforation of a diverticulum, resulting in intramural and/or localised pericolonic inflammation with all the expected symptoms of diverticulitis: local pain and tenderness, left lower quadrant mass, fever, and leukocytosis.

Plain abdominal radiographs are usually normal. Some patients with diverticulitis present with colonic obstruction. Small bowel obstruction can occur either from localized paralytic ileus or from true obstruction if the small bowel is caught up in the edema or fibrotic scarring surrounding the inflammatory mass.

CT is the modality of choice in acute diverticulitis. It will establish the diagnosis by demonstrating the abnormal segment of colon (colonic wall thickening, presence of diverticula) and the presence of inflammatory changes in the pericolic fat (see figures). Complications such as abscess and fistula formation can be seen.

Barium enema is useful in chronic diverticular disease. It is used for operative decision making and planning, to assess the length of colon involved, and to assess the degree of colonic narrowing (see figures).

Some patients experience episodic bleeding. Colonic diverticular hemorrhage is usually painless and occurs unrelated to diverticulitis. The site of bleeding is usually the right colon (75%) owing to the larger neck and dome of these diverticula. The bleeding may be torrential and life threatening.

Notes

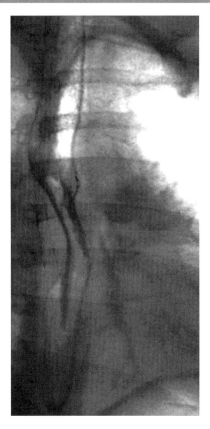

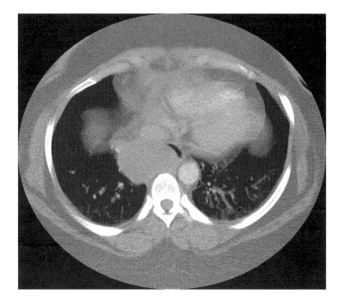

History: A patient without relevant symptoms, with an incidental abnormality noted on chest x-ray, was referred for further imaging.

1. Which of the following should be included in the differential diagnosis of the imaging findings shown for this patient? (Choose all that apply.)
   A. Aortic aneurysm
   B. Bronchogenic carcinoma
   C. Congenital foregut cyst
   D. Lymphoma
   E. Esophageal carcinosarcoma

2. All of the following are foregut congenital cysts *except:*
   A. Neurogenic cysts
   B. Bronchogenic cysts
   C. Pericardial cysts
   D. Enteric duplication cysts

3. What is the most common symptom of an esophageal duplication cyst?
   A. Asymptomatic
   B. Dyspnea
   C. Chest pain
   D. Dysphagia
   E. Arrhythmia

4. Which of the following statements about imaging of esophageal duplication cysts is true?
   A. Radionuclide scanning with ^{99m}Tc pertechnetate is positive in half of the cases.
   B. On barium swallow, the cyst typically appears as an intramural diverticulum.
   C. On CT, the appearance is identical to the bronchogenic cyst except that the wall of the lesion is thinner.
   D. On MRI, the lesion typically has short T1 and long T2 relaxation times.

C A S E   6

Duplication Cyst of the Esophagus

1. A, C, and D

2. C

3. A

4. A

Reference

Jeung MY, Gasser B, Gangi A, et al: Imaging of cystic masses of the mediastinum. *Radiographics* 2002;22:S79-S93.

Cross-Reference

Gastrointestinal Imaging: *THE REQUISITES,* 3rd ed, p 10.

Comment

The barium swallow discloses an extrinsic impression on the
lower esophagus (see figures). The angles of the impression
are obtuse, the mucosa is smooth and intact, and the lumen is
somewhat compromised. There is no evidence of ulceration
or mucosal destruction. All these findings suggest an extrinsic
origin. In fact, the lesion is a noncommunicating duplication
cyst of the esophagus. A small percentage of cysts communicate with the esophagus and can act like an epiphrenic diverticulum if the cyst is located in the lower esophagus. Esophageal
duplication cysts of the gut are the most common enteric cyst
(25%). Duplication cysts are one of the cystic manifestations
of foregut malformations.

CT demonstrates a paraesophageal cystic mass, which usually is not communicating with the lumen (see figures). A small
percentage communicate. Bronchogenic and neurogenic cysts
are the other two foregut malformation cysts, and all can affect
the esophagus. These cysts tend to be unilocular and bear a
close embryologic relationship to congenital cystic adenoma-
toid malformation of the lung. Duplication cysts are usually
lined with squamoid cells with some columnar elements and
are usually seen in the lower esophagus.

Bronchogenic cysts are usually indistinguishable and are
most commonly seen in the mediastinum in a subcarinal location. They usually contain some ciliated columnar epithelium
and are thought to be the result of abnormal bronchial bud-
ding during lung development. They never communicate with
the esophagus. Neurogenic cysts are usually located in the
posterior mediastinum and in a more posterior position than
either duplication or bronchogenic cysts. They are thought to
be an embryologic abnormality associated with incomplete
separation from the notochordal structures. Neurogenic cysts
are commonly associated with vertebral abnormalities such as
hemivertebrae or butterfly vertebrae.

Notes

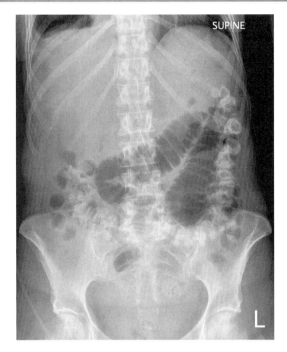

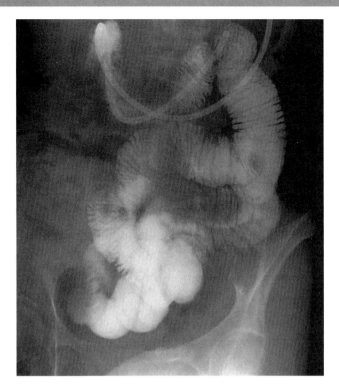

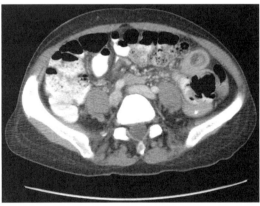

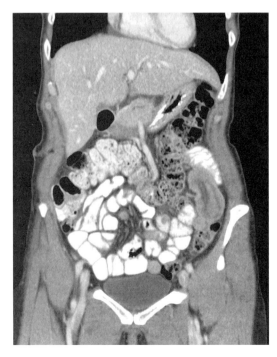

History: A 56-year-old woman underwent resection of small bowel melanoma metastases. Nine days after surgery, she developed nausea and vomiting.

1. Which of the following should be included in the differential diagnosis of the imaging findings shown for this patient? (Choose all that apply.)
   A. Polyp
   B. Lipoma
   C. Intussusception
   D. Bowel wall thickening

2. Which of the following statements regarding small bowel tumors is true?
   A. Small bowel tumors most commonly manifest with intussusception.
   B. Small bowel tumors are usually benign.
   C. The most common malignancy of the distal small bowel is carcinoid.
   D. The most common site of small bowel lymphoma is proximal jejunum.

3. What is the most common tumor of the small bowel?
   A. Gastrointestinal stromal tumor
   B. Lymphoma
   C. Carcinoid
   D. Melanoma

4. Which of the following polyposis syndromes is associated with an increased risk of small bowel cancer?
   A. Lynch syndrome
   B. Peutz-Jeghers syndrome
   C. Cronkhite-Canada syndrome
   D. Cowden syndrome

Small Bowel Intussusception

1. A and C

2. C

3. A

4. B

References

Buckley JA, Fishman EK: CT evaluation of small bowel neoplasms: spectrum of disease. *Radiographics* 1998;18:379-392.

Kim YH, Blake MA, Harisinghani MG, et al: Adult intestinal intussusception: CT appearances and identification of a causative lead point. *Radiographics* 2006;26:733-744.

Cross-Reference

Gastrointestinal Imaging: *THE REQUISITES,* 3rd ed, p 145.

Comment

Tumors of the small bowel are not commonly encountered because they tend to occur with less frequency than esophageal, gastric, or colonic lesions; are harder to detect; and are often asymptomatic. Except for the polyposis syndromes, they are usually seen in the older population and can manifest with bleeding, intussusception, and bowel obstruction. The most common benign small bowel tumor is the gastrointestinal stromal tumor (GIST), followed by lipomas. Both lesions, as well as other benign and malignant polypoid processes, can result in a bowel intussusception. Lymphoid hyperplasia can act as the nidus for intussusception in small children.

Most cases are seen in children; only 5% to 15% of all cases of intussusception are seen in adults. Intussusceptions in adults are commonly seen when they are symptomatic and obstructed (see figure). However, most intussusceptions are probably transient, causing chronic vague abdominal symptoms that usually subside over time. Of course, when the intussusceptum (the telescoping part of the bowel) becomes locked into the intussuscipiens (the receiving part of the bowel), the symptoms are immediately evident and the situation is worsened by edema and vascular congestion, making reduction difficult (see figures). In children especially, most intussusceptions are ileocolonic and often can be reduced by slow and careful distention of the colon via a barium enema. In adults the intussusceptions tend to be ileoileum and require surgical intervention. Invariably, an adult intussusception has a polyp, benign or malignant, as the leading nidus of the intussusception (see figures).

Notes

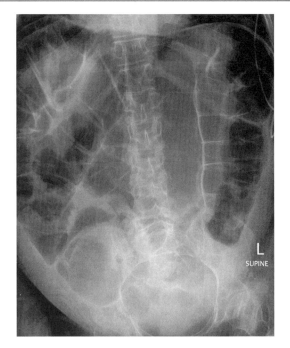

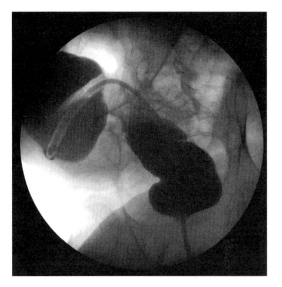

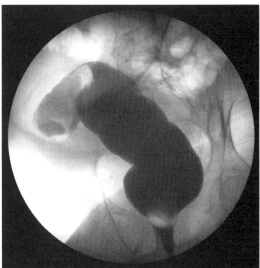

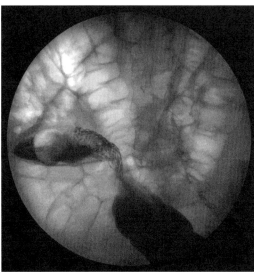

History: A 24-year-old man with muscular dystrophy developed acute abdominal distention 18 hours ago.

1. Which of the following should be included in the differential diagnosis for this patient? (Choose all that apply.)
   A. Normal variant
   B. Small bowel obstruction
   C. Cecal volvulus
   D. Sigmoid volvulus
   E. Colonic ileus (Ogilvie syndrome)

2. What is the most common form of volvulus seen in the colon?
   A. Sigmoid
   B. Bascule
   C. Cecal
   D. Ogilvie
   E. Hirschsprung

3. What is the name of the radiologic sign seen at the site of torsion on contrast enema?
   A. Apple core sign
   B. Bird beak sign
   C. Coffee bean sign
   D. Whirl sign
   E. Kidney bean sign

4. All of the following statements about sigmoid volvulus are true *except:*
   A. Volvulus is the third most common cause of colonic obstruction, sigmoid is the most common type of volvulus.
   B. Laparotomy and sigmoidopexy are the therapy of choice.
   C. A redundant sigmoid colon is a predisposing factor.
   D. The development of gangrene is suggested by clinical signs of peritonism or imaging signs of pneumoperitoneum or pneumatosis.

CASE 8

Sigmoid Volvulus

1. D

2. A

3. B

4. B

References

Feldman D: The coffee bean sign. *Radiology* 2000;216:178-179.
Kerry RL, Lee F, Ransom HK: Roentgenologic examination in the diagnosis and treatment of colon volvulus. *Am J Roentgenol* 1971;113:343-348.

Cross-Reference

Gastrointestinal Imaging: *THE REQUISITES,* 3rd ed, p 310.

Comment

Sigmoid volvulus is the most common type of volvulus seen in the gastrointestinal tract, accounting for 8% to 10% of cases of large bowel obstruction. The incidence is higher in areas of the world where roundworm infestation is endemic. In the West, the condition tends to occur in older patients (slightly higher rate in men), with a mortality rate of about 20%. Ultimately the mortality rate depends upon the degree of torsion and the time between the onset of symptoms and diagnosis and treatment. The amount of torsion around the sigmoid mesentery can vary from 180 to 540 degrees and usually occurs about 20 to 25 cm from the anal verge. The torsion is counter-clockwise. Patients commonly present with abdominal distention and pain and inability to pass stool or gas.

Plain films of the abdomen are often enough to make the diagnosis in 70% of patients (see figures). They show a grossly dilated sigmoid colon in the well-known coffee bean configuration arising out of the pelvis. The sigmoid haustra is effaced and there may be evidence of proximal obstruction if the amount of torsion is so great as to become an obstruction above the volvulus. Most of the time the torsion allows proximal air to pass into the volvulus but does not permit retrograde or distal escape of air, and evidence of proximal obstruction might not be present in such cases. If no free air is present and there is no evidence of pneumatosis or clinical evidence of peritonitis, a water-soluble enema is the best choice among contrast examinations. Contrast material will demonstrate a normal-caliber distal sigmoid and rectum, but will taper to the diagnostic bird beak sign at the site of torsion (see figures).

Notes

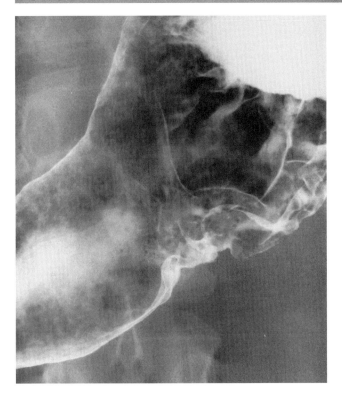

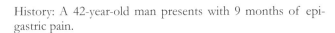

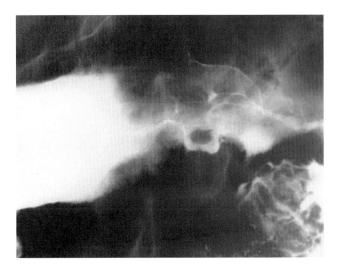

History: A 42-year-old man presents with 9 months of epi-gastric pain.

1. Which of the following describes the abnormalities shown in the images? (Choose all that apply.)
   A. Ulcer along the greater curvature
   B. Mass surrounding the ulcer
   C. Ulcer projects into the gastric lumen
   D. Ulcer edge ragged and heaped up
   E. Clubbed surrounding rugal folds

2. Which of the following features of a gastric ulcer is most suspicious for a malignant ulcer?
   A. Ulcer is located in the gastric antrum.
   B. Ulcer projects outside the gastric lumen.
   C. There are clubbed surrounding rugal folds.
   D. There is an associated duodenal ulcer.
   E. Hampton's line is apparent.

3. Which of the following does *not* have an association with gastric malignancy?
   A. AIDS
   B. Benign gastric ulcer
   C. *Helicobacter pylori* infection
   D. Nitrites and nitrates
   E. Partial gastrectomy

4. Of the following imaging modalities, which provides the best assessment of gastric cancer staging?
   A. MRI
   B. Barium upper GI study and follow-through
   C. CT
   D. Bone scan
   E. Endoscopic ultrasound (EUS)

Malignant Ulcer of the Stomach

1. A, B, C, and D

2. C

3. B

4. C

References

Iyer R, Dubrow R: Imaging upper gastrointestinal malignancy. *Semin Roentgenol* 2006;41(2):105-112.
Low VHS, Levine MS, Rubesin SE, et al: Diagnosis of gastric carcinoma: sensitivity of double-contrast barium studies. *Am J Roentgenol* 1994;162:329-334.

Cross-Reference

Gastrointestinal Imaging: *THE REQUISITES*, 3rd ed, p 82-85.

Comment

Today, potential gastric malignancy is almost exclusively evaluated by endoscopy and CT. However in asymptomatic screening situations, high-quality double-contrast barium studies are still quite useful. Superficial spreading mucosal lesions with little or no mass can be missed on CT. Lesions such as those shown in the images from an upper GI study included with this case (see figures) are best augmented with CT evaluation, which allows much more accurate grading of the lesions. Perigastric involvement as well as lymph node spread and metastatic spread are well evaluated on multidetector computed tomography (MDCT) of the thorax, abdomen, and pelvis.

Some of the characteristics of benign gastric ulcer include the following:

- Hampton's line, a well-defined thin lucency seen at the base of the ulcer, an ulcer collar
- Ulcer crater projected outside the gastric lumen
- Ulcer symmetrically placed on a gastric mass such as might be seen in surrounding edema of a gastrointestinal stromal tumor (GIST)
- Gastric folds flowing right up to the crater edge; although there may be thickening of the fold due to inflammation, there is no evidence of clubbing (with clubbing, the termination of a fold swells into a clublike configuration)

Notes

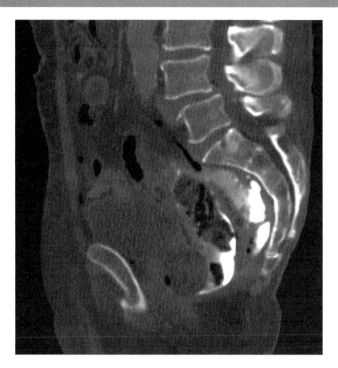

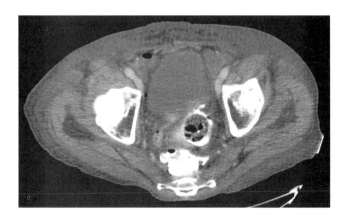

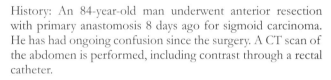

History: An 84-year-old man underwent anterior resection with primary anastomosis 8 days ago for sigmoid carcinoma. He has had ongoing confusion since the surgery. A CT scan of the abdomen is performed, including contrast through a rectal catheter.

1. Which of the following could be included in the differential diagnosis for widening of the presacral space? (Choose all that apply.)
   A. Ascites
   B. Rectal perforation
   C. Sacral chordoma
   D. Anorectal carcinoma
   E. Pelvic lipomatosis

2. Which of the following structures is the most likely to be disrupted in this patient?
   A. Rectal anastomosis
   B. Urinary bladder
   C. Pelvic veins
   D. No disruption present

3. Which of the following presacral space lesions is *not* an indication for percutaneous intervention?
   A. Presacral abscess
   B. Hematoma
   C. Hemorrhage
   D. Tumor recurrence

4. What is the most common primary retrorectal tumor?
   A. Adrenal rest tumor (pheochromocytoma)
   B. Osteogenic sarcoma
   C. Chordoma
   D. Congenital developmental cysts
   E. Ependymoma

CASE 10

Presacral Widening

1. B, C, D, and E

2. A

3. B

4. D

References

Bullard Dunn K: Retrorectal tumors. *Surg Clin North Am* 2010;90(1):163-171.
Dahnert W: *Radiology Review Manual*, 6th ed. Philadelphia: Lippincott Williams & Wilkins; 2007, p 786.

Cross-Reference

Gastrointestinal Imaging: *THE REQUISITES,* 3rd ed, pp 315-316.

Comment

The presacral space between the midrectum and sacral bone (measured below the peritoneal reflection) can be variable and sometimes is a dilemma for radiologists. This space is taken up with fascia and some fatty tissue in most people. The measurement is valid only when the rectum is fully distended, and the lack of distention in inflammatory disease involving the rectum is usually what accounts for the widening. In Crohn's disease, perirectal inflammatory changes are also present.

Widening can be due to processes that involve the rectum (most common), causes that affect the sacral bone, and processes that affect the retroperitoneum. Rectal causes can be both inflammatory (see figures) and neoplastic. Retroperitoneal causes can include retroperitoneal lipomatosis or fibrosis. Sacral diseases that can result in widening include sacral bony tumors (metastatic disease, as well as chordomas and neurofibromas) and sacral inflammation such as osteomyelitis.

Notes

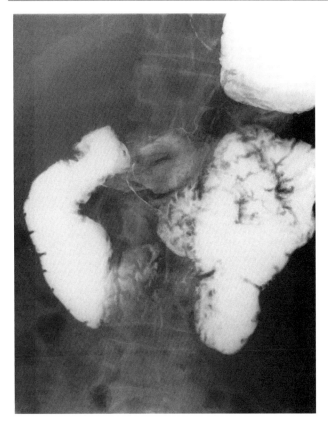

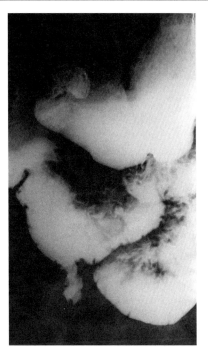

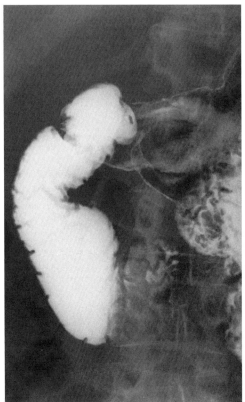

History: A 30-year-old woman with weight loss of unknown etiology presents with symptoms of bloating and abdominal distention soon after eating.

1. Which of the following should be included in the differential diagnosis for this lesion? (Choose all that apply.)
   A. Superior mesenteric artery (SMA) syndrome
   B. Postbulbar peptic scarring
   C. Abdominal aortic aneurysm
   D. Intramural hematoma
   E. Lymphadenopathy

2. The duodenal obstruction is worse with the patient in the supine position, and relieved when the patient is placed erect or prone. What syndrome does she have?
   A. Superior mesenteric artery (SMA) syndrome
   B. Bouveret syndrome
   C. Chagas syndrome
   D. Mirizzi syndrome
   E. Ogilvie syndrome

3. There are types of patients who are most susceptible to this condition. Which of the following is *not* a predisposing condition?
   A. Young women with eating disorders
   B. Burn patients
   C. Patients in body casts
   D. Spinal scoliosis
   E. Severe illness and sudden weight loss

4. Regarding the SMA syndrome, which of the following statements is *true*?
   A. The normal aortomesenteric angle is at least 25 to 30 degrees.
   B. Females are affected more than males.
   C. The treatment of choice is surgical bypass.
   D. The Wilkie maneuver (applying pressure inferior to the umbilicus in a dorsal and superior direction) helps to relieve the obstruction.

CASE 11

Superior Mesenteric Artery Syndrome

1. A, C, D, and E

2. A

3. D

4. B

Reference

Dahnert W: *Radiology Review Manual*, 5th ed. Philadelphia: Lippincott Williams & Wilkins; 2003, p 861.

Cross-Reference

Gastrointestinal Imaging: *THE REQUISITES*, 3rd ed, p 90.

Comment

The transverse retroperitoneal portion of the duodenum is nestled in an angle created by the aorta posteriorly and the superior mesenteric artery anteriorly (see figures). This angle can vary in size, and hence this condition is sometimes controversial. Some refuse to accept that SMA syndrome is a real condition. Given the narrowness of the angle we are now able to measure on multidetector computed tomography (MDCT) sagittal images in asymptomatic patients, this is quite understandable. However, from time to time we are faced with the so-called SMA syndrome, and its symptoms and findings cannot be denied. Patients complain of abdominal pain, nausea, weight loss, and especially vomiting. Imaging of the abdomen often shows a dilated stomach and proximal duodenum. The duodenum is narrowed at the level of the aortic-SMA angle and the distal duodenum has a normal caliber.

MDCT sagittal imaging now permits us to measure the angle. An abnormal angle of less than 25 degrees is required to establish a diagnosis of SMA syndrome. In severe unremitting cases, surgical intervention, such as gastrojejunostomy, may be required.

Notes

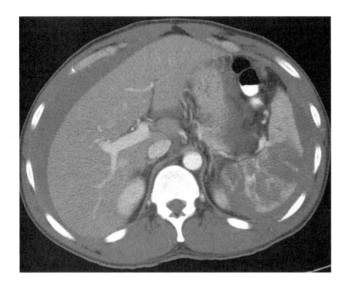

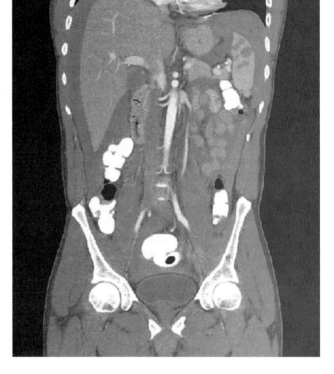

History: A young man is involved in a motor vehicle accident.

1. What is the grade of splenic injury shown on this CT scan?
   A. Grade I
   B. Grade II
   C. Grade III
   D. Grade IV
   E. Grade V

2. In a patient who had trauma with splenic injury, what findings will increase the urgency of surgical intervention?
   A. Preexisting splenomegaly
   B. Multiple left rib fractures
   C. Demonstration of continued bleeding
   D. Presence of subcapsular hematoma

3. Which of the following complications has been reported to be associated with splenic injury and splenectomy?
   A. Page spleen
   B. Encapsulated bacterial sepsis
   C. Thrombocytopenia
   D. Left diaphragm injury

4. Which of the following is most often associated with splenic injury in blunt trauma?
   A. Other abdominal viscera
   B. Lower rib fractures
   C. Left kidney
   D. Left diaphragm

Splenic Laceration

1. C

2. C

3. B

4. B

Reference

Dahnert W: *Radiology Review Manual*, 6th ed. Philadelphia: Lippincott Williams & Wilkins; 2007, p 807-809.

Cross-Reference

Gastrointestinal Imaging: *THE REQUISITES,* 3rd ed, p 211.

Comment

The spleen is the most commonly injured organ in the abdomen as a result of blunt abdominal trauma, with an incidence of 25%. Historically, the treatment of choice for splenic injury was surgical, commonly splenectomy. However, splenectomy is associated with a life-long risk for potentially fatal sepsis due to encapsulated bacteria. This has led to an evolution in the management of splenic injuries to appropriately triage patients toward operative versus nonoperative management. Currently, nonoperative management of isolated blunt splenic injury is considered the standard of care for hemodynamically stable children. Patients who are hemodynamically unstable should proceed directly to surgical exploration.

Patients who are hemodynamically stable routinely receive a CT examination (see figures). The degree of splenic injury is assessed and assigned a grade. The grade will help in determining whether the patient will or will not require intervention and the need for continued evaluation of the spleen. The grading method depends on size, depth, and number of the lacerations and hematomas; amount of extravasation; and whether there is continued bleeding (see figures).

Splenic trauma is commonly graded using the Organ Injury Scaling system (American Association for the Surgery of Trauma). A grade I injury is the least-severe injury and is a subcapsular hematoma less than 10% of splenic surface area and/or a small capsular tear no deeper than 1 cm, nonexpanding, not actively bleeding. A grade V injury is a shattered spleen with involvement of the splenic vascular pedicle.

Notes

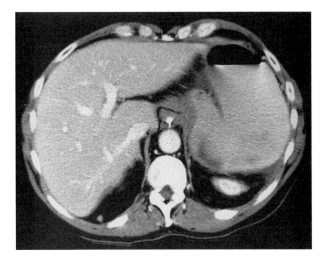

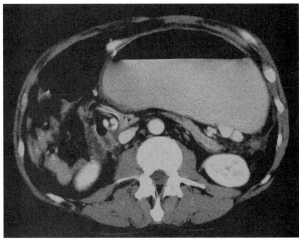

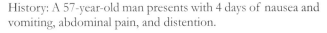

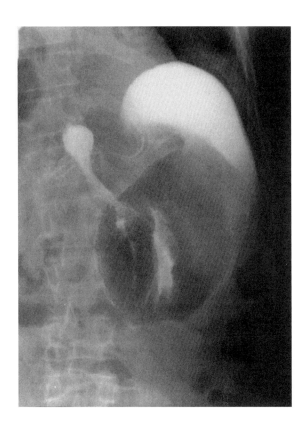

History: A 57-year-old man presents with 4 days of nausea and vomiting, abdominal pain, and distention.

1. Which of the following should be included in the differential diagnosis for this abnormality (gastric distention)? (Choose all that apply.)
   A. Gastric atony
   B. Gastric outlet obstruction
   C. Gastric pneumatosis
   D. Gastroparesis
   E. Gastric volvulus

2. Review the provided images. What is the single best diagnosis?
   A. Diaphragmatic incarcerated hernia
   B. Organoaxial gastric volvulus
   C. Mesenteroaxial gastric volvulus
   D. Para-esophageal hiatal incarcerated hernia

3. What is the treatment for the condition demonstrated in the provided images?
   A. Endoscopy
   B. Nasogastric tube
   C. Surgery
   D. Nothing, the condition is self-limiting and reversible

4. Which of the following statements about gastric volvulus is true?
   A. Occurs more commonly in female patients.
   B. The Borchardt triad (pain, nonproductive retching, and inability to pass a nasogastric tube), although diagnostic of acute volvulus, occurs in only 25% of cases.
   C. If diagnosed and managed promptly, the mortality rate from acute gastric volvulus is less than 5%.
   D. The most common anatomic defect associated with gastric volvulus is abnormal laxity of gastric ligaments.

Gastric Volvulus

1. A, B, D, and E

2. C

3. C

4. D

Reference

Peterson CM, Anderson JS, Hara AK, et al: Volvulus of the gastrointestinal tract: appearances at multimodality imaging. *Radiographics* 2009;29:1281-1298.

Cross-Reference

Gastrointestinal Imaging: *THE REQUISITES,* 3rd ed, p 54-55.

Comment

To understand gastric volvulus, it is useful to consider the anatomy of the stomach and its attachments. The stomach is fixed to the diaphragm just above the gastroesophageal junction proximally and to the retroperitoneum at the first duodenal flexure distally. In between, the stomach is attached posteriorly by a fan-shaped mesentery (the mesogastrum).

There are two varieties of gastric volvulus. The axis of the organ is the long axis of the stomach, an imaginary line drawn between the gastroesophageal junction and the cardia to the pylorus. Organoaxial volvulus refers to rotation of the stomach upward along this long axis. In this condition, the greater curvature is thrown up cephalad to the lesser curvature, a horizontal-lie stomach. This is the most common type; it is usually chronic and asymptomatic and seen in older patients. Strangulation and necrosis have been reported in 5% to 25% of patients with this type.

The axis of the mesentery is the middle of the mesenteric fan, the gastrohepatic omentum, a line passing through the middles of the lesser and greater curvatures. Mesenteroaxial volvulus refers to left-to-right or right-to-left rotation of the stomach about this axis. This brings the pylorus close to the cardia, and the antrum is thrown cephalad to the fundus (see figures). This type of volvulus is more serious and more likely to be incarcerated.

Mesenteroaxial volvulus can occur, albeit infrequently, with stomachs in the normal epigastric location. Variations of mesenteroaxial volvulus is more often seen when the stomach has migrated (usually owing to massive hiatal herniation) or where the stomach has been displaced by left diaphragm elevation. In these scenarios, the gastric mesentery has been considerably distorted and/or disrupted with the migration.

Some patients have few or no symptoms and have the condition a long time. However, when the torsion begins to obstruct or affect the vascular supply (see figures), the patient presents with symptoms ranging from nausea and vomiting to severe pain to cardiovascular collapse from gastric necrosis. Because of these potential risks, it is imperative that the referring service be made aware of an asymptomatic or minimally symptomatic gastric volvulus.

Notes

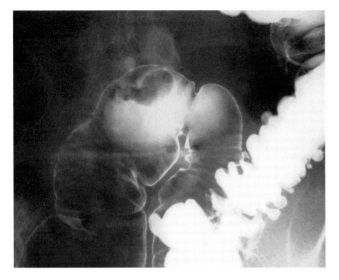

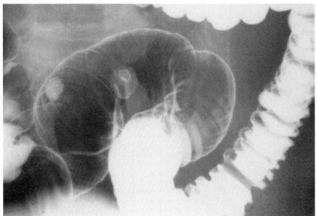

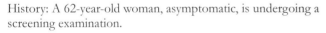

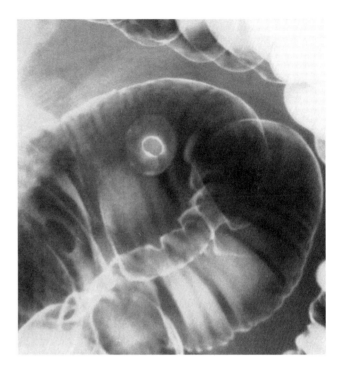

History: A 62-year-old woman, asymptomatic, is undergoing a screening examination.

1. Which of the following should be included in the differential diagnosis? (Choose all that apply.)
   A. Adenoma
   B. Ulcer
   C. Cancer
   D. Diverticulum
   E. Fecal debris

2. What is the treatment for the lesion demonstrated in the provided images?
   A. Staging CT scan
   B. Surgery
   C. Colonoscopy
   D. No specific treatment is necessary

3. Which is the most common histological subtype of colonic adenomatous polyp?
   A. Filiform
   B. Tubular adenoma
   C. Tubulovillous adenoma
   D. Villous adenoma

4. What is the typical clinical presentation of a patient with a colonic polyp?
   A. Anemia
   B. Bright rectal bleeding (hematochezia)
   C. Occult rectal bleeding
   D. Mucorrhea
   E. Asymptomatic

Adenoma of the Colon

1. A, C, D, and E

2. C

3. B

4. E

References

O'Brien MJ, Winawer SJ, Zauber AG, et al: The National Polyp Study: patient and polyp characteristics associated with high-grade dysplasia in colorectal adenomas. *Gastroenterology* 1990;98:371-379.

Thompson WM, Foster WL, Paulson EK, et al: Causes of errors in polyp detection at air-contrast barium enema examination. *Radiology* 2006;239:139-148.

Cross-Reference

Gastrointestinal Imaging: *THE REQUISITES,* 3rd ed, p 268-271.

Comment

Colonic adenomas are found in the colons of 15% to 30% of patients older than 60 years, with the prevalence very dependent on age, heredity, and risk factors. Polyps come in three histologically identifiable forms. The first, and most common (80%), is the tubular adenoma. These polyps are usually small and carry very little risk for malignant degeneration. They can be on long stalks (see figures). However, the fact that the stalk permits the polyp to move with the patient can occasionally make detection on both air contrast barium enema (ACBE) and CT quite difficult.

The other two types are tubovillous adenomas and villous adenomas. Villous adenomas have the greatest risk for developing into a malignancy. Some researchers and clinicians consider a colonic villous adenoma a low-grade malignancy regardless of what the histologic picture shows. Polyps less than 0.5 mm (diminutive polyps) have little or no malignant potential. Polyps 1 to 2 cm in size carry about a 10% risk. Polyps greater than 2 cm are generally thought to have a 30% to 40% risk of malignancy.

The anatomic distribution of colonic adenomas seems to be an equal distribution throughout the colon. However, the larger the polyp, the more likely it will be in the distal colon. Moreover, in patients older than 60 years, the number of polyps detected in the right colon is on the rise.

Notes

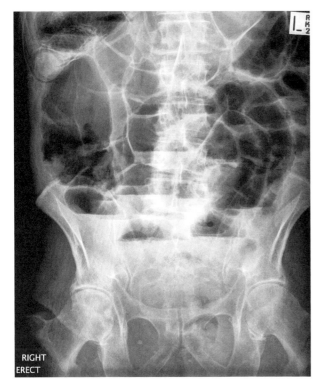

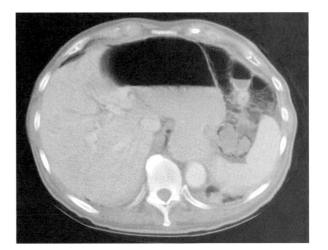

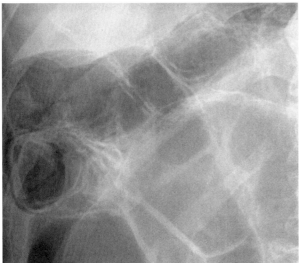

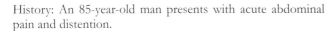

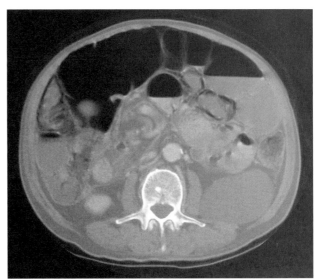

History: An 85-year-old man presents with acute abdominal pain and distention.

1. Review the provided images. Which of the following findings are present? (Choose all that apply.)
   A. Gastric distension
   B. Small bowel distention
   C. Colonic distention
   D. Pneumoperitoneum
   E. Pneumatosis

2. Which of the following is an iatrogenic cause of pneumatosis intestinalis?
   A. Oxygen therapy
   B. Hyperbaric therapy
   C. Chemotherapy
   D. Dialysis

3. In an older patient with abdominal pain found to have pneumatosis intestinalis, what condition must be considered first?
   A. Acute bowel obstruction
   B. Bowel ischemia and necrosis
   C. Colonic diverticulitis
   D. Duodenal ulceration

4. What imaging procedure should *not* be performed in a patient with suspected acute bowel ischemia?
   A. Angiography
   B. Barium small bowel study
   C. MRI
   D. Ultrasound

Pneumatosis Intestinalis

1. A, B, D, and E

2. C

3. B

4. B

References

Scheidler J, Stabler A, Kleber G, Neidhardt D: Computed tomography in pneumatosis intestinalis: differential diagnosis and therapeutic consequences. *Abdom Imaging* 1995;20:523-528.

Kim AY, Ha HK: Evaluation of suspected mesenteric ischemia: efficacy of radiologic studies. *Radiol Clin North Am* 2003;41:327-342.

Cross-Reference

Gastrointestinal Imaging: *THE REQUISITES*, 3rd ed, p 335-338.

Comment

Pneumatosis intestinalis of the bowel describes a condition in which air collects in the layers of the wall of the bowel (see figures). The most plausible cause for this condition is a breakdown of the mucosal integrity, allowing bowel air to pass through the mucosa into the submucosa. To gain access to the bowel wall, there must be some disruption of the mucosal integrity, such as mucosal tears or ischemic or necrotic disease of the bowel.

Ischemia is a common and most serious cause. Inflammatory conditions, such as necrotizing enterocolitis, pseudomembranous colitis, Crohn's disease, and even infectious agents also are known to produce pneumatosis. It can affect patients who take steroids. Also, obstruction, trauma, prior endoscopy, malignancies, chemotherapy, and bowel surgery are associated with the development of pneumatosis. CT is a wonderful method for demonstrating even minor amounts of pneumatosis (see figures).

The radiologic appearance may be one of multiple linear submucosal air lucencies in nature. Portal venous gas in a patient with pneumatosis often indicates the presence of bowel necrosis, which is probably the most significant associated finding. A benign form of pneumatosis, referred to *as pneumatosis intestinalis cystica,* is a condition in which subserosal blebs are seen in the distal bowel, usually having no clinical significance. The patients are asymptomatic and the condition has been associated with air tracking along bronchovascular pathways into the retroperitoneum, out the mesentery, and finally to the subserosal layer of the distal bowel (Macklin's pathway).

Notes

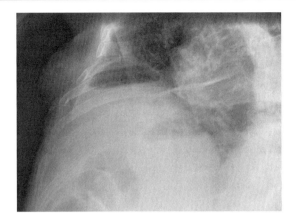

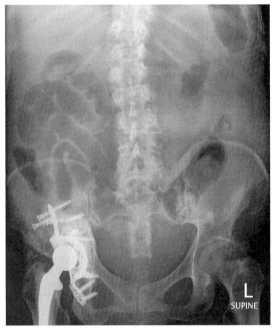

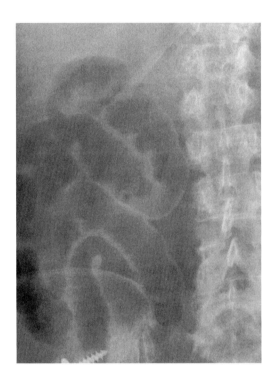

History: A 71-year-old woman presents with melena, nausea, vomiting, and abdominal pain.

1. What is the minimal amount of free intraperitoneal gas visible on an upright chest film?
   A. 1 to 2 mL
   B. Approximately 5 mL
   C. 10 to 20 mL
   D. Approximately 50 mL
   E. 100 to 150 mL

2. What is Rigler's sign?
   A. A differential diagnosis for free intraperitoneal gas due to a loop of bowel interposed between the liver and the right diaphragm.
   B. A sign of free intraperitoneal gas on a supine abdominal radiograph where both sides of the bowel wall are visible owing to gas on both sides.
   C. A sign of free intraperitoneal gas on a supine abdominal radiograph where the inferior surface of the central tendon of the diaphragm is visible.
   D. A sign of free intraperitoneal gas on a supine abdominal radiograph where there is an oval central lucency.

3. What imaging procedure is best for demonstrating free intraperitoneal gas?
   A. Abdominal radiograph, erect
   B. Abdominal radiograph, left decubitus
   C. Chest radiograph, erect
   D. CT scan

4. What is the usual amount of time for air that is introduced into the abdomen during surgery to be reabsorbed?
   A. 0 to 1 day
   B. 1 to 3 days
   C. 3 to 10 days
   D. 10 to 20 days

Pneumoperitoneum

1. A

2. B

3. D

4. C

References

Miller RE, Nelson SW: The roentgenologic demonstration of tiny amounts of free intraperitoneal gas: experimental and clinical studies. *Am J Roentgenol* 1971;112:574-585.

Rigler LG: Spontaneous pneumoperitoneum: a roentgenologic sign found in the supine position. *Radiology* 1941;37:604-607.

Cross-Reference

Gastrointestinal Imaging: *THE REQUISITES,* 3rd ed, p 332-335.

Comment

Intraperitoneal gas is often encountered in the abdominal cavity. The most common cause of the free gas is surgery or surgical laparoscopy. Air that is introduced into the abdomen during surgery usually takes 3 to 10 days to reabsorb. Under certain circumstances, this process can take several weeks. The more air introduced, the longer it takes to reabsorb. Thin patients take longer to reabsorb air. This finding might relate to the fact that obese patients usually have more omental fat, which decreases the amount of air that can be introduced. If the patient has postoperative ileus or peritonitis, the ability of the peritoneum to absorb the air is also reduced.

For many years, the upright chest film (see figures) and the left lateral decubitus view of the abdomen were considered the best for demonstrating even minute amounts (1 to 2 mL) of gas. However, CT has been shown to demonstrate free gas even when these views cannot. Multidetector computed tomography (MDCT) is now considered, by far, the best modality for demonstrating even the tiniest amounts of free gas.

Several signs have been described regarding the appearance of free intraperitoneal gas on a conventional supine abdominal image. Often the patient is too sick for upright or decubitus views to be obtained, and the only view that can be obtained is a supine film (see figures). In this situation one or more of these signs may be seen.

Rigler's sign refers to the ability to see both sides of the bowel wall because there is gas on both sides. What we routinely see on abdominal images when we see intestinal gas is actually a tissue-gas interface, specifically a mucosal-gas interface. The serosal side of the bowel cannot be seen without the presence of free gas in the peritoneum. Thus, when we are seeing both a mucosal-gas interface and a serosal-gas interface, we are seeing Rigler's sign. When three loops of bowel touch each other we may see a lucent triangle in the center representing three serosal-gas interfaces; this is known as Rigler's triangle. This sign is difficult to see unless there is a sufficient amount of free gas. Ability to see the patient's falciform ligament is another sign indicating free gas. Also, free gas beneath the liver margin in Morrison's pouch results in a tissue-gas interface with the liver margin as well as lucency that typically is not present on a supine film. Occasionally we see the lateral pelvic ligament, which becomes visible with the presence of sufficient amounts of free gas. CT is considerably more sensitive in the detection of free intraperitoneal gas.

Notes

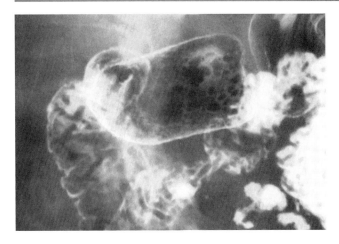

History: A 70-year-old woman presents with gastroesophageal reflux symptoms.

1. Which of the following should be included in the differential diagnosis of this case? (Choose all that apply.)
   A. Benign lymphoid hyperplasia
   B. Brunner's gland hyperplasia
   C. Heterotopic gastric mucosa
   D. Duodenitis
   E. Ectopic pancreatic rests

2. What can occur as a response to increased acidity in the duodenal bulb?
   A. Benign lymphoid hyperplasia
   B. Brunner's gland hyperplasia
   C. Heterotopic gastric mucosa
   D. Ectopic pancreatic rests

3. Which of the following polyposis syndromes does *not* involve the duodenum?
   A. Familial adenomatous polyposis
   B. Peutz-Jeghers syndrome
   C. Cronkhite-Canada syndrome
   D. Filiform polyposis

4. What is the most common benign tumor of the duodenum?
   A. Adenoma
   B. Brunner gland hamartoma
   C. Carcinoid
   D. Mesenchymal tumors

Heterotopic Gastric Mucosa of the Duodenum

1. A, B, C, and E

2. B

3. D

4. D

References

Levine MS, Rubesin SE, Herlinger H, et al: Double-contrast upper gastrointestinal examination: technique and interpretation. *Radiology* 1988;168:593-602.
Op den Orth JO: Use of barium in evaluation of disorders of the upper gastrointestinal tract: current status. *Radiology* 1989;173:601-608.

Cross-Reference

Gastrointestinal Imaging: *THE REQUISITES,* 3rd ed, p 96.

Comment

It is not uncommon to encounter nodular filling defects within the duodenal bulb. These may be solitary or multiple and are of variable size. Certain distinguishing features can help differentiate the conditions that are known to produce this radiologic appearance.

Heterotopic gastric mucosa in the duodenal bulb occurs more commonly than most radiologists recognize, occurring in up to 20% of patients in some pathologic series but seen in less than 1% of patients in radiologic series. The radiologic appearance is that of slightly elevated lesions of varying sizes measuring only a few millimeters in diameter and often clustered in a mosaic pattern in the base of the duodenal bulb (see figure). A distinguishing feature is their sometimes angulated or plaque-like margins. These lesions are believed to have no clinical significance.

Benign lymphoid hyperplasia of the bulb and proximal duodenum is characterized by multiple tiny (1- to 2-mm), smooth filling defects, which are usually diffuse throughout the region. Often there is no known reason for their appearance, but they occur more commonly in patients with decreased immune competence, such as those with hypogammaglobulinemia or agammaglobulinemia.

Brunner's gland hyperplasia has a different radiologic appearance than the two aforementioned entities. The filling defects in this condition are larger, often ranging up to 1 cm. These lesions are smooth and diffuse, often producing a cobblestone appearance. They may be associated with hyperacidity, although this belief is not universally accepted, given the high incidence of hyperacidity disease and the low incidence of Brunner's gland hypertrophy. However, acidity might be a contributing factor.

The possibility of pancreatic rests, either single or multiple, giving rise to a polypoid filling defect in the duodenal bulb, should also be considered. A tiny barium collection, which can at times be seen in the center of these filling defects, is the orifice of a duct, and such a finding is an extremely important diagnostic finding.

Benign tumors of the duodenum, such as leiomyomas (GIST), adenomas, and neurofibromas, occur more commonly in the proximal duodenum, particularly the duodenal bulb.

Also, polyposis syndromes, such as Peutz-Jeghers, Cronkhite-Canada, and familial polyposis syndromes, are known to cause multiple polyps in the duodenum.

Notes

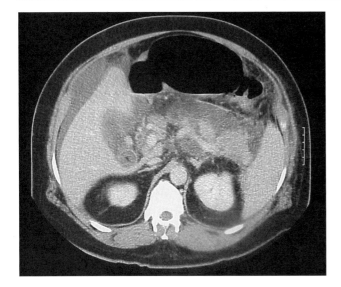

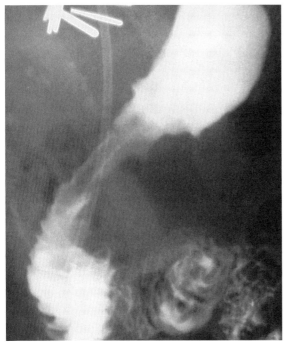

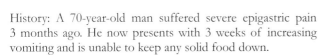

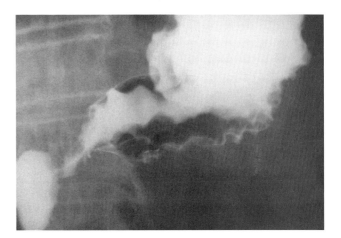

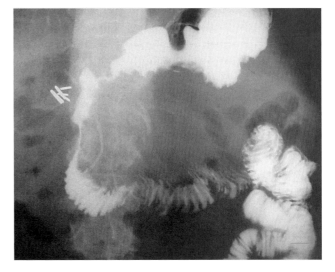

History: A 70-year-old man suffered severe epigastric pain 3 months ago. He now presents with 3 weeks of increasing vomiting and is unable to keep any solid food down.

1. Which of the following should be included in the differential diagnosis of the dominant imaging finding? (Choose all that apply.)
   A. Superior mesenteric artery (SMA) syndrome
   B. Pancreatic head disease
   C. Right renal disease
   D. Duodenal ulceration
   E. Normal

2. What is the most common primary malignant lesion of the duodenum?
   A. Adenocarcinoma
   B. Lymphoma
   C. Carcinoid
   D. Sarcoma

3. Several viscera are related to the descending duodenum; therefore, a disease process in these viscera can involve the descending duodenum. Conversely, a disease process arising in the descending duodenum can spread to these viscera. Which of these viscera are *not* related to the descending duodenum?
   A. Aorta
   B. Gallbladder
   C. Common bile duct
   D. Right kidney
   E. Pancreas

4. What is the most common cause for duodenal inflammation?
   A. Hyperacidity and peptic ulcer disease
   B. Pancreatitis
   C. Crohn's disease
   D. Duodenal diverticulitis

Duodenal Narrowing Secondary to Pancreatitis

1. B, C, D, and E

2. A

3. A

4. A

References

Bilimoria KY, Bentrem DJ, Wayne JD, et al: Small bowel cancer in the United States: changes in epidemiology, treatment, and survival over the last 20 years. *Ann Surg* 2009;249(1):63-71.

Levine MS, Turner D, Ekberg O, et al: A reliable radiologic diagnosis? *Gastrointest Radiol* 1991;16:99-103.

Cross-Reference

Gastrointestinal Imaging: *THE REQUISITES,* 3rd ed, p 99.

Comment

Thickened folds and spasm of the duodenal bulb and sweep can be seen in a number of conditions both primary in the duodenum or in the adjacent structures in the periduodenal area. In the duodenum the commonest is the result of peptic ulcer disease. Although spasm is not always a component, thickened fold can be seen in such conditions as Zollinger-Ellison syndrome, eosinophilic enteritis, Crohn's disease, Whipple's disease, and amyloid, as well as intramural bleeding and hypoproteinemia. Also to be considered are malignancies.

Pancreatitis affecting the pancreatic head almost always affects the folds of the second portion of the duodenum (see figures). The folds appear thick and irregular, especially on the pancreatic side (see figures). There may be tethering of folds (Selleck's folds), also seen on the same side (see figures).

The most common primary malignancy of the duodenum is adenocarcinoma, which accounts for 64% of tumors. The distribution of other primary tumors comprises carcinoid, 21%; lymphoma, 10%; and sarcoma, 4%. Elsewhere in the small bowel, the proportion of patients with carcinoids has increased, and carcinoid is now the most common tumor in the ileum. Sarcomas and lymphomas can develop throughout the entire small bowel.

Besides the pancreas, the right kidney bears a close and, in many patients, a contiguous relationship to the duodenum. It is not unusual to see a large right-sided upper pole renal malignancy affecting the adjacent duodenum.

Notes

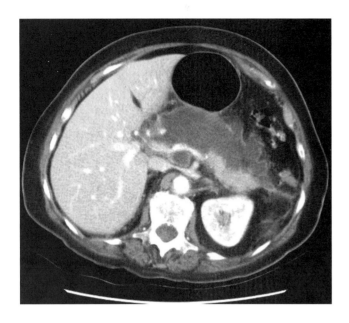
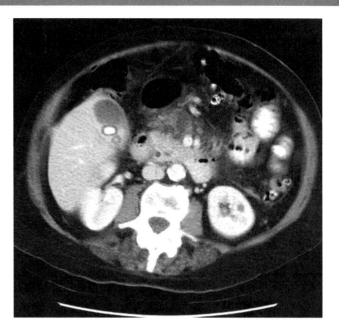

History: A 69-year-old woman with epigastric pain has now been in the hospital for 10 days.

1. Which of the following should be included in the differential diagnosis for this patient? (Choose all that apply.)
   A. Pancreatic abscess
   B. Pancreatic pseudocyst
   C. Pancreatic mucinous cystadenoma
   D. Pancreatic serous cystadenoma
   E. Pancreatic hematoma

2. What is the *most common* cause of acute pancreatitis (in Western society)?
   A. Alcohol
   B. Trauma
   C. Cholelithiasis
   D. Metabolic
   E. Drugs

3. Which of the following signs on contrast-enhanced CT indicates pancreatic necrosis?
   A. Mesenteric stranding
   B. Gas bubbles
   C. Lack of contrast enhancement of pancreatic parenchyma
   D. Enlargement of pseudocyst with high-density content

4. All of the following are potential complications of severe acute pancreatitis *except:*
   A. Infection
   B. Biliary obstruction
   C. Death
   D. Diabetes insipidus
   E. Malabsorption

Acute Pancreatitis

1. A, B, C, and E

2. A

3. C

4. D

References

Balthazar EJ, Ranson JHC, Naidich DP, et al: Acute pancreatitis: prognostic value of CT. *Radiology* 1985;156:767-772.

Dahnert W: *Radiology Review Manual*, 6th ed. Philadelphia: Lippincott Williams & Wilkins; 2007, pp 727-731.

Cross-Reference

Gastrointestinal Imaging: *THE REQUISITES,* 3rd ed, p 171-172.

Comment

Acute pancreatitis (see figures) is a serious condition whose frequency varies from country to country. The incidence has slowly declined in the United States since the turn of the 21st century. The disease is associated with a 10% to 15% mortality rate, is more common in the black population, and affects male more than female patients. Alcoholic pancreatitis is seen in younger adults, and biliary related etiologies are more commonly seen in an older population. Pancreatitis also results from trauma, drugs, and iatrogenic (endoscopic retrograde cholangiopancreatography [ERCP]) and idiopathic causes. These patients present with abdominal tenderness and guarding as well as fever and tachycardia.

In hemorrhagic pancreatitis both the Cullen sign (a bluish discoloration around the umbilicus) and the Grey Turner sign (discoloration along the flanks) may be seen as blood collects in the peritoneum and dissects along tissue planes. Associated with virtually every case of pancreatitis is some change at the left lung base. The change may be prominent or minimal, depending on the severity of the case. The inflammatory process in the right upper quadrant results in diminished diaphragmatic excursion on the left and hypoventilation of the left lung base, with resultant degrees of atelectasis, effusions, and air-space disease.

Passed gallstones lodged in the sphincter of Oddi is a common cause of pancreatitis (see figures). The size of the stone and duration of occlusion determine the severity of the pancreatitis. Approximately 5% of post-ERCP patients will develop some degree of pancreatitis.

Notes

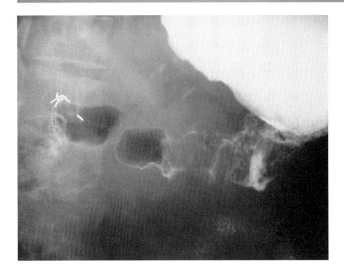

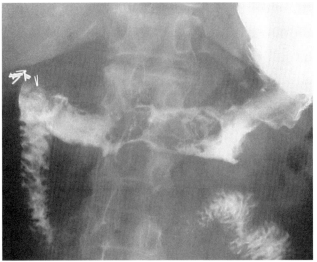

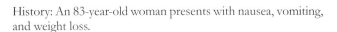

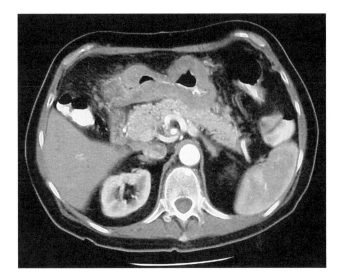

History: An 83-year-old woman presents with nausea, vomiting, and weight loss.

1. Which of the following should be included in the differential diagnosis of the imaging findings shown? (Choose all that apply.)
   A. Gastric adenocarcinoma
   B. Gastric lymphoma
   C. Hematogenous breast cancer metastasis
   D. Direct spread from pancreatic mucinous cystadenocarcinoma
   E. Peritoneal ovarian cancer seeding

2. What is the single best diagnosis?
   A. Gastric adenocarcinoma
   B. Gastric lymphoma
   C. Hematogenous breast cancer metastasis
   D. Direct spread from pancreatic mucinous cystadenocarcinoma
   E. Peritoneal ovarian cancer seeding

3. What is the most common type of primary lymphoma of the stomach?
   A. T-cell non-Hodgkin's
   B. B-cell non-Hodgkin's
   C. Mucosa-associated lymphoid tissue (MALT)
   D. Hodgkin's lymphoma
   E. Burkitt's lymphoma

4. Which of the following is *not* a known risk factor for gastrointestinal lymphoma?
   A. AIDS
   B. *Helicobacter pylori*
   C. Celiac disease
   D. Ulcerative colitis
   E. Epstein-Barr virus (EBV)

Gastric Lymphoma

1. A, B, C, and E

2. A

3. C

4. D

Reference

Dahnert W: *Radiology Review Manual*, 6th ed. Philadelphia: Lippincott Williams & Wilkins; 2007, pp 851-852.

Cross-Reference

Gastrointestinal Imaging: *THE REQUISITES*, 3rd ed, p 60.

Comment

The stomach is the area of the gastrointestinal tract most commonly affected by lymphoma. It may be part of generalized lymphoma involving other portions of the body and lymph system, or it may be primary, involving only the stomach and associated lymph nodes. Approximately half of all cases are primary lymphoma, and half are associated with generalized disease.

Lymphoma accounts for only 5% or less of primary gastric malignant neoplasms. Most lymphomas of the stomach are of the non-Hodgkin's variety, with Hodgkin's disease being the least common. Hodgkin's lymphoma typically accounts for less than 10% of cases. The disease predominantly affects men and is typically seen in an older age group (50 years and older).

Lymphoma has a variety of presentations in the stomach. It can appear as thickened gastric folds and be indistinguishable from gastritis and other causes of rugal fold thickening. It can also occur as a solitary mass or as multiple masses and polyps. These masses are known to ulcerate. Rarely, it infiltrates the entire stomach and produces more of a linitis plastica appearance, but this is more typically seen with Hodgkin's lymphoma because of the cellular desmoplastic reaction associated with it (see figures). Lymphoma readily crosses the pylorus into the duodenum, somewhat more readily than does carcinoma. However, both are known to cross the pylorus, carcinoma in greater numbers because of its greater incidence. It is not a specific distinguishing feature.

Surgical resection of the involved stomach is still the best treatment and may be supplemented by chemotherapy, depending on the situation. Patients with advanced primary disease or systemic lymphoma are best treated by chemotherapy first.

Notes

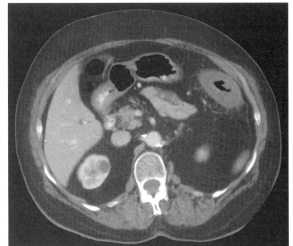

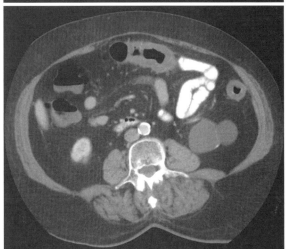

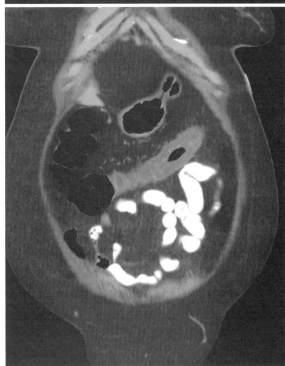

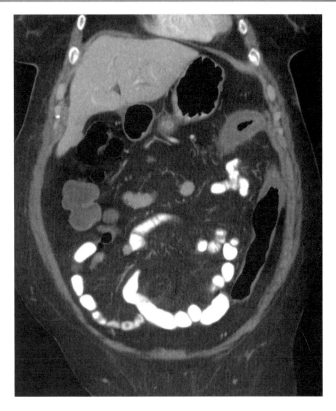

History: A 77-year-old woman had undergone transvaginal uterine polypectomy 2 days ago. She complains of nausea, syncope, and hematochezia.

1. Which of the following should be included in the differential diagnosis of the imaging findings shown? (Choose all that apply.)
   A. Crohn's colitis
   B. Pseudomembranous colitis
   C. Colon carcinoma
   D. Hemorrhage
   E. Lymphoma

2. What is the most likely diagnosis in this case?
   A. Typhlitis
   B. Radiation
   C. Diverticulitis
   D. Ischemia

3. All of the following CT findings may be associated with ischemic colitis *except:*
   A. Pneumatosis
   B. Hemorrhage
   C. Fistula
   D. Edema

4. Which of the following describes the prognosis of ischemic colitis?
   A. Most patients improve and fully recover.
   B. Most patients develop progressive colonic gangrene.
   C. Most patients develop a stricture.
   D. Patients are at high risk for developing colon carcinoma.

CASE 21

Ischemic Colitis of the Transverse Colon

1. A, B, D, and E
2. D
3. C
4. A

References

Rha SE, Ha HK, Lee SH, et al: CT and MR imaging findings of bowel ischemia from various primary causes. *Radiographics* 2000;20:29-42.

Taourel P, Aufort S, Merigeaud S, et al: Imaging of ischemic colitis. *Radiol Clin North Am* 2008;46:909-924.

Cross-Reference

Gastrointestinal Imaging: *THE REQUISITES,* 3rd ed, p 298.

Comment

Ischemic bowel disease is a common clinical problem, especially in the elderly. Most often it is produced by low flow to the intestines, which occurs in patients who are in hypotensive states, those who are experiencing cardiac failure, and patients who have just had surgery, and in patients with other conditions. Arterial obstruction is less common but can affect elderly patients with atherosclerotic disease that obstructs mesenteric vessels or those with embolic disease who have cardiac abnormalities. Also, a small percentage of patients have ischemia caused by venous obstruction.

Arteriography is being used less commonly with the advent of high-quality multidetector computed tomography (MDCT) in patients with ischemia. Angiography often does not demonstrate obstructing vessels. CT is probably the best modality for defining the involved segments and identifying underlying pathologic conditions or complications (see figures).

Ischemic disease of the colon is often segmental and rarely involves the entire colon (see figures). The different regions of the colon have separate blood supplies, although they are interconnected to some extent. The watershed regions are defined as the areas of transition between the superior and inferior mesenteric blood supplies. This term often applies to the splenic flexure (see figures), although sometimes it can include parts of the rectosigmoid junction as well. The splenic flexure is thought by some to be the most susceptible area for ischemia in patients with low flow-states because it is the most distal point of arterial flow to the colon. On the other hand, some think that being supplied by two arterial systems confers some protection.

Interestingly, most disease seems to occur in the descending and sigmoid regions. The right colon also is commonly involved because it is prone to ischemia resulting from pathologic distention. The right colon is the most distended segment of colon under most conditions.

Radiologically, ischemia first can be identified as thickening and edema of the bowel wall. Nodularity of the bowel wall could be the result of either multiple areas of focal edema or hemorrhage (thumbprinting). The mucosa may become shaggy and begin to resemble inflammatory bowel disease. As the ischemic area heals, the colon may become fibrotic, with loss of haustral pattern and even with formation of pseudodiverticula. This fibrosis can be multifocal. However, in at least 50% of cases healing is complete without stricture.

Notes

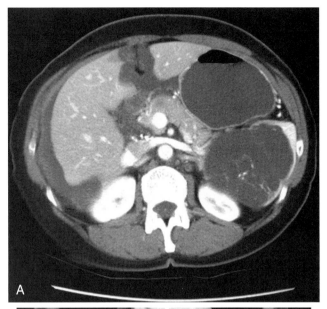

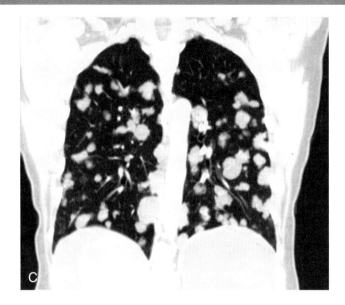

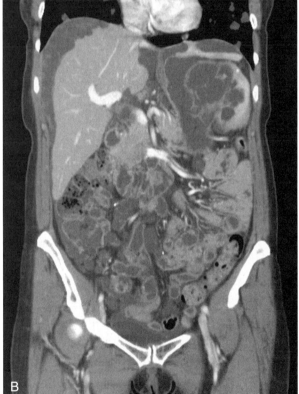

History: A 62-year-old woman presents with dyspnea and abdominal distention; she has a history of ovarian carcinoma.

1. Which of the following should be included in the differential diagnosis of the dominant imaging finding on figure A? (Choose all that apply.)
   A. Acquired (post-traumatic) pseudocyst
   B. Hemangioma
   C. Cystic metastasis
   D. Hydatid cyst
   E. Epidermoid cyst

2. What is the most common cause for benign splenic cysts?
   A. Lymphangioma
   B. Echinococcal cyst
   C. Congenital epidermoid cyst
   D. Post-traumatic pseudocyst

3. Which of the following is true about metastatic disease involving the spleen?
   A. Lymphomas are the most common splenic malignancy.
   B. Metastatic ovarian cancer is cystic owing to central necrosis.
   C. The most common origin of splenic metastases is melanoma.
   D. 25% to 50% of patients with terminal disease owing to metastatic malignancy have splenic lesions.

4. What is the most common benign neoplasm of the spleen?
   A. Angiomyolipoma
   B. Lymphangioma
   C. Hemangioma
   D. Hamartoma

Metastatic Disease to the Spleen

1. A, C, D, and E

2. D

3. A

4. C

References

Kamaya A, Weinstein S, Desser TS: Multiple lesions of the spleen. *Semin Ultrasound CT MRI* 2006;27:389-403.

Warshauer DM, Hall HL: Solitary splenic lesions. *Semin Ultrasound CT MRI* 2006;27:370-388.

Cross-Reference

Gastrointestinal Imaging: *THE REQUISITES,* 3rd ed, p 215.

Comment

The most common cystic lesions that affect the spleen are the acquired lesions and epidermoid cysts. Acquired cysts are thought to be mostly traumatic in origin (the small splenic laceration that heals, leaving a hematoma, seroma, and finally a cystic fluid collection that can remain indefinitely). These cysts are without a well-defined lining and calcify over the years. They account for about 80% of benign cystic lesions of the spleen and are best left alone. Epidermoid cysts have a well-defined epithelial lining and are probably congenital in origin. These cysts are also often an incidental finding on CT examinations. Occasionally a pseudocyst in the pancreatic tail can be confused with a splenic cyst. However, with multidetector computed tomography (MDCT) and multiplanar evaluation of the abdomen, these can usually be sorted out.

Primary neoplasms of the spleen are rare, with hemangioma being the most common. Metastatic disease involving the spleen is also very uncommon. However, as seen in the images, it should not be neglected in the differential diagnosis for splenic defects in patients with known primary neoplasms (see figures). In this case, the primary cancer is ovarian carcinoma, and there has been widespread dissemination of tumor throughout the peritoneal cavity with ascites (see figures) and invasion of the spleen as well as involvement of the thoracic cavity (see figures).

Notes

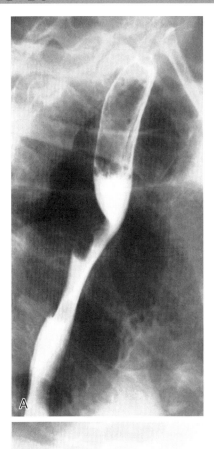

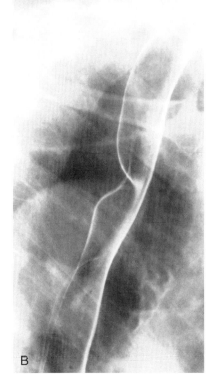

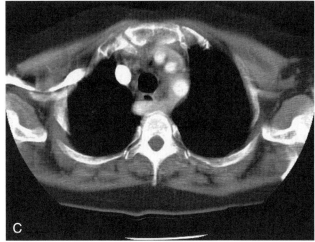

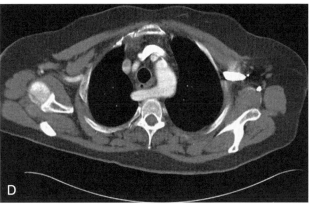

History: An 82-year-old woman presents with heartburn.

1. Which of the following should be included in the differential diagnosis of the dominant imaging finding on figure A? (Choose all that apply.)
   A. Aberrant vessel
   B. Esophageal leiomyoma
   C. Esophageal cancer
   D. Thoracic osteophyte
   E. Neurofibroma

2. Review the figures. What is the most likely diagnosis?
   A. Aberrant left subclavian artery
   B. Aberrant right subclavian artery
   C. Anomalous superior vena cava
   D. Double aortic arch

3. How does a patient with an aberrant right subclavian artery usually present?
   A. Asymptomatic
   B. Stridor
   C. Mediastinal mass
   D. Dysphagia

4. Which of the following is *not* an extrinsic impression normally seen during a barium swallow?
   A. Aortic arch
   B. Left main bronchus
   C. Right atrium
   D. Diaphragmatic hiatus

Aberrant Right Subclavian Artery

1. A, B, D, and E

2. B

3. A

4. C

References

Berdon WE: Rings, slings, and other things: vascular compression of the infant trachea updated from the midcentury to the millennium—the legacy of Robert E. Gross, MD, and Edward B.D. Neuhauser, MD. *Radiology* 2000;216:624-632.

Freed K, Low VHS: The aberrant subclavian artery. *Am J Roentgenol* 1997;168(2):481-484.

Cross-Reference

Gastrointestinal Imaging: *THE REQUISITES,* 3rd ed, p 12-14.

Comment

The normal extrinsic impressions one expects to see on the esophagus are the aortic arch, the left main bronchus, and the left atrium of the heart. Congenital malplaced right subclavian artery originating from the distal aspect of the aortic arch (instead of its usual origin off the right common carotid artery) is seen in slightly less than 1% of the population. In crossing back from left to right across the mediastinum to reach the right limb, the aberrant right subclavian artery passes behind the esophagus. The posterior-crossing artery shown here impressed the posterior wall of the upper esophagus and may produce dysphagia.

A barium esophagogram is the simplest and least expensive way of making the diagnosis (see figures). However, if necessary, multidetector computed tomography (MDCT) can demonstrate the anomaly, as in the images presented in this case (see figures). Here one can see the aberrant subclavian artery cross to the right of the mediastinum behind the esophagus. The term *dysphagia lusoria* historically applied to the impression of a greatly enlarged left atrium of rheumatic heart disease. However, today it is generally used to describe dysphagia caused by any impression by any vascular structure.

Notes

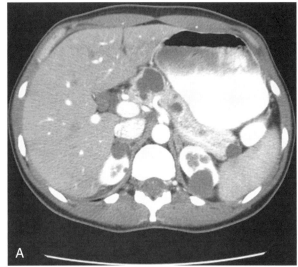

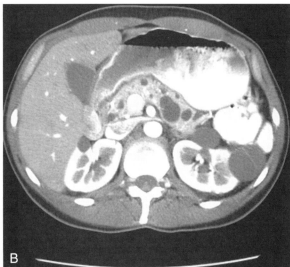

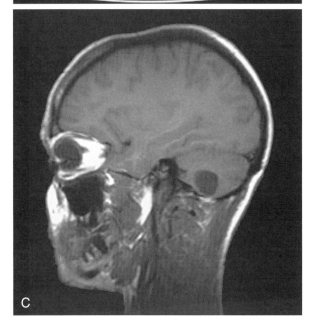

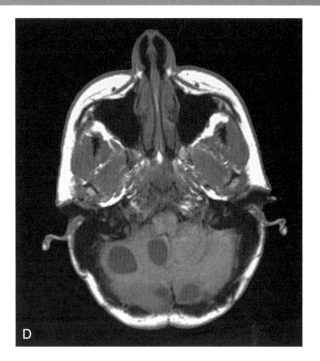

History: A 29-year-old man presents with dizziness and dyspepsia.

1. Which of the following should be included in the differential diagnosis of the dominant imaging finding on figures A and B? (Choose all that apply.)
   A. Trauma
   B. Cystic fibrosis
   C. Cystic metastases
   D. Multiple congenital cysts
   E. Postinflammatory pseudocysts

2. Several abdominal lesions have been reported to be associated with von Hippel–Lindau disease (VHL). Which of the following is *not* a recognized association?
   A. Pheochromocytoma
   B. Renal cell carcinoma
   C. Mesenteric carcinoid
   D. Pancreatic islet cell tumor

3. Which of the following studies would be most appropriate in the work-up of this patient?
   A. CT of the orbits
   B. Radionuclide bone scan
   C. Chest plain radiographs
   D. Spinal MRI

4. Regarding VHL disease, which of the following statements is true?
   A. Cerebellar hemangioblastomas are usually multiple and aggressive.
   B. Pheochromocytoma in VHL disease occurs in older patients and is usually multiple.
   C. The renal malignancies associated with VHL disease are clear cell tumors.
   D. The scrotal lesions associated with VHL disease are testicular cystadenomas.

von Hippel–Lindau Disease

1. C, D, and E

2. C

3. D

4. C

Reference

Choyke, PL, Glenn, GM, Walther, MM, et al: von Hippel-Lindau disease: genetic, clinical and imaging features. *Radiology* 1995;194:629-642.

Cross-Reference

Gastrointestinal Imaging: *THE REQUISITES,* 3rd ed, p 168.

Comment

The images in this case show multiple pancreatic cysts of varying size (see figures). The CT images are from a patient with von Hippel–Lindau (VHL) disease. VHL disease is an autosomal dominant inherited disease of capillary angiomatous hamartomas with CNS involvement of the brain and retina. In the brain, the lesion is usually a hemangioblastoma of the posterior fossa (see figures). Visceral abdominal tumors also seen in this condition include renal cell carcinoma, pheochromocytoma, and increased incidence of cystic malignancy of the pancreas.

Multiple pancreatic cysts are seen in almost three quarters of patients with VHL disease and are highly suggestive of the diagnosis. Solid islet cell tumors may be seen in VHL disease. Most of the cases are discovered in the third and fourth decades of life. If malignancy is present at the time of diagnosis, the prognosis is usually poor. Thus, suspicion should be aroused when any patient undergoing a CT of the abdomen demonstrates multiple pancreatic cysts, and the abdomen should be carefully searched for such neoplasms as pheochromocytomas and renal cell cancers.

Notes

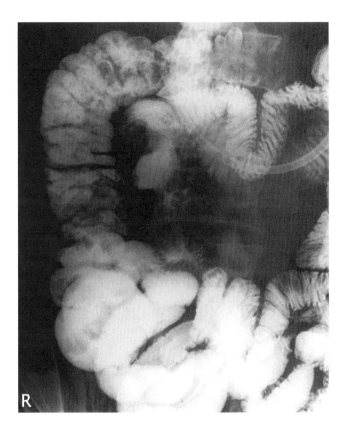

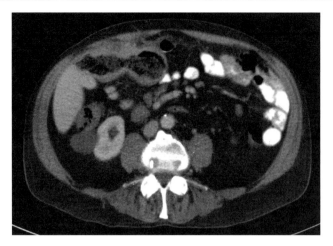

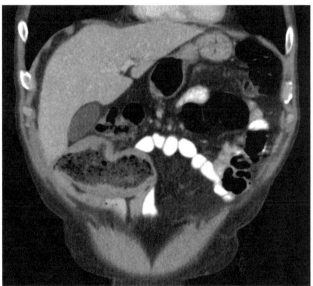

History: A 35-year-old man presents with 3 weeks of upper abdominal pain.

1. Which of the following should be included in the differential diagnosis of the dominant imaging findings? (Choose all that apply.)
   A. Adenocarcinoma
   B. Lymphoma
   C. Stromal tumor
   D. Dermoid tumor
   E. Metastatic melanoma

2. What is the most likely lesion to cause large masses involving the gut without bowel obstruction?
   A. Adenocarcinoma
   B. Lymphoma
   C. Desmoid tumor
   D. Metastatic melanoma

3. Which of the following correctly describes *aneurysmal dilation* of the small bowel?
   A. A large mass encasing the small bowel, in which the gut lumen is channeled through the lesion, leaving a false channel surrounded by tumor but without obstruction
   B. Dilation of the superior mesenteric artery
   C. Dilation of the small bowel proximal to a segment of narrowing
   D. A diverticulum greater than 10 cm in diameter

4. What small bowel lesion results in elevated levels of 5-hydroxyindoleacetic acid (5-HIAA) in the urine?
   A. VIPoma
   B. Pheochromocytoma
   C. Carcinoid
   D. Insulinoma

Small Bowel Lymphoma

1. A, B, C, and E

2. B

3. A

4. C

References

Dahnert, W. *Radiology Review Manual*, 6th ed. Philadelphia: Lippincott Williams & Wilkins, 2007, pp 851-852.

Yoo CC, Levine MS, McLarney JK, et al: Value of barium studies for predicting primary versus secondary non-Hodgkin's gastrointestinal lymphoma. *Abdom Imaging* 2000;25:368-372.

Cross-Reference

Gastrointestinal Imaging: *THE REQUISITES,* 3rd ed, p 133.

Comment

Lymphoma is a common malignancy of the small bowel. It can grow to large masses, which, quite often, do not obstruct the bowel. This phenomenon is due to a particular characteristic of lymphoma called aneurysmal dilation, in which the gut lumen is channeled through the lesion, leaving a false channel surrounded by tumor but without obstruction (see figures). This condition may be rarely seen in other small cell lesions of the gut, such as melanoma, but it most commonly indicates lymphoma. It does not seem to occur in Hodgkin's disease, and the mechanism is not understood. As a result, patients can present with large abdominal masses, possibly with constitutional symptoms, but no complaints related to bowel obstruction. CT findings include large masses involving the bowel, most often with large foamy lymphomatous nodes in the peritoneum, in the retroperitoneum, and at the base throughout the mesentery (see figures).

Notes

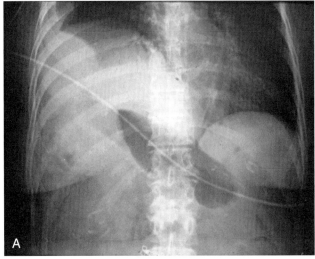

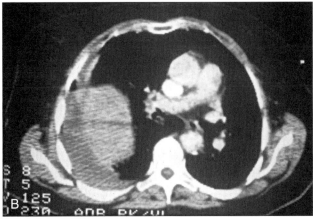

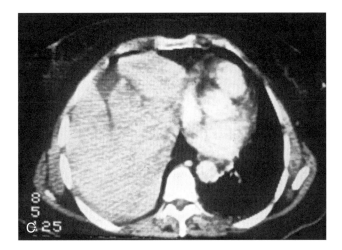

History: A 70-year-old woman was injured in a motor vehicle accident.

1. Which of the following should be included in the differential diagnosis of the dominant imaging finding on figure A? (Choose all that apply.)
   A. Morgagni hernia
   B. Bochdalek hernia
   C. Spigelian hernia
   D. Traumatic diaphragmatic hernia
   E. Diaphragmatic eventration

2. What other abdominal or pelvic injury is most commonly involved with this abnormality?
   A. Aorta
   B. Fractures
   C. Hepatic and splenic laceration
   D. Hollow organ perforation

3. What is the most commonly herniated organ in patients with traumatic diaphragmatic injury?
   A. Stomach
   B. Colon
   C. Liver
   D. Spleen

4. What is the most common sign of a diaphragmatic hernia on CT (including coronal and sagittal reformats)?
   A. Abdominal viscera in the thorax
   B. Elevated hemidiaphragm
   C. The collar sign, a waistlike constriction of viscera at the level of the diaphragm
   D. Discontinuity of the diaphragm

C A S E   2 6

Traumatic Diaphragmatic Injury

1. A, B, D, and E

2. B

3. A

4. D

References

Eren S, Kantarci M, Okur A: Imaging of diaphragmatic rupture after trauma. *Clin Radiol* 2006;61:467-477.

Low V, Kelsey P: CT demonstration of traumatic ventral hernia and diaphragmatic rupture. *Austral Radiol* 1990;34:172-174.

Cross-Reference

Gastrointestinal Imaging: *THE REQUISITES,* 3rd ed, p 193.

Comment

Most traumatic diaphragmatic ruptures are associated with high-velocity, high-impact motor vehicle accidents (85%), and the remainder are usually associated with falling from ladders and roofs or from penetrating trauma. Diagnosis of diaphragmatic trauma is often delayed or missed, even with the current advances in imaging. This is often the case with penetrating injuries. The more severe the diaphragmatic trauma, the easier the diagnosis. However, the more severe the trauma, the less likely is survival. This is especially true of right-sided trauma because of the increased incidence of aortic tears associated with it. The size of the diaphragmatic tear can vary from 1 cm to almost the entire diaphragm (about 15 cm), such as in this case (see figures).

Notes

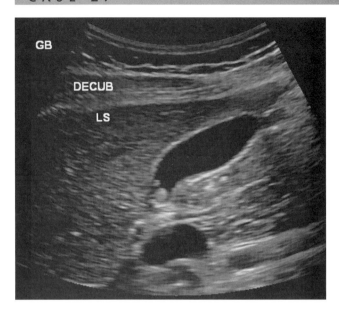

History: A 33-year-old woman, 12 weeks pregnant, underwent routine ultrasound, with an incidentally noted finding in the gallbladder.

1. Which of the following should be included in the differential diagnosis of the imaging finding? (Choose all that apply.)
   A. Polyps
   B. Adherent calculi
   C. Adenomyomatosis
   D. Primary gallbladder cancer
   E. Hematogenous metastatic deposits

2. What is the most common type of gallbladder polyp?
   A. Adenoma
   B. Papilloma
   C. Cholesterol
   D. Hyperplastic

3. What types of tumors can produce multiple mural nodules?
   A. Klatskin tumor
   B. Lymphoma
   C. Metastases
   D. Primary cancer

4. What benign condition can produce gallbladder wall nodularity?
   A. Adenomyomatosis
   B. Emphysematous cholecystitis
   C. Intramural hemorrhage
   D. Intramural pseudodiverticulosis

Gallbladder Polyps

1. A, B, C, and E

2. C

3. C

4. A

References

Lee KF, Wong J, Li JCM, Lai PBS: Polypoid lesions of the gallbladder. *Am J Surg* 2004;188:186-190.

Terzi C, Sokmen S, Seckin S, et al: Polypoid lesions of the gallbladder: report of 100 cases with special reference to operative indications. *Surgery* 2000;127:622-627.

Cross-Reference

Gastrointestinal Imaging: *THE REQUISITES,* 3rd ed, pp 246-252.

Comment

Although calculi are by far the most common cause of filling defects within the gallbladder, several noncalculous lesions can produce filling defects within the gallbladder lumen. One of the more common noncalculous causes is a gallbladder polyp. Polyps in the gallbladder produce echogenic filling defects within the lumen but are fixed, often along the nondependent surface of the gallbladder (see figure). They do not move with changes in position. Polyps of the gallbladder, particularly when they are multiple, are most often cholesterol polyps. The patient with multiple cholesterol polyps is considered to have a type of cholesterolosis. If the polyp is solitary, it could be cholesterol, an adenoma, or a papilloma.

Rarely, other conditions produce multiple mural nodules or protrusions that simulate gallbladder polyps. Adenomyomatosis with prominence of the Rokitansky-Aschoff sinuses sometimes results in some mural nodularity. Adherent stones can also produce polyp-like lesions that can be difficult to differentiate from true polyps. Metastases are quite uncommon in the gallbladder, but when they occur, they can produce mural polyps. Melanoma, breast cancer, and lymphoma infiltrating the gallbladder can cause gallbladder metastases. Primary gallbladder carcinoma can result in the formation of a solitary polypoid lesion but rarely results in multiple mural polyps. Potentially, blood clots, hemorrhage, and even varices could produce mural polyps or nodularity, but this is quite uncommon.

Notes

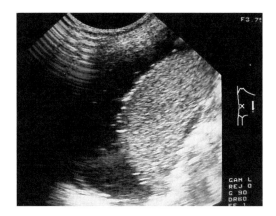

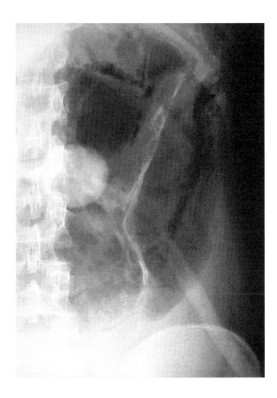

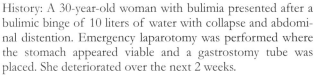

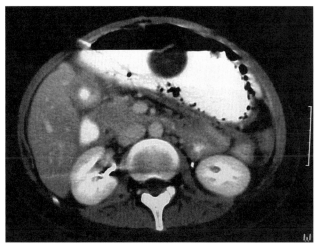

History: A 30-year-old woman with bulimia presented after a bulimic binge of 10 liters of water with collapse and abdominal distention. Emergency laparotomy was performed where the stomach appeared viable and a gastrostomy tube was placed. She deteriorated over the next 2 weeks.

1. What conditions can be associated with this finding? (Choose all that apply.)
   A. Pulmonary disease
   B. Peptic ulcer disease
   C. Gastric outlet obstruction
   D. Gastroparesis
   E. Endoscopy (especially with intervention)

2. Some infectious processes are recognized to produce this abnormality. Which of these agents is *not* known to cause this abnormality?
   A. Hemolytic streptococci
   B. *Clostridium* species
   C. Coliform bacteria
   D. *Helicobacter pylori*

3. Ingestion of what type of substance can cause this problem?
   A. Alcohol
   B. Antibiotics
   C. Corrosives
   D. Corticosteroids

4. What is the most common location for intramural gas to occur in the gastrointestinal tract?
   A. Stomach
   B. Small bowel
   C. Colon
   D. Multiple sites

Emphysematous Gastritis

1. A, B, C, and E

2. D

3. C

4. C

References

Lee S: Gastric emphysema. *Am J Gastroenterol* 1984;79(11):899-904.
Low VHS, Thompson RI: Gastric emphysema due to necrosis from massive gastric distention. *Clin Imaging* 1995;19(1):34-36.

Cross-Reference

Gastrointestinal Imaging: *THE REQUISITES,* 3rd ed, p 88.

Comment

The finding of air in the wall of the stomach is quite often an ominous sign (see figures). Although air in the stomach wall can be a sequela of recent endoscopy or gastric surgery, it is a rare complication. Despite the thousands of endoscopic procedures performed, a radiologist rarely encounters air in the gastric wall as a result of them.

Most commonly the occurrence of air in the wall represents a severe infection of the stomach, a type of phlegmonous gastritis. Although many organisms have been isolated in these infections, the most common are hemolytic streptococci, *Clostridium welchii,* and coliform bacteria. Infection may be slightly more common in severe diabetes, relating to the overall systemic disease process as well as local diabetes-induced vasculitides. Infection has been identified in otherwise healthy patients, as well as in those with a variety of chronic, debilitating conditions (e.g., transplant recipients, postoperative patients, those with AIDS). The process by which the infection develops is uncertain, but it is believed that ulcers or other breaks in the mucosa allow bacteria access to the submucosal tissue, with resultant spread of infection. Discovery of phlegmonous gastritis probably indicates impending necrosis of the gastric wall. Prompt therapy, including gastrectomy and antibiotics, is necessary because the mortality rate is quite high.

Emphysematous gastritis also can be encountered in patients with gastric outlet obstruction, in whom elevated intraluminal pressures can force air into the gastric wall. Rarely, the condition is seen in patients with pulmonary disease who also develop pneumatosis in other parts of the gastrointestinal tract.

Patients who ingest corrosive agents in an attempt to commit suicide also can develop this complication, which heralds necrosis of the gastric wall. As is true of other radiologic findings, the clinical history is the most important factor in establishing the correct diagnosis.

Notes

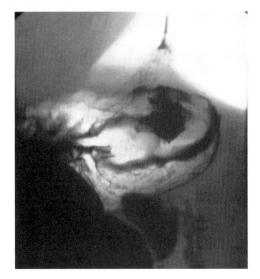

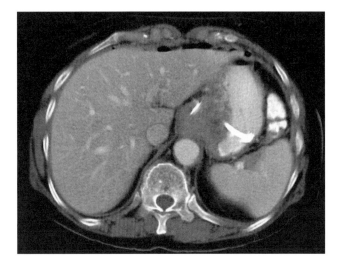

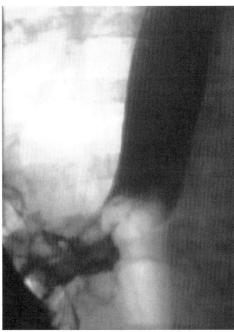

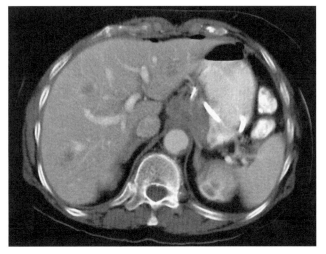

History: A 44-year-old man presents with dysphagia.

1. Which of the following should be included in the likely differential diagnosis of the imaging findings? (Choose all that apply.)
   A. Esophageal adenocarcinoma
   B. Esophageal squamous cell carcinoma
   C. Primary esophageal lymphoma
   D. Gastric adenocarcinoma
   E. Gastric squamous cell carcinoma

2. What is the most common type of malignancy seen at the gastroesophageal junction?
   A. Adenocarcinoma
   B. Lymphoma
   C. Squamous cell carcinoma
   D. Metastatic melanoma

3. There are non-neoplastic processes that could give this appearance of a mass at the gastro-esophageal junction. Which of the following would *not* be expected to give this appearance?
   A. Reflux
   B. Bezoar
   C. Normal
   D. Surgery
   E. Varices

4. What inflammatory process is a predisposing factor associated with this lesion?
   A. Alcoholic esophagitis
   B. Barrett's metaplasia
   C. Crohn's disease
   D. *Helicobacter pylori* gastritis

Adenocarcinoma of the Gastroesophageal Junction

1. A, B, and D

2. A

3. A

4. B

References

Iyer R, Dubrow R: Imaging upper gastrointestinal malignancy. *Semin Roentgenol* 2006;41:105-112.
Rudiger Siewert J, Feith M, et al: Adenocarcinoma of the esophagogastric junction: results of surgical therapy based on anatomical/topographic classification in 1,002 consecutive patients. *Ann Surg* 2000;232:353-361.

Cross-Reference

Gastrointestinal Imaging: *THE REQUISITES,* 3rd ed, pp 23-26.

Comment

A tumor at the gastroesophageal (GE) junction may have arisen from the stomach or from the esophagus. The gastric tumors are nearly always adenocarcinomas. Of the tumors arising from the esophagus, squamous cell carcinoma was by far the most common (80% to 90%). However, the incidence of adenocarcinoma of the esophagus has increased almost 500% in the Western world since 1980.

This change is due directly to the increased incidence of Barrett's metaplasia, now seen in the distal esophagus. Patients with Barrett's metaplasia have a 40% or greater risk of malignancy, and almost all adenocarcinomas of the distal esophagus and gastroesophageal junction are a result of pre-existing Barrett's metaplasia. These patients are usually younger than those with the typical squamous cell lesion of the esophagus. They often have a long history of heartburn symptoms and present with dysphagia to solid foods. The correlating factors of smoking and alcohol seen with squamous cell carcinoma might not apply to this lesion. Although almost all adenocarcinomas arise from underlying dysplastic disease (Barrett's), a tiny percentage might arise from the sparse adenomatous glands of the esophagus directly. In general, the more distal the lesion, the more lightly the predisposing factor is Barrett's metaplasia.

The 5-year survival rate in general for this lesion is 10% to 12%, but this, too, is to a great extent related to the spread of the disease. It can be very local, it can spread via the adjacent lymph node chain (upper celiac in the gastrohepatic ligament), or it can occur with distal metastatic disease to the lung and elsewhere.

Radiologic findings include mass, narrowing, and irregularity at the GE junction (see figures). This may be associated with some chronic inflammatory changes on barium studies. CT images reveal a thickened esophageal wall (greater than 5 mm) as well as the possibility of nodes in the mediastinum and paragastric areas (see figures).

Notes

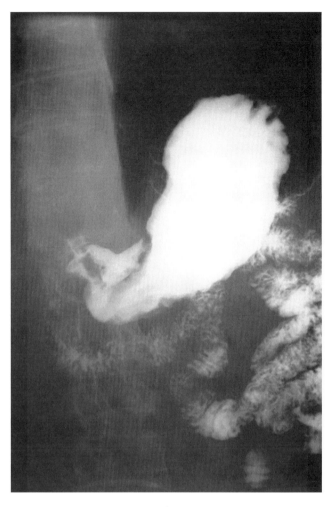

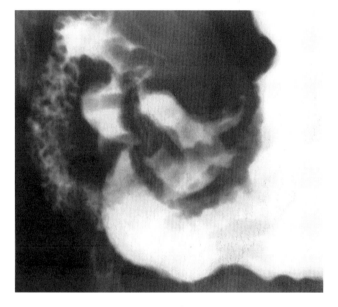

History: A 70-year-old man presents with epigastric pain and weight loss.

1. In what condition is the Carmen meniscus sign (CMS) found?
   A. Linitis plastica
   B. Hypertrophic gastritis
   C. Ulcerated gastric cancer
   D. Giant gastric peptic ulcer

2. What is the Kirkland complex?
   A. The central excavated collection of barium due to ulceration
   B. The concave lucent margin around the ulceration
   C. The distorted rugal folds around the ulceration
   D. The mass effect surrounding the ulceration

3. Where must the lesion be located for the CMS to be seen?
   A. The lesion may occur anywhere in the stomach
   B. The lesion must occur on the lesser curvature of body or antrum
   C. The lesion must obliterate the cardiac rosette at the gastroesophageal junction
   D. The lesion must invade the pylorus, causing gastric outlet obstruction

4. How is the CMS best seen?
   A. It is best seen with 3D ultrasonography
   B. It is best seen with CT virtual gastrography
   C. It is best seen on single-contrast or biphasic studies
   D. It is best seen on double-contrast barium studies

Carmen Meniscus Sign

1. C

2. B

3. B

4. C

Reference

Low V H S , Levine M S , Rubesin S E , et al: Diagnosis of gastric carcinoma: sensitivity of double-contrast barium studies. *Am J Roentgenol* 1994; 162:329-334.

Cross-Reference

Gastrointestinal Imaging: *THE REQUISITES,* 3rd ed, p 82-85.

Comment

The Carmen meniscus sign was first described by Dr. Carmen in the late 1930s before double-contrast studies were in routine use. It is a sign that is considered to be pathognomic for an ulcerated gastric malignancy. The sign is confusing and not well understood. This is because certain conditions must be present for the sign to occur. First, the lesion must be a flat infiltrating ulcerative lesion with heaped-up margins. Second, the lesion must be in the saddle region of the stomach, the lesser curve of the body or antrum (see figures). The examination should be a single-contrast or at least a biphasic study (when both single-contrast and double-contrast evaluation are used). The sign may be seen on a double-contrast study but is often not recognized. Finally, compression must be applied to the stomach so that the ulcerated margins of the ulcer are forced together to entrap barium in a curved semilunar configuration, with the convexity directed toward the lumen of the stomach. The lucency that results from the heaped-up walls of the ulcer touching each other is called the Kirkland complex (see figures).

Notes

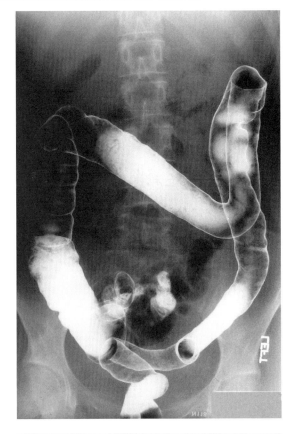

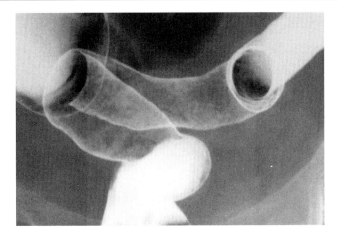

History: A 26-year-old woman presents with a 3-year history of crampy abdominal pain and bloody diarrhea.

1. Which of the following should be included in the differential diagnosis of the imaging findings? (Choose all that apply.)
   A. Pseudomembranous colitis
   B. Ulcerative colitis
   C. Crohn's disease
   D. *Salmonella* colitis

2. Which of the following is characteristically *absent* in patients with acute ulcerative colitis?
   A. Terminal ileal disease
   B. Loss of colonic haustra
   C. Granular mucosal pattern
   D. Distal colonic distribution

3. Which inflammatory bowel disease (IBD) is most likely to cause fistulas to form?
   A. Pseudomembranous colitis
   B. Ulcerative colitis
   C. Crohn's disease
   D. Ischemic colitis

4. Which IBD has the greatest risk for malignancy?
   A. Pseudomembranous colitis
   B. Ulcerative colitis
   C. Crohn's disease
   D. Irritable bowel disease

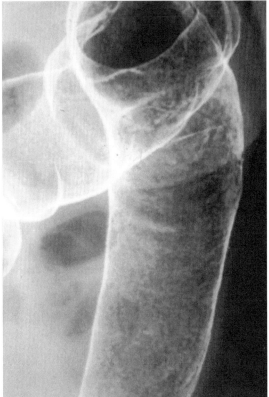

CASE 31

Acute Ulcerative Colitis

1. B, C, and D

2. A

3. C

4. B

References

Gore RM, Balthazar EK, Ghahremani GG, Miller FH: CT features of ulcerative colitis and Crohn's disease. *Am J Roentgenol* 1996;167:3-15.

Thoeni RF, Cello JP: CT Imaging of colitis. *Radiology* 2006;240:623-638.

Cross-Reference

Gastrointestinal Imaging: *THE REQUISITES,* 3rd ed, p 291-294.

Comment

Ulcerative colitis (UC) is a superficial inflammatory disease usually affecting the distal colon. It begins as a granularity, hyperemia, and edema of the mucosa and progresses to multiple widespread evenly distributed tiny ulcerations (see figures). The patient presents with abdominal pain, diarrhea, and blood per rectum. The disease can disappear spontaneously, in which case one ought to reconsider the diagnostic possibilities, or it can go on to simmering chronic disease with occasional flare-ups. The entire colon may be involved in about a third of patients presenting with severe disease.

Differentiating between ulcerative colitis and Crohn's disease can sometimes be very difficult clinically and histologically. Radiologic examinations can sometimes be more specific. In ulcerative colitis the disease starts distally and progresses proximally. The terminal ileum is never involved with UC, although it can appear patulous (backwash ileitis). The skip lesions and asymmetry seen in Crohn's disease are not present in UC. The fistula formation commonly seen in Crohn's disease is not seen with UC. Involvement of other parts of the gut, such as may be seen with Crohn's disease, is never seen in UC. Extracolonic manifestations can be seen in both diseases. The risk for malignancy is much higher in UC than in Crohn's disease.

Notes

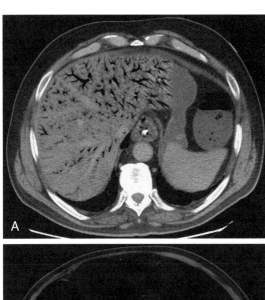

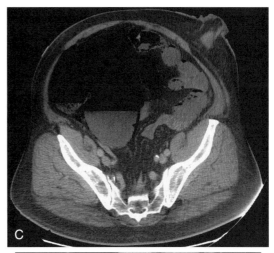

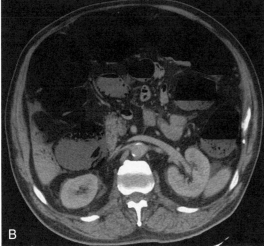

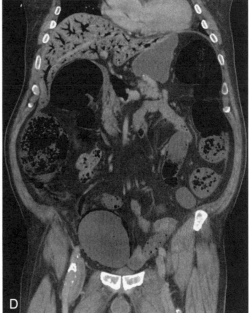

History: A 69-year-old man presents with acute abdominal pain and tenderness, nausea, and vomiting.

1. Which of the following should be included in the differential diagnosis of the dominant imaging finding on figure A? (Choose all that apply.)
   A. Hepatic arterial gas
   B. Aerobilia
   C. Portal venous gas
   D. Periportal edema

2. What other finding on figures B to D is linked to the finding in figure A?
   A. Pneumoretroperitoneum
   B. Pneumoperitoneum
   C. Pneumatosis
   D. Pneumothorax

3. Some benign conditions (not catastrophic bowel necrosis) are recognized as causes for gas in the portal venous system. Which of these is *not* an explanation for gas in the portal venous system?
   A. Bowel obstruction
   B. Gallstone erosion
   C. Instrumentation
   D. Bowel surgery

4. How does one distinguish gas in the portal venous system of the liver from other abnormal gas collections?
   A. Gas in the periphery of the liver
   B. Gas centrally in the liver
   C. Gas-forming bubbles
   D. Gas-forming streaks

Portal Venous Gas

1. A, B, and C

2. C

3. B

4. A

References

Gore RM, Yaghmai V, Thakrar KH, et al: Imaging in intestinal ischemic disorders. *Radiol Clin North Am* 2008;46:845-875.

Scheidler J, Stabler A, Kleber G, Neidhardt D: Computed tomography in pneumatosis intestinalis: differential diagnosis and therapeutic consequences. *Abdom Imaging* 1995;20:523-528.

Cross-Reference

Gastrointestinal Imaging: *THE REQUISITES,* 3rd ed, p 209-210.

Comment

Gas in the portal venous system can be a serious finding, especially in the elderly (see figures). There are benign causes for this finding. Nevertheless, the identification of potential gas in the portal venous system always requires immediate communication with the clinical service to consider the catastrophic issue of bowel necrosis. A careful evaluation of the bowel for pneumatosis is also required. Occasionally gas can be seen in the mesenteric vessels, as in this case (see figures).

Gas in the biliary system is almost never a life-threatening event. The only exception might be gas in the biliary system due to gas-forming pyogenic infection. This is exceedingly rare and the patient would be extremely ill. Most gas in the biliary system is the result of surgery (choledocho-enterostomies), erosion of gallstones through the wall of a chronically inflamed gallbladder into adjacent hollow viscus, or endoscopic retrograde cholangiopancreatography (ERCP) and papillotomy.

Notes

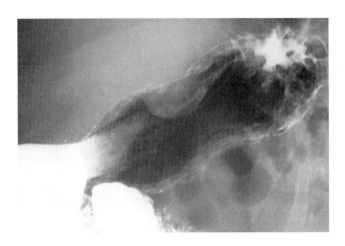
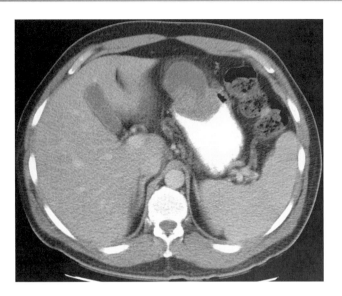

History: A 48-year-old man presents with epigastric pain.

1. Which of the following should be included in the differential diagnosis of the dominant imaging finding? (Choose all that apply.)
   A. Lipoma
   B. Lymphoma
   C. Neurofibroma
   D. Stromal tumor
   E. Duplication cyst

2. What is the most common benign submucosal tumor of the stomach?
   A. Lipoma
   B. Neurofibroma
   C. Stromal tumor
   D. Duplication cyst

3. How is a malignant tumor (leiomyosarcoma) distinguished from a benign stromal tumor (leiomyoma)?
   A. Tumor size
   B. Metastases
   C. Mucosal surface ulceration
   D. Mitotic activity on pathology

4. What congenital abnormality can mimic a leiomyoma?
   A. Gastric fundal diverticulum
   B. Heterotopic gastric mucosa
   C. Gastric mucosal prolapse
   D. Ectopic pancreatic rest

Large Gastrointestinal Stromal Tumor of the Stomach

1. B, C, and D

2. C

3. B

4. D

References

Darnell A, Dalmau E, Pericay C, et al: Gastrointestinal stromal tumors. *Abdom Imaging* 2006;31:387-399.

Levy AD, Remotti HE, Thompson WM, et al: Gastrointestinal stromal tumors: radiologic features with pathologic correlation. *Radiographics* 2003;23: 283-304.

Cross-Reference

Gastrointestinal Imaging: *THE REQUISITES,* 3rd ed, pp 76-77.

Comment

Smooth muscle or gastrointestinal stromal tumors (GISTs) are among the more commonly encountered tumors of the stomach. They account for almost half of all benign stomach tumors. Only a small percentage (less than 10%) are malignant. Benign GISTs occur equally among men and women, whereas malignant GISTs are more common in men. There tends to be a slight increase in the number of tumors with increasing age.

It is difficult to radiologically distinguish between benign and malignant GISTs and other submucosal tumors (see figures). The benign GIST can be found anywhere in the stomach, whereas its sarcomatous counterpart is usually more proximal. The pattern of growth is variable. The majority of both types of lesions grow endogastrically, or into the lumen. However, a small but significant percentage grow exophytically, or into the perigastric abdominal cavity, creating only a mild extrinsic mass impression on the stomach. This growth is fairly unusual but should be considered whenever a large intra-abdominal mass with growth into the abdominal cavity is encountered in the vicinity of the stomach. The tumors that grow into the lumen can ulcerate and can be large or even, rarely, multiple. Because these tumors are vascular, ulceration over the stretched and thinned mucosa can occur, and patients can present with a GI bleed.

Distinguishing benign from malignant smooth muscle tumors is difficult even for the pathologist. The classic criterion has been the number of mitotic figures visible per high-power field (more than 10 for malignant GIST). However, the nature of the histologic activity of the tumor is variable in different parts, and sampling can have a significant impact on the mitotic activity and pleomorphism viewed by the pathologist. Some believe that size of the tumor is just as important. Tumors less than 5 cm in diameter are more likely to be malignant.

Finally, the absolute criterion is evidence of metastatic disease. If the lesion is indeterminate based on pathologic findings, CT often becomes an absolute necessity to determine the exact nature of the tumor (see figures).

Notes

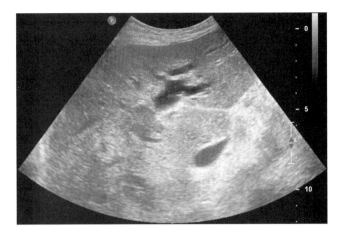

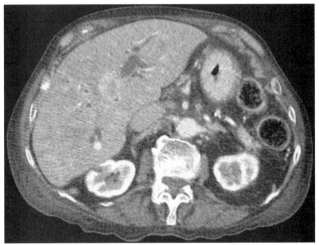

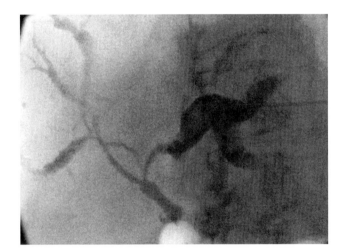

History: A 93-year-old woman presents with painless jaundice.

1. Which of the following should be included in the differential diagnosis of the dominant imaging findings? (Choose all that apply.)
   A. Amebic abscess
   B. Biliary cystadenoma
   C. Cholangiocarcinoma
   D. Metastatic breast cancer
   E. Hepatocellular carcinoma

2. What is this condition called?
   A. Chilaiditi's syndrome
   B. Mirizzi's syndrome
   C. Klatskin's tumor
   D. Caroli's malformation

3. Which of these conditions is a known predisposing factor for a patient to develop cholangiocarcinoma?
   A. Postviral hepatitis fibrosis
   B. Recurrent bacterial infection
   C. Echinococcal cyst
   D. Sclerosing cholangitis

4. This tumor is known to appear in a range of forms. Which of these choices is *not* a recognized form?
   A. Biliary stricture
   B. Biliary polyp
   C. Biliary cyst
   D. Liver mass

CASE 34

Bile Duct Malignant Stricture (Klatskin's Tumor)

1. C, D, and E

2. C

3. D

4. C

References

Bloom CM, Langer B, Wilson SR: Role of US in the detection, characterization, and staging of cholangiocarcinoma. *Radiographics* 1999;19:1199-1218.

Lee HY, Kim SH, Lee JM, et al: Preoperative assessment of resectability of hepatic hilar cholangiocarcinoma: combined CT and cholangiography with revised criteria. *Radiology* 2006;239:113-121.

Cross-Reference

Gastrointestinal Imaging: THE REQUISITES, 3rd ed, p 232.

Comment

Cholangiocarcinomas are adenomatous tumors that arise from the lining of the bile ducts. Because they can arise from any portion of the biliary system (even the tiniest branches in the liver), the appearance of cholangiocarcinomas can be quite variable. They most often form nontumorous strictures, which are malignant cells spreading down the walls of the bile duct in a scirrhous pattern. They can also form polypoid masses that project into the lumen of the ducts. In the liver parenchyma itself, cholangiocarcinomas are often identified as liver masses and are indistinguishable from other liver tumors. Patients in whom these growths arise in the extrahepatic bile ducts have the best prognosis.

Cholangiocarcinomas can produce jaundice or other symptoms before they spread to adjacent structures. Cholangiocarcinoma is often fatal because it invades adjacent critical structures in the region, such as the bile ducts and portal vein. Distant metastases are not common.

Ultrasound and CT inspection of the bile ducts reveals proximal ductal dilation (see figures), an area of narrowing, or a polypoid lesion in the duct lumen. Proximal ductal dilation is often evident. On CT examination, the tumors themselves are typically evident only when they are in the liver parenchyma and mass effect is visible. Approximately one third of cholangiocarcinomas manifest as liver masses because they grow exophytically into the liver parenchyma.

The type of cholangiocarcinoma that arises at the confluence of the right and left bile ducts is termed a Klatskin tumor. This tumor is typically scirrhous cholangiocarcinoma that grows along the ducts, producing thickening of the wall of the ducts and progressive narrowing of the lumen. As the tumor grows, focal lobar atrophy can become evident. CT can demonstrate a mass in the region. Direct cholangiography (either by percutaneous transhepatic cholangiography or by endoscopic retrograde cholangiopancreatography) demonstrates the extent and severity of biliary obstruction (see figures). The access achieved to the bile ducts also allows therapeutic maneuvers such as stenting to provide relief from jaundice. The condition is almost invariably fatal within 6 to 8 months because critical structures in the region, such as the portal vein, are often invaded. Enlarged lymph nodes in the porta hepatis and Mirizzi syndrome caused by an impacted stone in the cystic duct can mimic this condition.

Notes

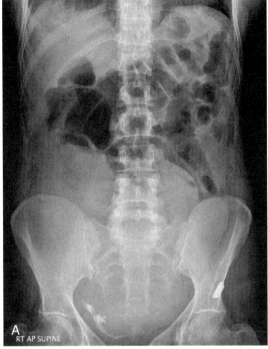

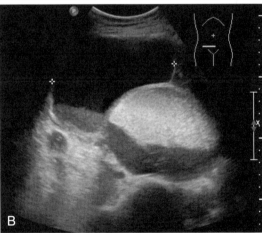

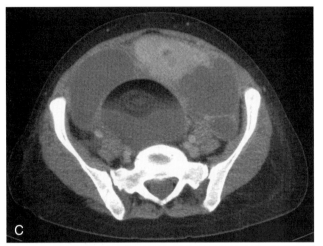

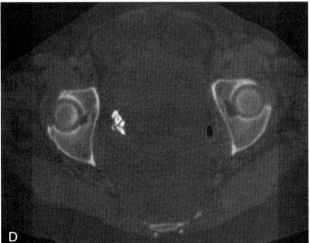

History: A 48-year-old woman presents with 5 days of constipation.

1. Which of the following should be included in the differential diagnosis of the dominant imaging finding on figure A? (Choose all that apply.)
   A. Tubo-ovarian abscess
   B. Lithopedion
   C. Appendiceal mucocele
   D. Ovarian dermoid
   E. Uterine fibroid

2. After reviewing all the provided images, what is the most likely diagnosis?
   A. Tubo-ovarian abscess
   B. Pelvic liposarcoma
   C. Adnexal endometrioma
   D. Ovarian dermoid
   E. Uterine fibroid

3. Which statement about ovarian dermoids is true?
   A. The usual clinical presentation is with abdominal pain.
   B. It is bilateral in 2% to 3% of cases.
   C. Malignant degeneration occurs in 1% to 2%, more commonly during pregnancy.
   D. Imaging finding of a fat-fluid level on imaging is diagnostic.
   E. Malignant transformation should be suspected if the cyst ruptures spontaneously.

4. A variety of tissues have been recognized in ovarian dermoids. Which of the following elements would you *not* expect to find in ovarian dermoids?
   A. Fat
   B. Skin
   C. Vesicles
   D. Teeth
   E. Hair

CASE 35

Pelvic Ovarian Dermoid

1. B, C, D, and E

2. D

3. D

4. C

References

Dill-Macky MJ, Mostafa A: Ovarian sonography. In Callen PW (ed): *Ultrasonography in Obstetrics and Gynecology*, 4th ed. Philadelphia: WB Saunders, 2000, pp 878-880.
Dodd D, Budzik R: Lipomatous tumors of the pelvis in women: spectrum of radiologic findings. *Am J Roentgenol* 1990;155:317-322.

Cross-Reference

Genitourinary Radiology: *THE REQUISITES,* 2nd ed, pp 288-290.

Comment

Benign dermoid cysts (also called mature cystic teratomas) are the most common pelvic masses in young women (see figures). They usually produce no symptoms and are bilateral in 10% to 15%, but they cause discomfort in some patients. The reasons are not clear. It might relate to a contiguous position of the lesion or possibly to degrees of torsion. On the other hand, it might also be a sign of possible malignancy. Fatty density is seen in almost 100% of ovarian dermoids along with hair and rudimentary teeth.

CT of the pelvis shows these findings, usually as an incidental finding in most patients (see figures). Extragonadal germ cell tumors, which include dermoid cysts, are not uncommon and are among the important diagnoses in the differential for upper anterior mediastinal masses. Malignant degeneration is rare but increases with the age of the patient. The size of the lesion and the amount of soft tissue and fatty material held by the lesion are variable. Torsion is the most common complication associated with these lesions.

Notes

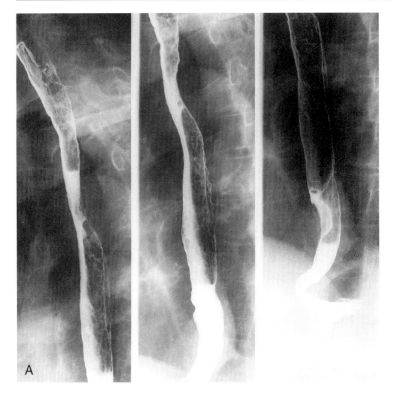

A

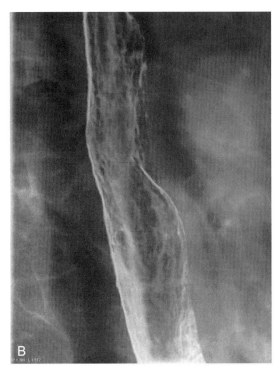

B

History: An 80-year-old man with oxygen- and steroid-dependent chronic obstructive airway disease develops dysphagia and odynophagia.

1. Which of the following should be included in the differential diagnosis of the dominant imaging finding on figure A? (Choose all that apply.)
   A. Glycogenic acanthosis
   B. Bubbles artifact
   C. Candidiasis
   D. Cytomegalovirus (CMV) esophagitis
   E. Papillomatosis

2. Which of the following distinguishes esophageal *Candida* infection in an immunocompromised patient from the same occurring in an immunocompetent host?
   A. Odynophagia occurs in the immunocompromised patient and dysphagia in the immunocompetent patients.
   B. Oral and pharyngeal involvement occurs in the immunocompromised and not in the immunocompetent patient.
   C. On barium swallow, the esophagus of the immunocompromised patient presents a "shaggy" appearance, and that of the immunocompetent patient presents a nodular appearance.
   D. The infection is identical in both the immunocompromised and the immunocompetent patient.

3. Which of the following statements about esophageal *Candida* infection is true?
   A. *Candida albicans* is the most common cause of infectious esophagitis.
   B. Most of the patients with *Candida* esophagitis also have clinically visible oropharyngeal thrush.
   C. The plaquelike nodules seen on double-contrast esophagography typically are orientated along circular folds with intervening normal mucosa.
   D. Patients with chronic esophageal motility disorders such as achalasia and scleroderma are more likely to develop esophageal *Candida* infection owing to deficient mucosal integrity.

4. Skin conditions may be associated with multiple tiny esophageal nodular lesions. Which of the following skin conditions is *not* associated with esophageal nodules?
   A. Acanthosis nigricans
   B. Bullous pemphigoid
   C. Pyoderma gangrenosum
   D. Dermatomyositis

CASE 36

Esophageal *Candida*

1. A, B, C, and E

2. C

3. A

4. D

References

Levine MS, Rubesin SE: Diseases of the esophagus: diagnosis with esophagography. *Radiology* 2005;237:414-427.

Pappas PG, Kauffman CA, Andes D, et al: Clinical practice guidelines for the management of candidiasis: 2009 update by the Infectious Diseases Society of America. *Clin Infect Dis* 2009;48:503-535.

Cross-Reference

Gastrointestinal Imaging: THE REQUISITES, 3rd ed, p 7.

Comment

Numerous small plaques or nodules of the esophageal mucosa are not an uncommon finding. A variety of conditions can produce these abnormalities. Often the correct diagnosis can be made based on the clinical information provided by the patient. These nodules are either diffuse or focal, and this determination has some bearing on the diagnostic possibilities.

The numerous filling defects commonly seen in the esophagus are usually a technical issue. Having the patient drink barium along with the CO_2 granules almost invariably yields this artifact. It is advisable to give the granules first, with a small amount of water immediately after.

Several infectious and inflammatory conditions can produce this true mucosal filling defect in the esophagus. The most important is *Candida* infection. These small, well-defined plaques, which are identified by the radiologist, correspond to the whitish ovoid or rounded plaques that are seen in the back of the pharynx of patients with thrush. Early on, they seem to line up on the longitudinal fold of the esophagus. This is usually referred to as the colonization stage. Later, as rhizoid extension into the mucosa and submucosa occurs, some ulceration may be detected (ulceration stage) and the patient experiences odynophagia. With progression of the ulceration stage, widespread diffuse ulceration and bleeding occur throughout the esophagus (the "shaggy" esophagus). Typically in the colonization phase the superficial plaques are only a few millimeters in diameter, but they can increase quickly to as large as 1 cm or more in diameter. In addition to immunocompromised patients, patients with scleroderma, achalasia, and other conditions associated with stasis of the esophageal contents can have *Candida* organisms visible on radiologic studies.

Reflux esophagitis can produce plaque-like elevations in the distal esophagus, and these growths correspond to areas of edema and inflammation without ulceration. Very rarely, herpetic esophagitis also produces multiple small nodular lesions. However, herpetic involvement is usually tiny punctuate ulcers rather than plaques.

A common benign condition of the esophagus is glycogenic acanthosis. This condition, which consists of swelling of the epithelium caused by increased cytoplasmic glycogen, predominantly affects the elderly. It is believed to be a degenerative phenomenon and of little or no clinical significance.

Some malignant and premalignant conditions also produce multiple plaques. Rarely, early esophageal cancer occurs as a focal area of irregular, variously sized raised plaques, without a discrete mass. Superficial spreading carcinoma of the esophagus can have more-diffuse nodules. Leukoplakia is a premalignant condition of the mouth that sometimes is found in the esophagus. Esophageal papillomatosis can be seen with acanthosis nigricans of the skin.

Notes

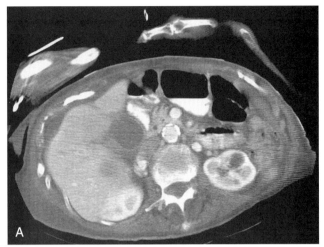

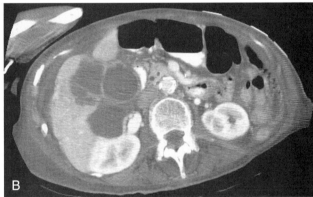

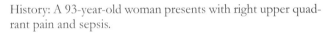

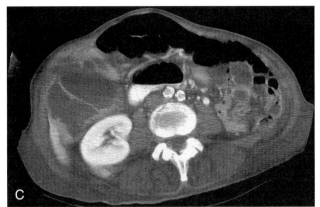

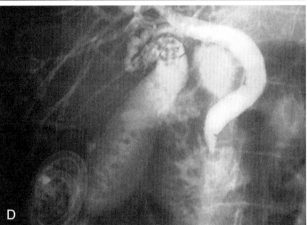

History: A 93-year-old woman presents with right upper quadrant pain and sepsis.

1. Which of the following should be included in the differential diagnosis of the dominant imaging finding on figures A to C? (Choose all that apply.)
   A. Acalculous cholecystitis
   B. Gallbladder perforation
   C. Gallbladder carcinoma
   D. Echinococcal cyst
   E. Emphysematous cholecystitis

2. Which of the following statements about acalculous cholecystitis is *true*?
   A. It accounts for less than 1% of all cases of acute cholecystitis.
   B. Apart from sepsis and shock, there are no physical signs.
   C. Ultrasonography is the investigation of first choice.
   D. Mortality is approximately 10%.

3. Which of the following is considered the definitive therapy for acalculous cholecystitis?
   A. Resuscitation and antibiotics
   B. Percutaneous cholecystostomy
   C. Cholecystectomy with drainage of any associated abscess
   D. Percutaneous abscess drainage

4. Conditions associated with acute acalculous cholecystitis include surgery, trauma, shock, ischemia, and mechanical ventilation. Which of these conditions is *not* known to be associated with acute acalculous cholecystitis?
   A. AIDS
   B. Burns
   C. Vasculitis
   D. Pregnancy
   E. Parenteral nutrition

Acute Cholecystitis and Perforation

1. A, B, and D

2. C

3. C

4. D

References

Kalliafas S, Ziegler DW, Flancbaum L, Choban PS: Acute acalculous cholecystitis: incidence, risk factors, diagnosis, and outcome. *Am Surg* 1998;64:471-475.

van Sonnenberg E, D'Agostino HB, Goodacre BW, et al: Percutaneous gallbladder puncture and cholecystostomy: results, complications and caveats for safety. *Radiology* 1992;183:167-170.

Cross-Reference

Gastrointestinal Imaging: *THE REQUISITES,* 3rd ed, p 252.

Comment

Acute cholecystitis is one of the most common of abdominal problems seen in patients presenting to the emergency department. About 90% of cases are associated with gallstones in younger patients, more often women. It is thought to occur as a result of occlusion of the cystic duct with a gallstone, resulting in biliary colic and inflammatory changes in the gallbladder and the famous Murphy sign. Most cases of acute cholecystitis spontaneously resolve in 7 to 10 days, and almost all patients have had prior episodes. A small number of patients go on to more severe disease such as gallbladder emphysema, perforation (see figures), and peritonitis. These conditions are life-threatening situations. Although the condition of acalculous cholecystitis is uncommon, it does tend to occur in older, and particularly in male, patients.

Notes

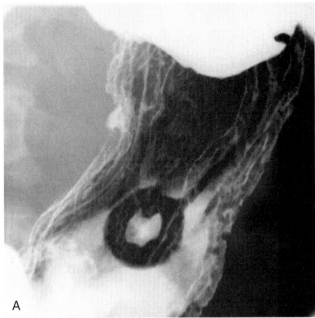

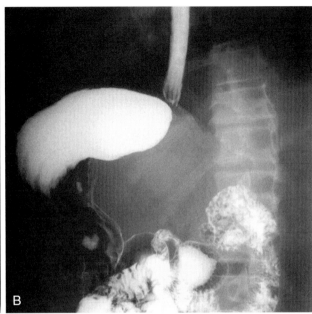

A

B

History: A 76-year-old man presents with hemoptysis and hematemesis.

1. Which of the following should be included in the differential diagnosis of the imaging finding shown in figure A? (Choose all that apply.)
   A. Villous adenoma
   B. Gastric stromal tumor
   C. Hematogenous metastasis
   D. Kaposi's sarcoma
   E. Lymphoma

2. Which of the following best describes a bull's-eye lesion?
   A. A rounded filling defect with a barium collection at its center owing to ulceration
   B. A round metastatic tumor deposit that is black owing to its melanoma origin
   C. A region of the stomach that is constricted, inelastic, and rigid
   D. A flat lobulated lesion with a reticular mucosal surface pattern

3. What is the most commonly encountered primary tumor resulting in hematogenous metastatic lesions to the stomach?
   A. Bronchogenic carcinoma
   B. Breast carcinoma
   C. Esophageal carcinoma
   D. Malignant melanoma

4. What is the most common site of melanoma metastasis to the gastrointestinal tract?
   A. Esophagus
   B. Stomach
   C. Small bowel
   D. Colon

Metastatic Lesions to the Stomach

1. B, C, D, and E

2. A

3. D

4. C

References

McDermott VG, Low VHS, Keogan MT, et al: Malignant melanoma metastatic to the gastrointestinal tract. *Am J Roentgenol* 1996;166:809-813.

Rubesin SE, Laufer I: Pictorial glossary of double contrast radiology. In Gore RM, Levine MS, editors: *Textbook of Gastrointestinal Radiology*, 2nd ed. Philadelphia: WB Saunders, 2000, pp 44-65.

Cross-Reference

Gastrointestinal Imaging: *THE REQUISITES,* 3rd ed, p 74.

Comment

Metastatic lesions to the stomach can take several forms. The form shown in this case is the classic bull's eye lesion; so named for the appearance of a rounded filling defect with a barium collection at its center. The mound is the metastatic mass arising from the intramural layer of the stomach and the displacement of barium. The bull's eye is the ulceration and resultant barium collection.

In this case the primary lesion is small cell carcinoma of the lung. However, hematogenous metastatic spread from other lesions can also cause a similar appearance. These lesions include breast cancer and melanoma. In addition, a smaller number of bull's eye lesions of the stomach can occur as a result of primary gastric tumors. These tumors include some presentations of lymphoma and Kaposi sarcoma. In recent decades the most common cause of bull's eye lesions in the stomach has been Kaposi's sarcoma seen in AIDS patients.

Another benign cause of a solitary bull's eye lesion of the stomach is a gastrointestinal stromal tumor (GIST) in which the mucosa over the center of the intramural lesion ulcerates. Occasionally bull's eye lesions are seen in the small bowel, but this location is uncommon.

Notes

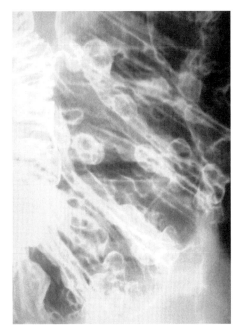

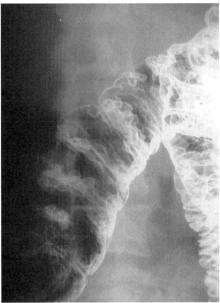

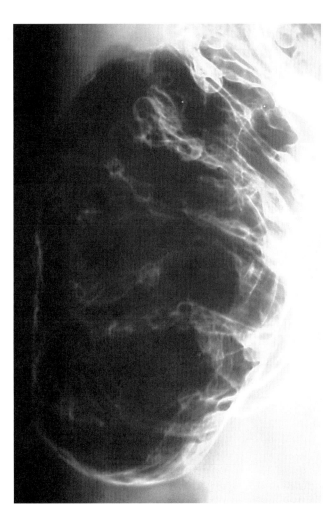

History: A 20-year-old man presents with a rectal discharge.

1. Which of the following should be included in the differential diagnosis of the imaging finding shown? (Choose all that apply.)
   A. Familial adenomatous polyposis
   B. Cronkhite-Canada syndrome
   C. Peutz-Jeghers syndrome
   D. Turcot's syndrome
   E. Filiform polyposis

2. Which polyposis syndrome is associated with osteomas and cortical hyperostosis?
   A. Familial adenomatous polyposis
   B. Cronkhite-Canada syndrome
   C. Peutz-Jeghers syndrome
   D. Turcot's syndrome
   E. Filiform polyposis

3. Several of the colonic polyposis syndromes have an autosomal dominant pattern of inheritance. Which of the following is the exception?
   A. Familial adenomatous polyposis
   B. Cronkhite-Canada syndrome
   C. Peutz-Jeghers syndrome
   D. Cowden's syndrome
   E. Gardner's syndrome

4. The patient imaged also has a rash, alopecia, and diarrhea. What is the likely diagnosis?
   A. Familial adenomatous polyposis (FAP)
   B. Cronkhite-Canada syndrome
   C. Peutz-Jeghers syndrome
   D. Turcot's syndrome
   E. Filiform polyposis

Colonic Polyposis

1. A, B, C, and D

2. A

3. B

4. B

Reference

Buck JL, Harned RK: Polyposis syndromes. In Gore RM, Levine MS, editors: *Textbook of Gastrointestinal Radiology*, 2nd ed. Philadelphia: WB Saunders, 2000, pp 1075-1088.

Cross-Reference

Gastrointestinal Imaging: *THE REQUISITES*, 3rd ed, p 284.

Comment

Innumerable adenomatous polyps of the colon, particularly in a young adult, usually indicate a polyposis syndrome. For years, these adenomatous polypoid conditions were classified as familial polyposis coli or (when fewer polyps) Gardner's syndrome. Patients with Gardner's syndrome were believed to develop the extracolonic manifestations. These conditions are inherited as autosomal dominant traits and cause the formation of numerous adenomatous colonic polyps. Many now believe that these two conditions represent variable penetrance of the same genetic defect and classify these entities as familial adenomatous polyposis syndrome (FAPS).

In patients with FAPS, polyps are seen primarily in the colon but can occur outside the colon, usually in the stomach or small bowel. There is also an associated increase of nonadenomatous polyps present in both colon and stomach. These growths usually are hyperplastic polyps or so-called fundic gland polyps. Adenomas also occur with slightly increased incidence in the stomach and duodenum, and there is an increased incidence of periampullary carcinoma (the second most common malignancy after colon carcinoma) among these patients. In some studies the incidence of small bowel adenomas has been notably increased.

Extraintestinal manifestations include bone abnormalities. Osteomas, although classically associated with Gardner's syndrome, occur in up to 50% of patients. There also is an increased incidence of cortical hyperostosis and dental abnormalities associated with FAPS. Epidermal cysts have been described, as have pigmented lesions of the retina. The incidence of thyroid carcinoma also is believed to be increased, particularly in women. Large intra-abdominal fibrous tumors, mesenteric fibromatosis, and desmoid tumors occur sporadically. Some believe that there is a slight increase in the incidence of pancreatic carcinoma and benign liver tumors. Tumors of the central nervous system (glioblastomas and medulloblastomas) are generally associated with Turcot's syndrome, but many claim that Turcot's is just another, more deadly, variation of FAPS.

Notes

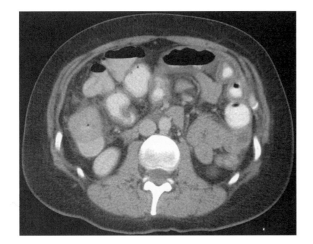

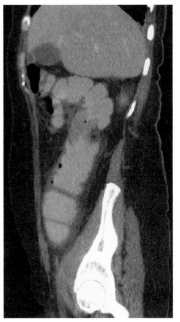

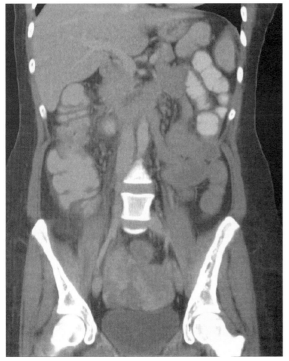

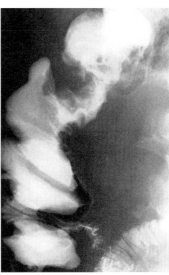

History: A 60-year-old woman presents with blood in her stools.

1. Which of the following should be included in the differential diagnosis of the imaging findings shown? (Choose all that apply.)
   A. Amoebic colitis
   B. Primary colon cancer
   C. Crohn's disease
   D. Ischemic stricture
   E. Pseudomembranous colitis

2. Several known and accepted risk factors are associated with colorectal cancer. Which of the following is *not* a risk factor?
   A. Adenomatous polyps
   B. Previous surgery
   C. Ulcerative colitis
   D. Diet
   E. Family history

3. What is the most common etiology for colorectal carcinoma?
   A. Adenoma
   B. Polyposis syndromes
   C. Chronic colitis
   D. Dysplastic colon

4. Which of the following correctly describes the apple core lesion?
   A. A short, sharply defined annular circumferential narrowing of a hollow viscus with overhanging margins.
   B. A partially thrombosed external hemorrhoid, the apple colors referring to the blue-green thrombosed areas against the red hemorrhoid.
   C. Nodularity seen in the base of an ulcerated mass referring to the appearance of the apple seeds exposed when the fruit is eaten to the core.
   D. The central channel cored out of an obstructive tumor, restoring patency to a hollow viscus

C A S E 4 0

Colonic Annular Carcinoma

1. A, B, C, and D

2. B

3. A

4. A

References

Dahnert W: *Radiology Review Manual*, 6th ed. Philadelphia: Lippincott Williams & Wilkins, 2007, pp 813-815.

Thoeni RF, Laufer I: Polyps and carcinoma of the colon. In Gore RM, Levine MS, (eds): *Textbook of Gastrointestinal Radiology*, 2nd ed. Philadelphia: WB Saunders, 2000, pp 1009-1048.

Cross-Reference

Gastrointestinal Imaging: *THE REQUISITES,* 3rd ed, p 272.

Comment

Although the incidence of colorectal carcinoma (CRC) has leveled off in the United States in recent years, it is still the fourth most common cancer after prostate, breast, and lung. Its mortality rate is exceeded only by lung cancer at this time. Survival depends on early detection, which in CRC means finding and removing polyps. In polyps between 5 mm and 10 mm there is about a 1% chance of malignancy. In polyps between 1 and 2 cm there is about a 10% risk. As the size of sessile polyps increases, the cancer risk increases; polyps larger than 2 cm have about a 40% risk. Diminutive polyps (less than 5 mm) have little or no risk of malignancy, and the search for diminutive polyps is probably a waste of time, expense, and effort. However, the screening for 1 cm or larger polyps is warranted. This can be done with colonoscopy, which has the added benefit of polyp removal at the time of discovery. However, the complication rate (perforation) is at least 10 times that of the air contrast barium enema (ACBE) and the cost is considerably higher than ACBE. If done by skilled radiologists, the detection rate of polyps 1 cm and larger, as well as CRC, approaches that of colonoscopy. Multidetector computed tomography (MDCT) is now especially useful in detection by evaluation for local, nodal and distant spread (figures 1 to 3). As the number of sites using CT colonoscopy increases, this holds promise as being an excellent screening method in the general population with minimal examination time, no sedation, and rapid results.

Notes

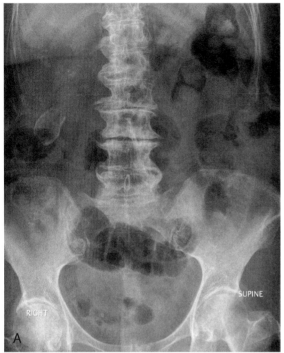

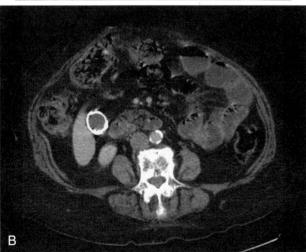

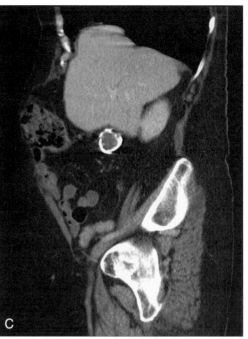

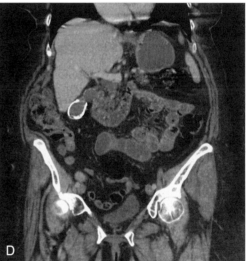

History: An 80-year-old woman presents with left-sided abdominal pain and vomiting.

1. What is your differential for the location and diagnosis of the large calcification seen in the right upper quadrant of the abdomen in figure A? (Choose all that apply.)
   A. Adrenal gland; e.g., tuberculosis
   B. Gallbladder; e.g., porcelain gallbladder
   C. Liver; e.g., hydatid cyst
   D. Kidney; e.g., calcified cyst
   E. Abdominal wall; e.g., old hematoma

2. Based on the figures, which of the following is the most likely diagnosis?
   A. Adrenal gland tuberculosis
   B. Porcelain gallbladder
   C. Hydatid cyst of the liver

D. Calcified renal cyst
E. Abdominal wall, old hematoma

3. What is the usual etiologic basis for this condition?
   A. Granulomatous reaction
   B. Systemic hypercalcemia
   C. Cystic duct obstruction
   D. Old hemorrhage

4. Name the major complication associated with this finding.
   A. Gallbladder abscess
   B. Gallbladder perforation
   C. Gallbladder carcinoma
   D. Emphysematous cholecystitis

Porcelain Gallbladder

1. B, C, D, and E

2. B

3. C

4. C

References

Kane RA, Jacobs R, Katz J, Costello P: Porcelain gallbladder: ultrasound and CT appearance. *Radiology* 1984;152:137-141.
Stephen AE, Berger DL: Carcinoma in the porcelain gallbladder: a relationship revisited. *Surgery* 2001;129:699-703.

Cross-Reference

Gastrointestinal Imaging: *THE REQUISITES,* 3rd ed, p 254.

Comment

It is thought that chronic cystic duct obstruction and subacute inflammation are the basis of gallbladder wall calcification. Quite often the calcified gallbladder is small and contracted (unlike the example in this case), and it is easy to confuse the finding with calcified gallstones (see figures). However, the porcelain gallbladder carries its own inherent risk, which much outweighs gallstones. The risk of developing carcinoma of the gallbladder in an untreated porcelain gallbladder is high, somewhere between 10% and 30%. Plain film and ultrasound can confuse calcified gallstones and a porcelain gallbladder. However, multidetector CT is much more adept at distinguishing the differences (see figures) and can show the cystic duct obstruction as well.

Notes

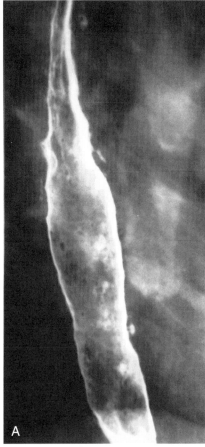

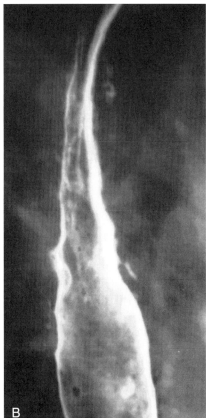

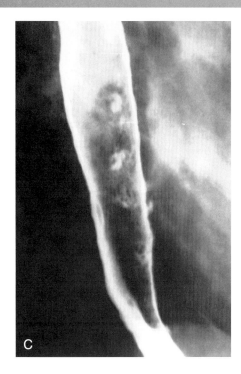

History: A 37-year-old man has recurrent episodes of dysphagia.

1. Which of the following should be included in the differential diagnosis of the imaging finding shown in figure A? (Choose all that apply.)
   A. Herpetic esophagitis
   B. *Candida* esophagitis
   C. Zenker's diverticula
   D. Esophageal diverticula
   E. Intramural pseudodiverticulosis

2. What structures are visible, filled by the barium?
   A. Chronic ulcerations
   B. Fibrosed traction diverticula
   C. Scarred pulsion diverticula
   D. Dilated excretory ducts of the esophageal mucous glands

3. What is the most common other esophageal abnormality seen with this condition?
   A. Ulcerative esophagitis
   B. Benign stricture
   C. Malignant stricture
   D. True diverticula

4. What pathogen has been associated with this condition?
   A. *Actinomyces* organisms
   B. Mixed oral flora
   C. *Candida* organisms
   D. *Helicobacter pylori*

Esophageal Intramural Pseudodiverticulosis

1. A, D, and E

2. D

3. B

4. C

References

Levine MS: Other esophagitides. In Gore RM, Levine MS (eds): *Textbook of Gastrointestinal Radiology*, 2nd ed. Philadelphia: WB Saunders, 2000, pp 381-384.

Cross-Reference

Gastrointestinal Imaging: *THE REQUISITES*, 3rd ed, p 30.

Comment

Intramural pseudodiverticulosis of the esophagus is a rare condition. Anatomically it represents barium filling the sparse adenomatous excretory ducts of the mucous glands of the esophagus. These mucous glands are normal anatomic structures of the esophagus but typically are not visible on radiologic studies. However, sometimes (thought to relate to chronic inflammation) these ducts become dilated, allowing barium to track into the ducts and glands.

Some type of inflammation must be present for these pathologic changes to occur, and the large majority of these patients have evidence of esophageal inflammation. A large proportion of patients with intramural pseudodiverticulosis also have strictures. The strictures are typically benign, but intramural pseudodiverticulosis has been reported in association with malignant strictures. *Candida* organisms have been found in patients with this condition, but the exact causal relationship is uncertain. More than likely, this finding represents a secondary infection of the glands and not a predisposing condition. Rarely this condition is found in patients with an otherwise normal esophagus. However, the very presence of intramural pseudodiverticulosis is abnormal.

Radiologically the intramural pseudodiverticulosis appears as small outpouchings, often with a flask shape. These outpouchings are most commonly mistaken for ulcers by those who are unfamiliar with the condition. Intramural pseudodiverticulosis may be either segmental or diffuse. Even intramural tracking and deep penetration may be evident. On CT, the condition produces changes of esophageal wall thickening and irregularity of the lumen, mimicking esophageal carcinoma. Because it is primarily a radiologic oddity, the condition's clinical course depends on treatment of the underlying condition.

Often, treatment of the stricture or inflammation results in a decrease or even disappearance of the pseudodiverticulosis. Slightly increased risks of adenocarcinoma of the esophagus have been associated with this condition.

Notes

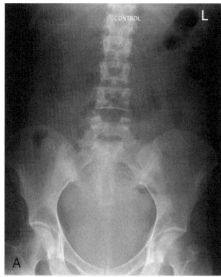

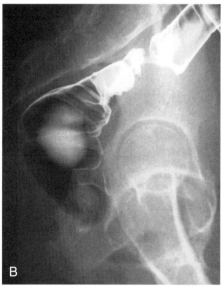

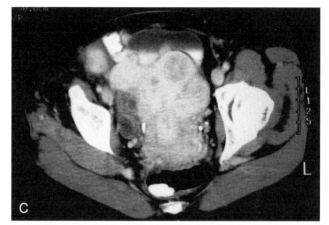

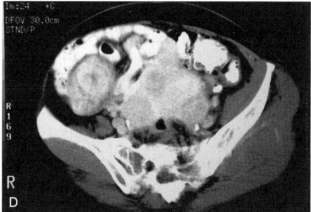

History: A 44-year-old woman presents with 1-year history of constipation and cramping lower abdominal pain.

1. Which of the following should be included in the differential diagnosis of the location and diagnosis in the imaging finding shown in figure A? (Choose all that apply.)
   A. Uterus; e.g., pregnancy
   B. Urinary bladder; e.g., outlet obstruction
   C. Ureter; e.g., obstruction
   D. Pelvic; e.g., abscess
   E. Ovary; e.g., tumor

2. Based on the figures, which of the following is the most likely diagnosis?
   A. Uterine fibroids
   B. Urinary bladder outlet obstruction
   C. Ureteric obstruction
   D. Pelvic abscess
   E. Ovarian carcinoma

3. Apart from her colon, what other organ system is most commonly compromised by a pelvic mass?
   A. Vascular
   B. Urinary tract
   C. Small bowel
   D. Lymphatic

4. How do malignant and benign pelvic lesions affect the bowel differently?
   A. Malignant masses obstruct the bowel, benign lesions do not.
   B. Malignant masses ulcerate and fistulate into the adjacent bowel, benign lesions do not.
   C. Benign lesions tend to incite a desmoplastic reaction, extending into surrounding tissues and bowel, but malignant lesions spread by local infiltration without reaction.
   D. Benign lesions tend to cause compression of bowel, but malignant lesions can result in contiguous invasion of the serosal surface of the bowel.

Pelvic Mass Impressing Rectum

1. A, B, D, and E

2. A

3. B

4. D

References

Szucs RA, Wolf EL, Gramm HF, et al: Extracolonic diseases involving the colon. In Gore RM, Levine MS (eds): *Textbook of Gastrointestinal Radiology*, 2nd ed. Philadelphia: WB Saunders, 2000, pp 1097-1102.

Cross-Reference

Gastrointestinal Imaging: *THE REQUISITES,* 3rd ed, p 291.

Comment

Large masses in the pelvis are quite common in women and are usually related to uterine fibroids. They can vary in size and appearance. Some can be solid, some have necrotic foci within them, and many have calcifications. If the mass is sufficiently large, it can compress the rectum, sigmoid, or descending colon, causing symptoms by its sheer bulk, such as in the images shown with this case. If the mass is malignant, it can invade the bowel from its serosal surface, causing narrowing, irregularity, and tethering of the bowel. Distention of such a segment of bowel is usually exceptionally painful, so keep this in mind when doing barium enemas as part of the workup on patients with possible malignant disease in the pelvis. The other issue (which is best addressed with CT) is the possibility of compression of one or both ureters and hydronephrosis.

Notes

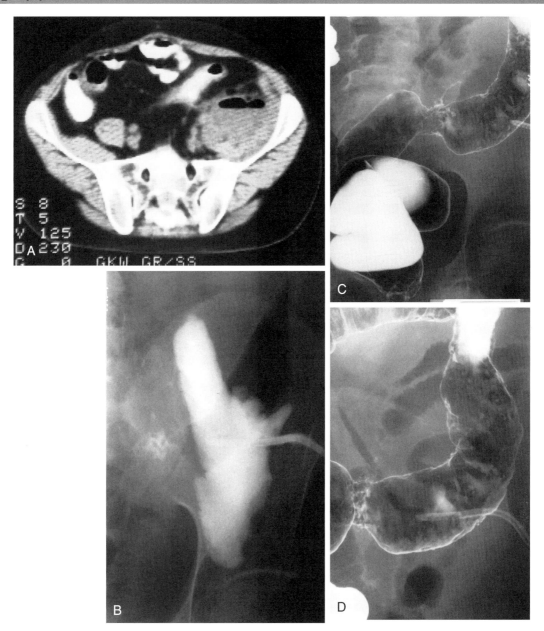

History: A 36-year-old man presents with fever and rigors, left flank and groin pain, and positive psoas sign on examination.

1. Which of the following should be included in the differential for the origin and diagnosis of the disease leading to the imaging finding shown in Figure A? (Choose all that apply.)
   A. Acute appendicitis
   B. Tuberculosis of the spine
   C. Crohn's disease of the small bowel
   D. Infected aortic aneurysm
   E. Idiopathic

2. What is the psoas sign?
   A. Palpation of the inferior iliopsoas muscle in the left iliac fossa of a patient's abdomen results in pain in the right iliac fossa.
   B. Leg lifting, or flexion of the hip, on the affected side elicits pain.

C. Abdominal pain is elicited by passive flexion and external rotation of the hip.
D. There is dullness to percussion in the left flank.

3. A decision is made to drain the psoas abscess by radiologic intervention. What is the optimal modality to use to undertake this procedure?
   A. CT
   B. Ultrasound
   C. Fluoroscopy
   D. No imaging required

4. Worldwide, what is the disease most closely associated with a psoas abscess?
   A. Pancreatitis
   B. Tuberculosis
   C. Crohn's disease
   D. Diverticulitis

Psoas Abscess

1. B, C, D, and E

2. B

3. A

4. B

References

Gore RM, Laufer I, Berlin JW: Ulcerative and granulomatous colitis: idiopathic inflammatory bowel disease. In Gore RM, Levine MS (eds): *Textbook of Gastrointestinal Radiology*, 2nd ed. Philadelphia: WB Saunders, 2000, pp 945-992.

Zissin R, Gayer G, Kots E, et al: Iliopsoas abscess: a report of 24 patients diagnosed by CT. *Abdom Imaging* 2001;26:533-539.

Cross-Reference

Gastrointestinal Imaging: *THE REQUISITES,* 3rd ed, pp 294-297.

Comment

In the modern setting, inflammation in the lower abdomen involving the bowel with extension through to the retroperitoneal psoas muscle has a limited differential diagnosis.

On the right, tuberculosis involving the terminal ileum and cecum is relatively uncommon, except perhaps in AIDS patients, and extension through the retroperitoneum would be unusual. Appendicitis might irritate the psoas, but violation of the retroperitoneum would be uncommon. Thus, the most likely diagnosis in a young patient with an inflammatory phlegmon in the right lower quadrant (RLQ) would be Crohn's disease with fistulous communication with the retroperitoneum. However, even with Crohn's disease, a breach of the retroperitoneum is not common.

A differential consideration should include actinomycosis, which, although uncommon, is known to routinely breach fascial and peritoneal barriers. Most of the fistulous communications seen in Crohn's disease are bowel to bowel, bowel to bladder, bowel to skin, and, on rare occasions, bowel to ureter.

Other conditions in which psoas infiltration can occur are metastatic disease, spinal diseases, and neuromuscular conditions such as neurofibromatosis.

Notes

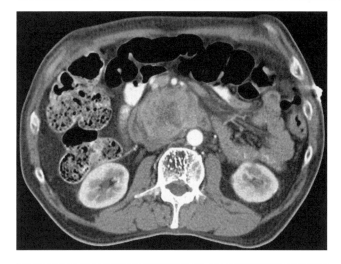

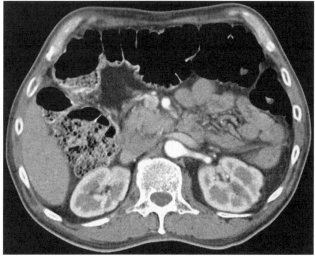

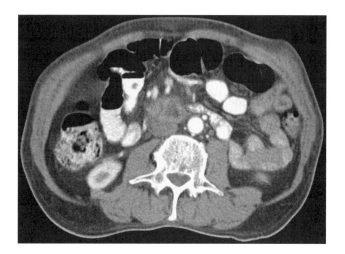

History: A 67-year-old man with melena. Upper GI endoscopy found an ulcerated extrinsic mass effect on the third part of the duodenum.

1. Which of the following should be included in the differential diagnosis of the case and imaging finding shown? (Choose all that apply.)
   A. Gastrinoma
   B. Lymphoma
   C. Carcinoma
   D. Pancreatitis
   E. Pseudocyst

2. What is the most common histologic type of pancreatic malignancy?
   A. Acinar epithelial adenocarcinoma
   B. Ductal epithelial adenocarcinoma
   C. Endocrine tumor
   D. Metastatic tumor
   E. Lymphoma

3. What is the most common clinical presentation of a patient with pancreatic cancer?
   A. Pain
   B. Jaundice
   C. Diabetes
   D. Weight loss

4. Where are most pancreatic cancers located?
   A. Head
   B. Body
   C. Tail
   D. Diffuse

Pancreatic Carcinoma

1. A, B, C, and D

2. B

3. A

4. A

References

Chezmar JL: Pancreatic neoplasms. In Gore RM, Levine MS (eds): *Textbook of Gastrointestinal Radiology*, 2nd ed. Philadelphia: WB Saunders, 2000, pp 1796-1811.

Horton KM, Fishman EK: Multidetector row CT with dual-phase CT angiography in the preoperative evaluation of pancreatic cancer. *Crit Rev Comput Tomogr* 2002;43:323-360.

Cross-Reference

Gastrointestinal Imaging: *THE REQUISITES,* 3rd ed, pp 159-165.

Comment

The CT images show a mixed-density pancreatic mass within the head and uncinate process. The adjacent superior mesenteric artery, superior mesenteric vein, and aorta remain separated by a fat plane, suggesting the tumor may be an operable lesion.

The clinical findings of jaundice and painless gallbladder enlargement (Courvoisier's gallbladder) are associated with this disease, as is Trousseau's syndrome (venous thrombotic disease) and occasionally new onset of diabetes mellitus. At the time of diagnosis, patients with symptoms have a median survival rate of about 20 months.

On occasion, and usually as an unexpected incidental finding, one can come across a small pancreatic head lesion, often in the uncinate process, that is asymptomatic. These fortunate patients may be candidates for resections and a Whipple procedure with an increased life expectancy.

Notes

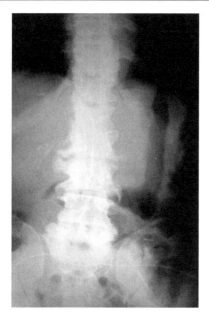

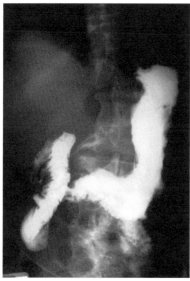

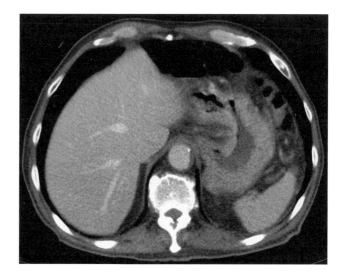

History: An 81-year-old man presents with confusion. His family reports also a history of 10 kg weight loss over 6 weeks. Initial investigations identified iron deficiency anemia.

1. Which of the following should be included in the differential diagnosis of the imaging finding shown? (Choose all that apply.)
   A. Lymphoma
   B. Pneumatosis
   C. Crohn's disease
   D. Adenocarcinoma
   E. Metastatic disease

2. What is the name of the association of gastric cancer metastatic to the left axilla?
   A. Irish node
   B. Virchow's node
   C. Krukenberg's node
   D. Sister Mary Joseph's node

3. Which is the most appropriate imaging modality to assess local spread of gastric cancer?
   A. Endoscopic ultrasound
   B. Barium upper GI study
   C. CT scan
   D. FDG PET scan

4. Which of the following statements about gastric cancer is *true*?
   A. Gastric cancer is the most common GI malignancy.
   B. About 10% of gastric cancers are of the linitis plastic type.
   C. Early gastric cancer is malignancy limited to the stomach, with no perigastric, lymph node or distant spread.
   D. Patients with the linitis plastica type of gastric cancer usually present with dysphagia.

Linitis Plastica of the Stomach

1. A, C, D, and E

2. A

3. A

4. B

References

Iyer R, Dubrow R: Imaging upper gastrointestinal malignancy. *Semin Roentgenol* 2006;41(2):105-112.

Low VHS, Levine MS, Rubesin SE, et al: Diagnosis of gastric carcinoma: sensitivity of double-contrast barium studies. *Am J Roentgenol* 1994;162:329-334.

Cross-Reference

Gastrointestinal Imaging: *THE REQUISITES,* 3rd ed, pp 57-59.

Comment

Close attention to the gas pattern of the stomach on plain film images can sometimes reveal diffuse abnormalities of the stomach, such as in this case (see figures). The gas pattern of the stomach in this patient suggests a narrow rigid stomach with loss of pliability, which is confirmed by barium upper GI study (see figures). A CT image shows diffuse thickening of the gastric wall (see figures). In this case, the findings (linitis plastica) are a result of diffuse scirrhous adenocarcinoma of stomach. However, other conditions can also give a similar appearance. Metastatic disease involving the stomach (especially from breast and lung) can result in an identical appearance, as can Hodgkin's type desmoplastic lymphoma of the stomach and inflammatory diseases such as severe diffuse peptic gastritis, corrosive gastritis, radiation gastritis, sarcoidosis, and Crohn's disease (ram's horn stomach), as well as some reported cases of syphilis.

Notes

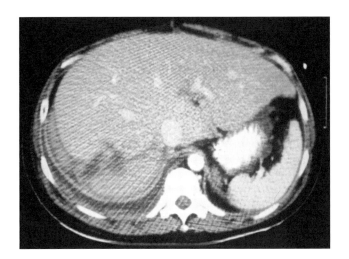 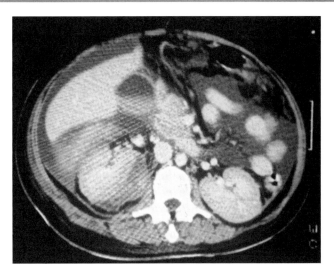

History: A 48-year-old man was involved in a motorcycle accident.

1. Which of the following show signs of a significant injury in the imaging presented? (Choose all that apply.)
   A. Bowel
   B. Kidneys
   C. Liver
   D. Lungs
   E. Spleen

2. What injury has the liver suffered?
   A. Laceration
   B. Biloma
   C. Contusion
   D. Subcapsular hematoma

3. What is the significance of the high density in the fluid adjacent to the liver?
   A. Artifact
   B. Bile leak
   C. Sentinel clot
   D. Active IV contrast extravasation

4. What is the artifact resulting in the alternating light and dark lines at the left base of the CT images?
   A. Movement by the patient
   B. Metallic foreign body
   C. Dealignment of detectors
   D. Scanning beyond the scanning circle

Liver Laceration

1. B, C, and D

2. A

3. C

4. B

References

Richards JR, Derlet RW: Computed tomography for blunt abdominal trauma in the ED: a prospective study. *Am J Emerg Med* 1998;16:338-342.

Shanmuganathan K, Mirvis SE, Reaney SM: CT appearance of contrast extravasations associated with injury sustained from blunt abdominal trauma. Pictorial essay. *Clin Radiol* 1995;50:182-187.

Cross-Reference

Gastrointestinal Imaging: THE REQUISITES, 3rd ed, p 207.

Comment

After the spleen, the liver is the next most common solid organ injured in blunt trauma to the abdomen. Liver traumas can be solitary, but most often they are seen with multiple injuries of the abdomen, abdominal wall, and thoracic wall as well as musculoskeletal and neurologic injuries elsewhere. By far the most common cause is trauma due to motor vehicle accidents. The injury to the liver is most serious when large blood vessels have been torn, such as the hepatic veins, the portal vessels, or the hepatic artery. Those with hepatic artery tears often do not make it to the emergency department.

Commonly what is seen in CT is a laceration with accompanying intrahepatic or subcapsular hematoma (see figures). Some degree of extrahepatic hematoma is seen in about 80% of cases. Hepatic contusion can manifest as a focal area of diminished density. However, these injuries are almost always self-limiting conditions for which no treatment is required. Survival of patients with intra-abdominal solid organ trauma has increased over the last few decades with improved on-site patient care and rapid transport to a trauma center. Without doubt, a major contributing factor has been the availability of CT imaging in or adjacent to the trauma center.

Blunt liver trauma has been categorized by organ injury scale, including contusion, hematoma, and laceration at one end of the scale, and major vascular injuries and hepatic avulsion at the other.

Notes

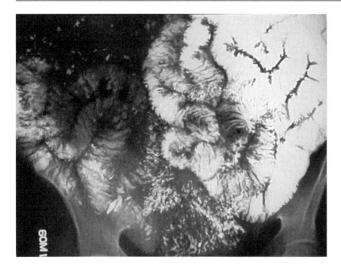

History: A 27-year-old woman presents with diarrhea.

1. Which of the following should be included in the differential diagnosis of the imaging finding shown in the figure? (Choose all that apply.)
   A. AIDS
   B. Giardiasis
   C. Celiac disease
   D. Crohn's disease
   E. Carcinoid disease

2. The figure shows the loops of distal ileum in the right abdomen displaying a fold density equal to or greater than that seen in the loops of jejunum in the left abdomen. What is the name and significance of this observation?
   A. Iliezation
   B. Jejunization
   C. Malrotation
   D. None, this is a normal variant

3. A sign on barium small bowel follow-through indicating malabsorption is described as "the barium forming smooth featureless elongated columns or clumps in the jejunum." What is the name of this sign?
   A. Flocculation
   B. Hypersecretion
   C. Effacement
   D. Moulage

4. What is the most common abnormality seen on barium small bowel studies in patients with celiac disease?
   A. Normality
   B. Intussusception
   C. Mosaic pattern
   D. Diffuse dilatation

Small Bowel Malabsorption

1. A, B, C, and D

2. B

3. D

4. D

References

Maglinte DD, Kelvin FM, O'Connor K, et al: Current status of small bowel radiography. *Abdom Imaging* 1996;21:247-257.

Rubesin SE, Grumbach K, Herlinger H, et al: Adult celiac disease and its complications. *Radiographics* 1989;9:1045-1066.

Cross-Reference

Gastrointestinal Imaging: *THE REQUISITES,* 3rd ed, pp 111-114.

Comment

There can be degrees of malabsorption seen in patients with diarrhea and various food intolerances. The best known of these is celiac disease, a form of gluten intolerance (also known as nontropical sprue). There appear to be varying degrees of intolerance. The cases that come to medical attention are in patients suffering from diarrhea, steatorrhea, and weight loss. The definitive diagnostic examination is small endoscopy with mucosal biopsy. Even with small ingested video capsules that can traverse the small bowel and provide video of the mucosal surface, the barium small bowel follow-through is the fastest and least expensive way of making a diagnosis. Patients with symptoms serious enough to motivate them to seek medical attention almost always have some or all of the findings of malabsorption on the barium examination (see figure). The classic appearance of flocculation, segmentation, and the famous moulage sign are infrequently seen owing to the continued improvement of modern barium suspensions. What is seen is dilation of bowel, atrophy and effacement of the fold pattern, particularly in the ileum, and hypersecretion.

Notes

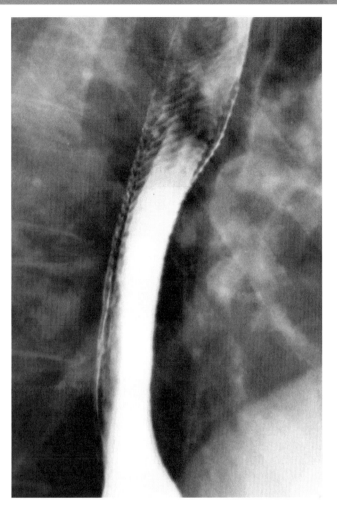

History: A 42-year-old man presents with heartburn.

1. Which of the following should be included in the differential diagnosis of the imaging finding shown in the figure? (Choose all that apply.)
   A. Shatzki rings
   B. Feline esophagus
   C. Ringed esophagus
   D. Fixed transverse folds
   E. Thickened folds of esophagitis

2. What is the cause of feline esophagus?
   A. Scarring of the longitudinal muscularis mucosa
   B. Membranous rings due to hypertrophied muscularis
   C. Transient spasm of the longitudinal muscularis mucosa
   D. Transient spasm of the circular muscularis mucosa

3. The ringed esophagus, a segment of fixed transverse folds, is a recognized finding in eosinophilic esophagitis. Which of the following statements regarding eosinophilic esophagitis is true?
   A. Resolves with antireflux therapy
   B. Cancer develops in 10% of patients
   C. Dysphagia is the most common presentation
   D. Usually associated with eosinophilic gastroenteritis

4. The patient in the figure complains of solid dysphagia, but there is little evidence of stricture or narrowing on the images. What should you do next?
   A. CT scan
   B. Endoscopy
   C. Solid bolus challenge
   D. Nothing further; a normal-appearing barium swallow excludes an esophageal stricture or other obstructive abnormality

Feline Esophagus, Eosinophilic Esophagitis

1. B, C, and D

2. C

3. C

4. C

References

Samadi F, Levine MS, Rubesin SE, et al: Feline esophagus and gastroesophageal reflux. *Am J Roentgenol* 2010;194:972-976.

Zimmerman SL, Levine MS, Rubesin SE, et al: Idiopathic eosinophilic esophagitis in adults: the ringed esophagus. *Radiology* 2005;236:159-163.

Cross-Reference

Gastrointestinal Imaging: *THE REQUISITES,* 3rd ed, p 31.

Comment

Most of the time the feline pattern of the esophagus (see figure) has been associated with gastroesophageal reflux disease (GERD). It can be seen with or without other findings of GERD, such as ulceration. It does not seem to have any connection to the presence of Barrett's metaplasia or esophageal carcinoma.

In recent years the condition of eosinophilic esophagitis (EOE) has become widely recognized and discussed in the medical literature. Among the endoscopic and radiographic findings associated with this condition is a corrugated pattern of the esophageal mucosa. This condition, once considered rare, is now being recognized more commonly. It seems to be a disease of Western industrialized nations, of younger patients (aged 20 to 40 years), with solid dysphagia being the most common symptom. The condition (EOE) seems to exist independent of the other eosinophilic infiltrative conditions seen in the stomach and small bowel of atopic patients. There have been no cases of esophageal cancer reported in these patients at this time.

Notes

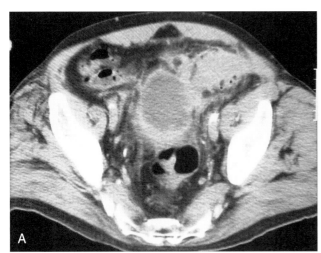

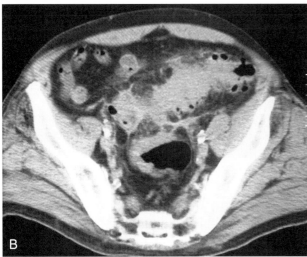

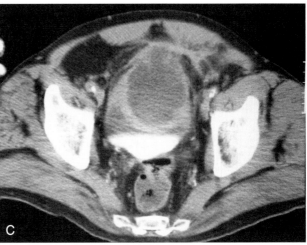

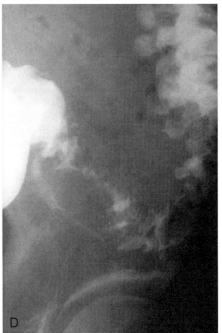

History: A 65-year-old woman presents with 4 weeks of lower abdominal pain, diarrhea, and fever; urine culture growing *Proteus mirabilis.*

1. Which of the following should be included in the differential diagnosis of the imaging finding shown in figure A? (Choose all that apply.)
   A. Ascites
   B. Appendicitis
   C. Cystitis
   D. Cancer
   E. Diverticulitis

2. Regarding colonic diverticula, which of the following statements is *false?*
   A. Colonic diverticula are true diverticula.
   B. Colonic diverticula align along the taenia coli.
   C. Colonic diverticula are pulsion lesions.
   D. Diverticula are most common in the sigmoid segment.
   E. The etiology of diverticulitis is similar to that of appendicitis.

3. Which of the following statements regarding colonic diverticular disease is true?
   A. Diverticular disease is a common worldwide condition.
   B. Most patients present with hemorrhage or diverticulitis.
   C. Diverticular disease is related to the modern Western diet high in animal fats.
   D. More than 60% of people in the United States older than 60 years have colonic diverticula.

4. Which of the following statements regarding imaging of colonic diverticulitis is *false?*
   A. The observation of narrowing means that there is or has been an episode of diverticulitis.
   B. A component of the narrowing is reversible.
   C. CT is a useful modality in diagnosing acute diverticulitis.
   D. Barium enema can be diagnostic.

Sigmoid Diverticulitis

1. B, C, D, and E

2. A

3. D

4. A

References

Birnbaum BA, Balthazar EJ: CT of appendicitis and diverticulitis. *Radiol Clin North Am* 1994;32:885-898.

Trenkner SW, Thompson WM: Since the advent of CT scanning, what role does the contrast enema examination play in the diagnosis of acute diverticulitis? *Am J Roentgenol* 1994;162:1493-1494.

Cross-Reference

Gastrointestinal Imaging: *THE REQUISITES,* 3rd ed, p 302.

Comment

Diverticular disease of the colon (diverticulosis coli) is a common disease of the Western world. The older the patient, the greater the likelihood of having the disease. However, in the last 3 or 4 decades there appears to be an increased incidence in younger patients. Diverticula formation is probably related to increased intraluminal pressures, decreased bowel transit times, and diminishing quantities of fiber in the diet in Western industrialized countries. Most of these patients are asymptomatic or manifest vague abdominal discomfort. A small group experience rectal bleeding, although a massive rectal bleed secondary to diverticulosis is uncommon (less than 5%). Very often the offending diverticulum is in the right colon.

About 15% of this population develops frank diverticulitis, such as shown in the images accompanying this case (see figures). The pathogenesis is thought to be infection secondary to impacted fecal matter within the diverticula, local peridiverticular inflammation, and finally, if untreated, frank diverticulitis with pericolonic abscess formation. Some of the abscesses spontaneously drain via communication with the colonic lumen, such as shown in the barium enema image (see figures). Most do not and will require surgical intervention or radiologic placement of an abscess drainage catheter. It is believed by some that the origin of the so-called giant sigmoid diverticulum is, in fact, the sequela of spontaneous drainage of a large diverticular abscess with the remaining cavity permanent, communicating with the sigmoid colon and epithelialized over time.

There is little doubt that CT of the abdomen is the best imaging method for diverticulitis. Not only can mild pericolic inflammatory changes be detected but also pericolic abscesses.

Notes

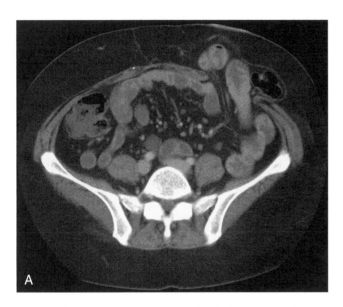

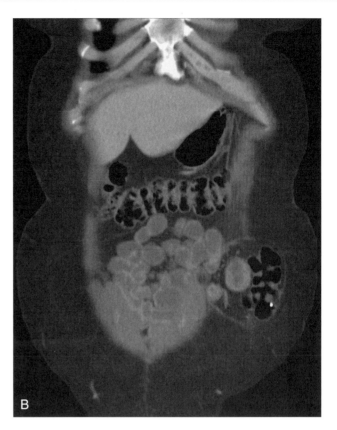

History: A 77-year-old woman with Crohn's disease and previous jejunal and colorectal resection presents with symptoms that suggest mild active inflammatory disease.

1. Which of the following should be included in the differential diagnosis of the imaging finding in figure A? (Choose all that apply.)
   A. Inguinal hernia
   B. Parastomal hernia
   C. Spigelian hernia
   D. Umbilical hernia
   E. Ventral hernia

2. This is a spigelian hernia. Through which anatomic area does this hernia pass?
   A. Linea alba
   B. Linea semilunaris
   C. Rectus abdominus
   D. Transversalis abdominus

3. What is the unusual type of hernia that contains only a portion of a loop of bowel wall and not the entire lumen?
   A. Littre's hernia
   B. Petit hernia
   C. Richter's hernia
   D. Valsalva hernia

4. Name the type of hernia that contains Meckel's diverticulum.
   A. Littre's hernia
   B. Petit hernia
   C. Richter's hernia
   D. Valsalva hernia

Ventral Hernia

1. B, C, and E

2. B

3. C

4. A

References

Aguirre DA, Santosa AC, Casola G, Sirlin CB: Abdominal wall hernias: imaging features, complications, and diagnostic pitfalls at multi-detector row CT. *Radiographics* 2005;25:1501-1520.

Zafar HM, Levine MS, Rubesin SE, Laufer I: Anterior abdominal wall hernias: findings in barium studies. *Radiographics* 2006;26:691-699.

Cross-Reference

Gastrointestinal Imaging: *THE REQUISITES,* 3rd ed, p 329.

Comment

Numerous types of hernias can be identified along the anterior abdominal wall. With the increased use of CT, some hernias are identified in patients who have no symptoms (see figures). In the adult population, incisional hernias are by far the most common. These develop in up to 5% of patients who have abdominal operations and typically occur within the first 6 months after the surgery. Affected patients might remain asymptomatic, however. Even though laparoscopic surgery is becoming increasingly popular, hernias can still occur through those small defects in the abdominal wall because they are not surgically closed. Richter's hernia is an unusual type of hernia that contains only a portion of a loop of bowel wall and not the entire lumen (e.g., the tip of the cecum caught in a right inguinal hernia).

Spigelian hernias are unusual. They occur in the lower abdomen, either in the right or left lower quadrant. The area through which the bowel herniates, termed the *linea semilunaris,* consists of a fibrous band of tissue joining the rectus sheath muscles with the transverse abdominal and internal oblique abdominal muscle. The hernia is probably the result of a weakness or congenital defect in the union of these muscles and fibrous bands. The hernia courses obliquely between these groups of muscles and can reside between bands of muscles, making it difficult to identify on clinical examination. Often, patients with spigelian hernias have intermittent or constant pain in the lower quadrant. The hernias contain either small bowel (right) or sigmoid colon (left), depending on where they are situated. They can have a large orifice, in which case there is less likelihood of obstruction or strangulation than with other types of hernias. They also can spontaneously reduce. Because they do not fully herniate through the abdominal wall, they are difficult to clinically diagnose, especially in obese patients. These hernias occur with similar frequency in men and women. They may be bilateral or associated with other abdominal wall defects. Quite often the defect in the abdominal wall contains fat and may be asymptomatic.

Notes

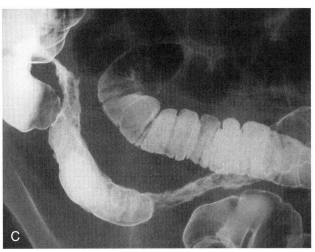

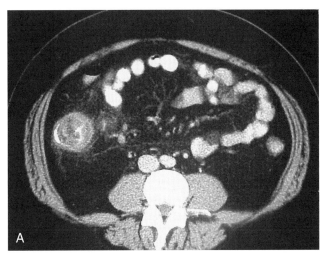

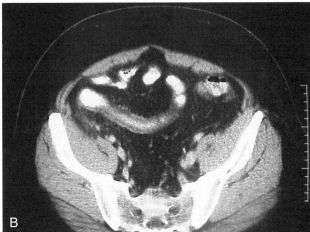

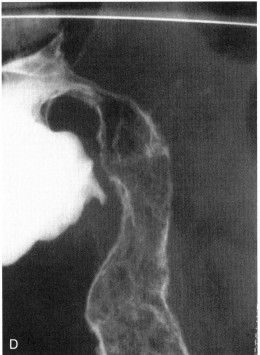

History: A 40-year-old man presents with right lower quadrant abdominal pain and fever.

1. Which of the following should be included in the differential diagnosis of the dominant imaging finding on figure A? (Choose all that apply.)
   A. Giardiasis
   B. Tuberculosis
   C. Crohn's disease
   D. Ulcerative colitis
   E. *Yersinia* infection

2. What is the most common clinical manifestation of Crohn's disease?
   A. Fistula formation
   B. Perianal disease
   C. Bleeding
   D. Diarrhea

3. Which of the following correctly describes the string sign?
   A. Sign on barium small bowel study where the small bowel lumen resembles a string
   B. Sign on an upright abdominal radiograph where the gas in the small bowel lines up as a string of small bubbles
   C. Sign on barium enema where the barium fills a string-like tract parallel to the lumen within a segment of bowel wall thickening
   D. Sign on barium small bowel study where the barium fills a string-like tract extending perpendicularly away from the bowel lumen

4. What parts of the gut are most commonly involved with Crohn's disease?
   A. Anus
   B. Small bowel
   C. Colorectum
   D. Stomach and duodenum

CASE 52

Crohn's Disease of the Terminal Ileum

1. B, C, D, and E

2. D

3. A

4. B

References

Horsthuis K, Bipat S, Bennink RJ, Stoker J: Inflammatory bowel disease diagnosed with US, MR, scintigraphy, and CT: meta-analysis of prospective studies. *Radiology* 2008;247:64-79.

Wills JS, Lobis IF, Denstman FJ: Crohn disease: state of the art. *Radiology* 1997;202:597-610.

Cross-Reference

Gastrointestinal Imaging: THE REQUISITES, 3rd ed, p 126.

Comment

Crohn's disease (or regional enteritis), as seen in the distal ileum of this patient (see figures), is one of the major idiopathic inflammatory bowel diseases (ulcerative colitis being the other). It is a transmural granulomatous inflammatory process and has been described in medical literature with various attached names for more than 200 years.

The cardinal clinical presentation includes diarrhea, abdominal pain, and weight loss. The incidence is higher in Europe and North America than in Asia. The incidence has increased steadily in the West until about the mid-1980s, when it began to stabilize. It tends to be a disease of young people (15 to 25 years old), although there is a second much smaller peak in the seventh decade. It has long been thought to be an immunologic response to some stimulating agent, although such an agent has never been identified.

Barium studies can be helpful with colonic involvement by identifying the specific pattern, which is usually quite different from that of ulcerative colitis. However, when only the terminal ileum alone is involved, all imaging studies are much less specific. The presence of fistulous communication, perianal fissuring, and extragastrointestinal manifestation may be helpful.

Notes

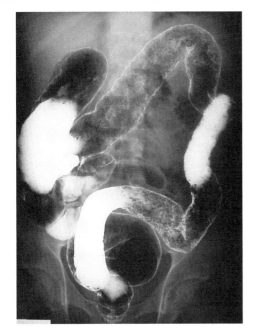

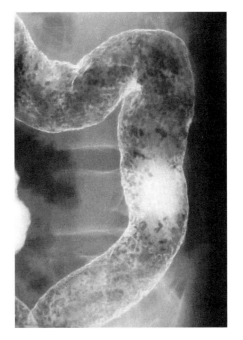

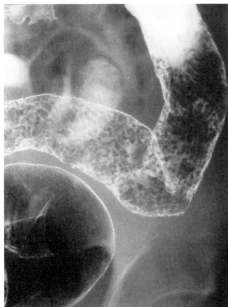

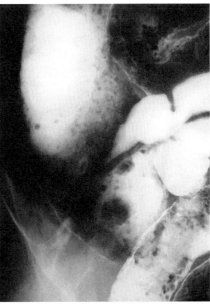

History: A 39-year-old man presents with 2-year history of intermittent bloody diarrhea.

1. Which of the following should be included in the differential diagnosis of the imaging findings shown in the figures? (Choose all that apply.)
   A. Familial adenomatous polyposis
   B. von Hippel–Lindau syndrome
   C. Peutz-Jeghers syndrome
   D. Turcot's syndrome
   E. Filiform polyposis

2. Noting the general appearance of the colon in figure 1, what disease has this patient suffered from previously?
   A. Melanosis coli
   B. Laxative abuse

C. Crohn's disease
D. Ulcerative colitis

3. What is the most common acute complication of severe acute ulcerative colitis?
   A. Stricture
   B. Hemorrhage
   C. Toxic megacolon
   D. Colovesical fistula

4. Patients with chronic ulcerative colitis undergo imaging or colonoscopic surveillance. What complication of chronic disease is being screened for?
   A. Stricture
   B. Carcinoma
   C. Sclerosing cholangitis
   D. Colovesical fistula

CASE 53

Chronic Ulcerative Colitis

1. A, C, D, and E

2. D

3. C

4. B

References

Roggeveen MJ, Tismenetsky M, Shapiro R: Ulcerative colitis. *Radiographics* 2006;26:947-951.

Zegal HG, Laufer I: Filiform polyposis. *Radiology* 1978;127:615-619.

Cross-Reference

Gastrointestinal Imaging: *THE REQUISITES,* 3rd ed, p 287.

Comment

Chronic or "burned out" ulcerative colitis can leave behind sequelae, such as the postinflammatory polyposis seen in this case (see figures). These defects are also known as filiform polyposis of the colon. In reality, they are not true polyps or even hyperplastic polyps (although a tiny number may be hyperplastic). They are, instead, mucosal tags, which have been left behind following the healing process. In the acute phase of severe ulcerative colitis there is marked ulcerative denouement of the colonic mucosal surface by the widespread ulcerative process. Not all the mucosa is ulcerated, and small islands of residual edematous mucosa remain (pseudopolyps). In the healing process, the colonic surface re-epithelializes. The small islands of residual mucosa that have survived the inflammatory process are re-epithelialized up to the base of the residual mucosal tags and in some cases beneath the tags, leaving them dangling in the bowel lumen and giving us the picture of filiform or postinflammatory polyposis. Although patients with ulcerative colitis who have suffered pancolitis continuously over 10 years have a 10% chance of malignancy, patients who have had limited involvement and healing will have a much lesser, but still increased risk. The patient shown has had pancolitis. Note the normal appearance of the terminal ileum (see figures).

Notes

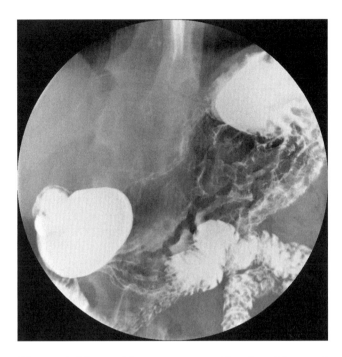

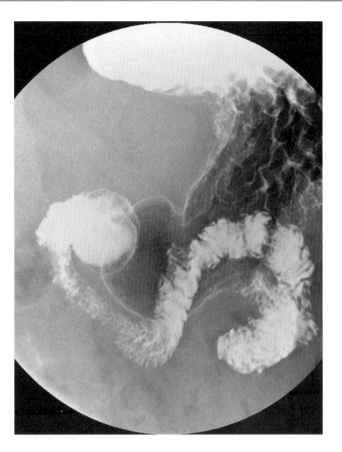

History: A 56-year-old man presents with a long history of heartburn and dyspepsia.

1. Which of the following should be included in the differential diagnosis of the imaging finding shown in the figures? (Choose all that apply.)
   A. Ménétrier's disease
   B. Hypergastrinemia
   C. Carcinoma
   D. Bezoar
   E. Normal

2. What neoplasm most commonly produces thickened gastric folds?
   A. Lymphoma
   B. Breast cancer metastasis
   C. Primary adenocarcinoma
   D. Gastric stromal tumor

3. What causes isolated fundal gastric varices?
   A. Fundoplication
   B. Portal hypertension
   C. Hypertrophic gastritis
   D. Splenic vein thrombosis

4. What is the most common infectious cause of thickened folds?
   A. *Mycobacterium avium-intracellulare*
   B. *Mycobacterium tuberculosis*
   C. *Treponema pallidum*
   D. *Helicobacter pylori*

CASE 54

Gastric Fold Thickening

1. A, B, C, and E

2. A

3. D

4. D

Reference

Levine MS: Stomach and duodenum: differential diagnosis. In Gore RM, Levine MS, editors: *Textbook of Gastrointestinal Radiology*, 2nd ed. Philadelphia: WB Saunders, 2000, pp 698-702.

Cross-Reference

Gastrointestinal Imaging: *THE REQUISITES*, 3rd ed, p 64.

Comment

It is extremely common to find thickened gastric folds on upper gastrointestinal examinations. The width of the gastric folds is usually about 3 to 5 mm in the distal prepyloric stomach and 8 to 10 mm proximally in the fundus. When the stomach is fully distended, normal gastric folds tend to run parallel to the lumen, whereas folds that are irregularly thickened, nodular, or serpiginous in appearance are usually considered abnormal.

Associated gastric wall thickening also may be visible on CT examination.

The presence of thickened rugal folds, gastric wall thickening, or both is a nonspecific finding. A variety of diseases can produce this radiologic finding, which can even be seen in healthy patients. The most common cause is some type of gastritis, such as alcoholic gastritis. *H. pylori* infection of the stomach is now recognized as an extremely common cause of inflammatory disease of the stomach and is by far the most common infectious process of the upper gastrointestinal tract. Zollinger-Ellison syndrome (gastrinoma) should always be considered, although it is rare. Numerous benign infiltrating processes, including eosinophilic gastritis, sarcoidosis, amyloidosis, Crohn's disease, and Ménétrier's disease, also can produce fold thickening. Of the neoplastic processes, lymphoma most typically manifests as thickened folds. Adenocarcinoma and even metastases also must be considered but are less common.

Varices of the stomach usually have associated esophageal varices and are related to increased portal venous pressure resulting from a variety of causes. Isolated fundal gastric varices, however, are a specific condition associated with splenic vein occlusion. The spleen normally drains via the splenic vein, but if this vein occludes, there are short gastric veins that act as collateral circulation in the fundal region of the stomach. These veins course over the proximal stomach and connect to the coronary vein, which then flows into the portal circulation. Splenic vein thrombosis is usually the sequela of pancreatitis or pancreatic carcinoma and less commonly the result of retroperitoneal processes, surgery, or hypercoagulability state.

Notes

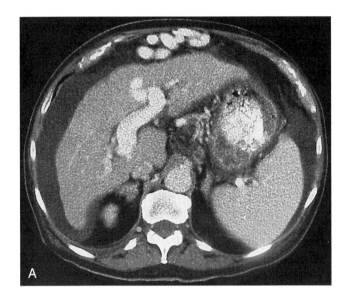

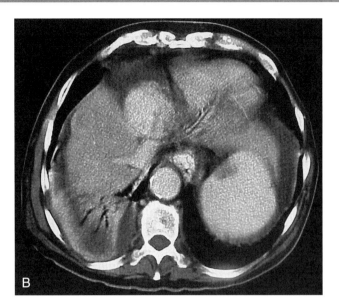

History: An 83-year-old man presents with lower limb pitting edema.

1. Which of the following should be included in the differential diagnosis of the imaging findings shown in figure A? (Choose all that apply.)
   A. Schistosomiasis
   B. Sickle cell disease
   C. Portal vein thrombosis
   D. Chronic left atrial failure
   E. Arteriovenous portal fistula

2. Name the leading cause for hepatic cirrhosis in North America.
   A. Alcoholism
   B. Wilson's disease
   C. Hemochromatosis
   D. Traumatic arteriovenous portal fistula

3. All of the following are some of the complications seen with portal hypertension *except:*
   A. Esophageal varices
   B. Portal vein thrombosis
   C. Hepatocellular carcinoma
   D. Right heart valvular fibrosis

4. With widespread cirrhotic involvement of the liver, what area may be spared or less affected?
   A. Liver hilum
   B. Caudate lobe
   C. Gallbladder bed
   D. Ligamentum teres

Portal Hypertension

1. A, B, and E

2. A

3. D

4. B

References

Baron RL, Gore RM: Diffuse liver disease. In Gore RM, Levine MS, editors: *Textbook of Gastrointestinal Radiology*, 2nd ed. Philadelphia: WB Saunders, 2000, pp1590-1638.

Sanyal AJ, Bosch J, Blei A, Arroyo V: Portal hypertension and its complications. *Gastroenterology* 2008;134:1715-1728.

Cross-Reference

Gastrointestinal Imaging: *THE REQUISITES,* 3rd ed, p 184.

Comment

Cirrhosis of the liver is the result of chronic liver hepatocyte toxicity resulting in fibrous tissue formation throughout the liver, with resultant tissue distortion and a smaller shrunken liver. The changes may initially be focal. However, when the entire liver is involved, the classic CT appearance of a small liver with nodular or irregular margins is seen. The caudate lobe may be partially spared. Although most of the liver's blood supply comes from the portal vein, the caudate lobe has a direct connection with the inferior vena cava in most patients. In the United States, most cirrhosis is alcohol induced (Laennec's cirrhosis) and is seen with splenomegaly, ascites, and esophageal varices (see figures). The falciform ligament may also be seen if there is sufficient ascites (see figures).

Other causes of cirrhosis include Wilson's disease and hemochromatosis. Portal vein hypertension is a form of relative occlusion of the portal vein. In some cases of cirrhosis a true portal vein thrombus may be seen. However, there also may be other causes of portal vein thrombosis apart from cirrhosis.

Notes

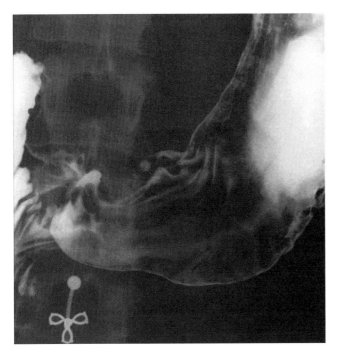 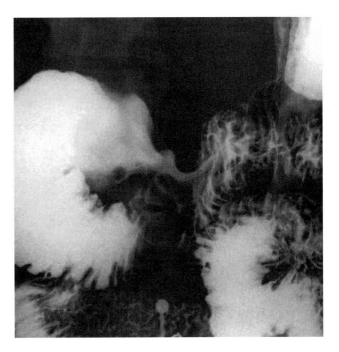

History: A 28-year-old woman presents with dyspepsia and vomiting and a history of alcohol and ibuprofen abuse.

1. Which of the following should be included in the differential diagnosis of an underlying disease resulting in the imaging finding shown in the figures? (Choose all that apply.)
   A. Gastric cancer
   B. Crohn's disease
   C. Zollinger-Ellison syndrome
   D. Atrophic gastritis
   E. Hypertrophic gastritis

2. Which choice is the most likely diagnosis?
   A. Normal variant
   B. Benign gastric ulcers
   C. Malignant gastric ulcers
   D. Gastritis
   E. Gastric polyps

3. Which of the following are features of a benign gastric ulcer?
   A. Hampton line sign
   B. Carmen meniscus sign
   C. Ulcer size less than 20 mm
   D. Ulcer in profile projects within the gastric lumen
   E. Radiating folds extending to surrounding edema mound

4. Which of the following is the most common cause of gastric and duodenal peptic ulcer disease in industrialized societies?
   A. Alcohol
   B. Smoking
   C. Use of nonsteroidal antiinflammatory drugs (NSAIDs)
   D. Steroid therapy
   E. *Helicobacter pylori* infection

CASE 56

Benign Gastric Ulcers

1. A, B, C, and E

2. B

3. A

4. E

References

Levine MS: Peptic ulcers. In Gore RM, Levine MS (eds): *Textbook of Gastrointestinal Radiology*, 2nd ed. Philadelphia: WB Saunders, 2000, pp 514-545.

Thompson G, Stevenson GW, Somers S: Benign gastric ulcer: a reliable radiologic diagnosis. *Am J Roentgenol* 1983;141:331-333.

Cross-Reference

Gastrointestinal Imaging: THE REQUISITES, 3rd ed, p 82.

Comment

Benign ulcers (see figures) can occur anywhere in the stomach, although they do have a propensity to occur in the lesser curvature, particularly in the middle of the body. This type of ulcer is often seen in the older patient, but the cause for this is uncertain. As a corollary, the majority of ulcers found in the fundus are malignant. The size of an ulcer has no bearing on its malignant potential, and giant gastric ulcers often represent a penetrating, walled-off, benign gastric ulcer. Also, the shape of the ulcer is usually round and well defined, but this is not always the case.

Much has been said about the gastric ulcer as seen in profile. Most benign gastric ulcers project outside the expected lumen of the stomach. However, if there is a great deal of edema or the ulcer is chronic, this might not be the case. Another common sign of a benign gastric ulcer is the Hampton line sign, which is a thin lucent line at the neck or base of the ulcer as it passes through the mucosal layer where undermining of the submucosa occurs. However, a very thick ulcer collar, particularly if it is asymmetrical, at the neck of the ulcer is not a Hampton line and may be seen in benign as well as malignant ulcers.

Often, radiating folds are seen extending toward an ulcer. If these folds pass all the way to the edge of the crater, the process is most likely benign. Infrequently, folds stop short as a result of a large collar of edema (in benign ulcers) or as a result of neoplastic tissue (in malignant ulcers); therefore, folds that stop short are a good but not absolute differential diagnostic feature. Also, the folds tend to be smooth and symmetrical in benign ulcers and more irregular, thickened, and fused in malignant ulcers. It has long been a part of gastric ulcer lore that malignant ulcers can show signs of healing.

Notes

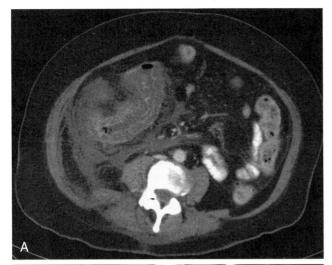

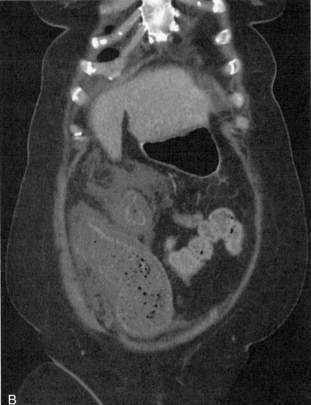

History: An immunocompromised 26-year-old woman presents with pain, rectal bleeding, and diarrhea.

1. Which of the following should be included in the differential diagnosis of the imaging finding shown in figure A? (Choose all that apply.)
   A. Ischemic colitis
   B. Bacterial colitis
   C. Crohn's disease
   D. Viral colitis
   E. Tuberculosis

2. Which of the following symptoms suggest that diarrhea occurring in a patient with AIDS is due to colitis?
   A. Watery, large-volume diarrhea
   B. Tenesmus, dyschezia, and urgency
   C. Frequent, small-volume, painful stools
   D. Bloating, nausea, and epigastric cramps

3. Which of the following statements regarding diarrhea in a patient with AIDS is *false*?
   A. Cytomegalovirus is the most common viral colitis.
   B. Cytomegalovirus colitis typically causes large, deep ulceration.
   C. Viral infections of the gastrointestinal tract tend to affect the small bowel.
   D. Pseudomembranous colitis results in clinical and imaging findings similar to those resulting from viral colitis.

4. When a patient with AIDS presents with diarrhea, what diagnostic study should be performed after history, examination, and routine blood tests?
   A. Stool examination
   B. Blood cultures
   C. Endoscopy
   D. CT scan

AIDS Colitis

1. B, C, D, and E

2. C

3. C

4. A

Reference

Glick S: Other inflammatory conditions of the colon. In Gore RM, Levine MS, editors: *Textbook of Gastrointestinal Radiology*, 2nd ed. Philadelphia: WB Saunders, 2000, pp 993-1008.

Cross-Reference

Gastrointestinal Imaging: *THE REQUISITES,* 3rd ed, p 297.

Comment

Cytomegalovirus (CMV) colitis is a type of colitis seen in AIDS patients and other immunocompromised patients. Both CT and barium studies can be quite helpful and suggestive. The discovery of large ulcers has been associated with CMV infection in AIDS patients. Ultimately the diagnosis is usually made when the virus is isolated in tissue specimens. Although CMV is probably the most common viral colonic infection seen today, other opportunistic infections are also seen, including *Cryptosporidium* infection and pseudomembranous colitis, both of which are more common in AIDS patients. Bacterial colitis must be included in the diagnosis; *Campylobacter* and even tuberculosis must be considered, although tuberculosis tends to affect the ileocecal area, as it would in patients without an impaired immune system.

Notes

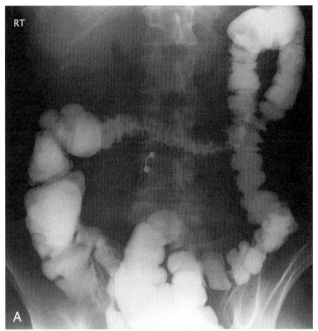

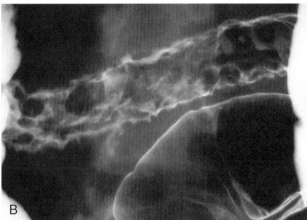

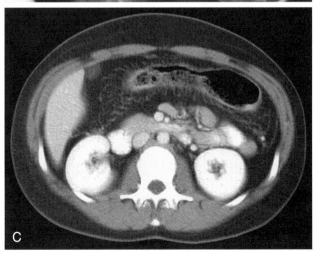

History: A 21-year-old woman presents with weight loss, diarrhea, and abdominal pain.

1. Which of the following should be included in the differential diagnosis of the imaging finding shown in figure A? (Choose all that apply.)
   A. AIDS
   B. Pancreatitis
   C. Cannon's point
   D. Crohn's disease
   E. Omental metastasis

2. Which of these findings are features more suggestive of Crohn's disease of the colon than of ulcerative colitis?
   A. Severe anorectal involvement is rare in Crohn's
   B. Granular mucosa in Crohn's colitis
   C. Contiguous and concentric disease in Crohn's colitis
   D. Discontiguous in ulcerative colitis
   E. Aphthous ulcers suggest Crohn's colitis

3. Which of the following statements regarding colonic ulceration is true?
   A. Collar button ulcers are typical in Crohn's disease
   B. Aphthous ulceration is pathognomonic of Crohn's disease
   C. Deep ulceration progressing to fistula formation suggests tuberculosis
   D. Crohn's disease is the most common cause of colovesical fistula.

4. Which of the following correctly describes the "cobblestone" sign?
   A. Mucosal ulceration with deep linear penetration
   B. Deep linear and serpiginous ulceration between lobules of edema
   C. Small superficial ulcers with a surrounding slightly elevated mound of edema
   D. Small mucosal ulcers that undermine the submucosa, resulting in a narrow neck leading to a larger round niche

Crohn's Disease of the Colon

1. A, B, D, and E

2. E

3. C

4. B

References

Horsthuis K, Bipat S, Bennink RJ, Stoker J: Inflammatory bowel disease diagnosed with US, MR, scintigraphy, and CT: meta-analysis of prospective studies. *Radiology* 2008;247:64-79.

Wills JS, Lobis IF, Denstman FJ: Crohn disease: state of the art. *Radiology* 1997;202:597-610.

Cross-Reference

Gastrointestinal Imaging: *THE REQUISITES,* 3rd ed, p 294.

Comment

Several types of ulcers are encountered with inflammation of the colon, and these ulcers can also affect all portions of the gastrointestinal tract because the bowel has only a limited number of ways to respond to inflammation of the mucosa. When ulceration extends through the mucosa and muscularis propria, it reaches the submucosa. The epithelium is relatively resistant, but the submucosa has difficulty containing the inflammatory process. Thus, ulcers tend to spread laterally when they reach the submucosa. With their thin necks and wide bases, the ulcers resemble collar buttons, hence the terminology.

Aphthous ulceration occurs in the colon as lymphoid follicles enlarge from inflammation and their overlying mucosa ulcerates. In other parts of the gastrointestinal tract, aphthous ulcers occur as focal ulcers, with surrounding edema. Either way, they produce a characteristic appearance of a tiny ulcer surrounded by edema (see figures). These ulcers were initially described in association with Crohn's disease but can be found in a variety of infectious processes, particularly viral infections. Amebiasis, salmonellosis, and even ischemia have also been known to produce aphthous ulcers.

Long, linear ulcers are rare and much more specific to Crohn's disease. Rarely do other inflammatory conditions cause this type of ulceration, although tuberculosis is also a consideration. Fistulas between bowel loops are a sequela of inflammation of the bowel, occurring with Crohn's disease or tuberculosis. Fistulas are never seen in patients with ulcerative colitis. The possibility of malignancy and the sequelae of radiation or surgery are other considerations when fistulas are encountered. Diverticulitis also can produce fistulas and is the most common cause of enterovesicular fistulas.

CT is fast becoming a valuable tool in the work-up of Crohn's disease (see figures). Only about 20% of Crohn's disease is limited to the colon. The classic findings of discontinuous disease (skip lesions) and asymmetrical involvement are usually evident.

Notes

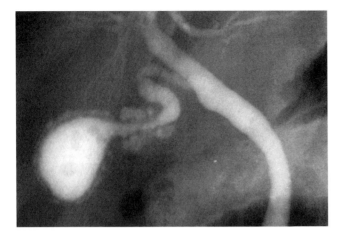

History: A 54-year-old man presents with right upper quadrant abdominal pain and an episode of jaundice.

1. Which of the following should be included in the differential diagnosis of the imaging finding shown in the figure? (Choose all that apply.)
   A. Adenyomatosis
   B. Gallbladder diverticulosis
   C. Adenomyomatous hyperplasia
   D. Intramural pseudodiverticulosis
   E. Cholecystitis glandularis proliferans

2. What is the underlying pathologic process in adenomyomatosis of the gallbladder?
   A. Benign glandular tumors derived from biliary tract epithelium
   B. Proliferation of the smooth muscle and infolding of the mucosa
   C. Granulation and fibrous tissue with plasma cells and lymphocytes
   D. Accumulation of lipids within macrophages in the gallbladder wall with enlarged villi

3. What is the long-term complication of adenomyomatosis of the gallbladder?
   A. Cancer
   B. Cholelithiasis
   C. Cholesterolosis
   D. None of the above

4. What is the name given to the tiny diverticula-like projections in the thickened gallbladder wall in adenomyomatosis?
   A. Tarlov cysts
   B. Virchov-Robin spaces
   C. Rokitansky-Aschoff sinuses
   D. Intramural pseudodiverticula

Adenomyomatosis of the Gallbladder

1. A, B, C, and E

2. B

3. D

4. C

References

Berk RN, van der Vegt JH, Lichtenstein JE: The hyperplastic cholecystoses: cholesterolosis and adenomyomatosis. *Radiology* 1983;146:593-601.

Boscak AR, Al-Hawary M, Ramsburgh SR: Adenomyomatosis of the gallbladder. *Radiographics* 2006;26:941-946.

Cross-Reference

Gastrointestinal Imaging: *THE REQUISITES,* 3rd ed, p 252.

Comment

Two conditions—adenomyomatosis and cholesterolosis—are grouped together as the hyperplastic cholecystoses. These conditions are not pathologically or physiologically related in any way, but both produce an abnormal thickening of the gallbladder wall. In adenomyomatosis there is abnormal thickening of the smooth muscle layer of the gallbladder, which results in exaggerated infolding of the mucosal folds and epithelium. Sometimes the epithelium becomes surrounded by the muscle layers and forms cysts. The exact reason that this condition develops is uncertain. Adenomyomatosis is unusual in that often only portions of the gallbladder wall become involved; other gallbladder conditions usually involve the entire gallbladder.

On contrast examinations of the gallbladder, these infoldings of the mucosal surface trap contrast material and appear as tiny diverticula-like projections in the wall (called Rokitansky-Aschoff sinuses). They become particularly pronounced when there is contraction of the gallbladder wall. If the proliferation is severe, there can be narrowing or deformity of the gallbladder lumen (see figure). A thickened gallbladder wall can be demonstrated on CT examination. If this thickening is focal, it can be impossible to distinguish the condition from gallbladder carcinoma. Thickening of the wall of the gallbladder also is apparent on ultrasound examination. Ring-down artifacts may be evident on the nondependent wall of the gallbladder. The wall of the gallbladder also can appear nodular or can appear to contain small polyps. Unlike other gallbladder conditions, there is little associated morbidity with adenomyomatosis, and there are no known long-term complications. Adenomyomatosis is not a precancerous condition.

Notes

Fair Game

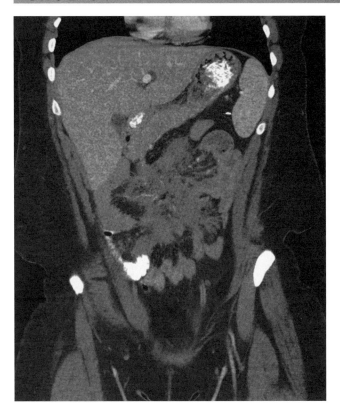

History: A 30-year-old woman presents with abdominal distention.

1. Which of the following should be included in the differential diagnosis of the imaging finding shown in the figure? (Choose all that apply.)
   A. Adhesions
   B. Tuberculosis
   C. Carcinoid
   D. Desmoid
   E. Mesenteric cyst

2. What polyposis syndrome is associated with mesenteric fibrosis?
   A. Turcot's syndrome
   B. Peutz-Jeghers syndrome
   C. Cronkhite-Canada syndrome
   D. Familial adenomatous polyposis

3. Some tumors can cause this appearance. Which of the following would *not*?
   A. Dermoid
   B. Lymphoma
   C. Carcinoid
   D. Peritoneal carcinomatosis

4. When mesenteric fibrosis occurs in a round mass, what is it called?
   A. Dermoid
   B. Desmoid
   C. Carcinoid
   D. Neurofibroma

Desmoid, Gardner's Syndrome

1. A, B, C, and D

2. D

3. A

4. B

References

Dahnert W: *Radiology Review Manual*, 6th ed. Philadelphia: Lippincott Williams & Wilkins, 2007, p 833.

Soravia C, Berk T, McLeod RS, Cohen Z: Desmoid disease in patients with familial adenomatous polyposis. *Dis Colon Rectum* 2000;43:363-369.

Cross-Reference

Gastrointestinal Imaging: *THE REQUISITES,* ed 3, p 284.

Comment

Various fibrous conditions, which represent a combination of fibrosis, inflammation, and fatty replacement, can affect the mesentery. These conditions have been given several names, which are somewhat dependent on which component of the disease predominates. Terms used for this condition include retractile mesenteritis, fibrosing mesenteritis, mesenteric panniculitis, mesenteric lipodystrophy, and desmoids. Many use the broad category of fibrosing mesenteritis to describe this condition. Most often this condition occurs in patients without any predisposing factors. Patients with familial adenomatous polyposis (Gardner's syndrome) are known to develop fibrotic lesions of the mesentery. The lesion may be an ill-defined fibrotic reaction, as in fibrosing mesenteritis, or it may be a more focal, rounded mass, which may be termed a desmoid. The modality that allows the best visualization of these changes is CT (see figure). The tissue is denser than the mesenteric fat, although areas of fat may be seen within it. The fibrous tissue travels along the tissue planes and tends to surround structures, such as vessels or bowel, and can encase them to some degree. It also may be a more localized, ovoid mass that appears well defined, which is what some tend to refer to as a desmoid. This infiltrating fibrous reaction also mimics neoplastic processes, and it may be difficult to distinguish the two. Lymphoma, serosal spread of tumor, and even carcinoid tumors can resemble fibrosing mesenteritis. On barium studies of the bowel, the loops of bowel may be displaced or fixed in position.

Notes

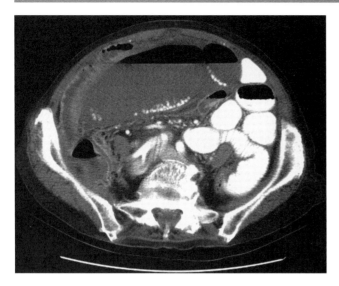

History: A 45-year-old woman presents with abdominal pain and sepsis.

1. Which of the following should be included in the differential diagnosis of the imaging finding shown in the figure? (Choose all that apply.)
   A. Renal cyst
   B. Hepatic cyst
   C. Cecal volvulus
   D. Xanthogranulomatous pyelonephritis
   E. Gallbladder hydrops

2. What is the likely state of the bile ducts?
   A. Obstructed common hepatic duct
   B. Obstructed common bile duct
   C. Obstructed cystic duct
   D. Patent bile ducts

3. What was the preceding pathology of the condition?
   A. Acute cholecystitis
   B. Acalculous cholecystitis
   C. Chronic cholecystitis
   D. Emphysematous cholecystitis

4. Untreated acute cholecystitis can progress to a variety of complications. Which of the following is *not* a complication of acute cholecystitis?
   A. Perforation
   B. Bile peritonitis
   C. Gallbladder hydrops
   D. Porcelain gallbladder

Gallbladder Hydrops

1. A, B, C, and E

2. C

3. A

4. D

References

Paulson EK: Acute cholecystitis: CT findings. *Semin Ultrasound CT MR* 2000;21:56-63.
Zeman RK: Cholelithiasis and cholecystitis. In Gore RM, Levine MS, (eds): *Textbook of Gastrointestinal Radiology*, 2nd ed. Philadelphia: WB Saunders, 2000, pp 1321-1345.

Cross-Reference

Gastrointestinal Imaging: *THE REQUISITES,* 3rd ed, p 245.

Comment

Patients with clinical findings of acute cholecystitis can be imaged either by ultrasound or CT. Ultrasound is very good at making the findings that confirm the diagnosis. However, CT provides additional information about what is happening not only in the right upper quadrant but also throughout the abdomen. In this case, the patient has developed a huge gallbladder (hydrops) with gallstones in the dependent position (see figure) as well as some fluid in the abdomen. Dilated loops of bowel secondary to bile peritonitis are seen nearby. This patient started with a case of acute cholecystitis and, owing to delay in seeking treatment, went on to develop a gangrenous gallbladder wall, perforation, and bile peritonitis.

Chronic cholecystis is relatively common and is seen on many abdominal CT studies, mostly as an incidental finding. Small contracted gallbladder with wall thickening and possibly increased enhancement and occasionally wall calcification are the usual signs. Acute cholecystitis is usually a surgical emergency. CT findings include wall thickening (3 to 4 mm) and wall enhancement. There may be fluid in the gallbladder fossa, and gallstones are usually present. High-resolution CT can often demonstrate the offending stone obstructing the cystic duct. One does have to remember that a small percentage of cases of acute cholecystitis are the acalculous type, with all these findings and no obvious stones.

Notes

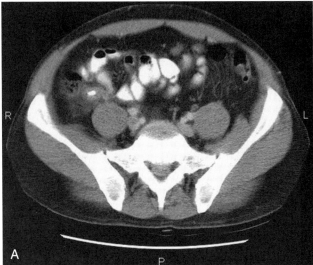

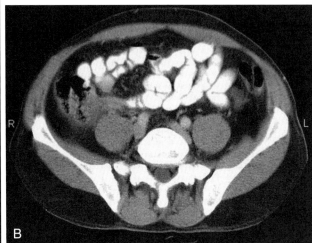

History: A 42-year-old man presents with acute right lower quadrant abdominal pain and tenderness.

1. Which of the following should be included in the differential diagnosis of the right lower quadrant calcification shown in Figure A? (Choose all that apply.)
   A. Phlebolith
   B. Diverticolith
   C. Appendicolith
   D. Ureteric calculus
   E. Lymph node calcification

2. Which of the following statements regarding appendicoliths is true?
   A. An appendicolith is visible in the majority of cases of appendicitis.
   B. Appendicitis occurs as a result of an appendicolith obstructing the appendix.
   C. The presence of an appendicolith is pathognomonic of appendicitis.
   D. They are composed of inspissated fecal debris, mucus, calcium phosphate, and inorganic salts.

3. Which of the following statements regarding appendicitis is true?
   A. The optimal management is surgical.
   B. The appendix is a considered to be a false diverticulum of the colon.
   C. The appendix is a continuation of and histologically similar to the cecum.
   D. The primary cause for clinical appendicitis is localized or free perforation of the appendix.

4. Which of the following statements regarding the imaging of appendicitis is true?
   A. Appendicitis is diagnosed when CT shows wall thickening more than 10 mm.
   B. Ultrasound is useful to diagnose appendicitis in less than 50% of cases.
   C. CT has an accuracy rate approaching 100% in the imaging diagnosis of appendicitis.
   D. The diagnosis of appendicitis by CT requires the presence of periappendiceal fluid collections.

Appendocolith with Appendicitis

1. A, B, C, and E

2. D

3. A

4. C

References

Birnbaum BA, Wilson SR. Appendicitis at the millennium. *Radiology* 2000;215:337-348.

Rao PM, Rhea JT, Novelline RA, et al. Helical CT technique for the diagnosis of appendicitis: prospective evaluation of a focused appendix CT examination. *Radiology* 1997; 202:139-144.

Cross-Reference

Gastrointestinal Imaging: *THE REQUISITES,* 3rd ed, p 318.

Comment

The advent of multidetector CT scanning (MDCT) in recent years has resulted in an enormous increase in anatomic and pathologic information available to the radiologist, with little change in the radiation dosage to patients. With the improved quality of multiplanar imaging, we are seeing the body with breathtaking clarity compared to previous years. We can now see small calcifications within an otherwise normal appendix. These small calcifications must begin at some time, and it is possible to image the normal appendix with a small appendolith within it. Is it a harbinger of impending appendicitis? That is not known with certainty, but it seems reasonable to assume that these patients are at a higher risk for appendicitis in the future. Currently MDCT has an accuracy rate approaching 100% in the imaging diagnosis of appendicitis. Ultrasound ranges between 70% and 90% in the current literature. Physical examination should be the primary examination of choice, and its role should not be diminished even as imaging becomes more important in the patient work-up. It would be presumptuous to think that everywhere a patient presents with abdominal pain, there will be sophisticated imaging available to make primary diagnosis.

Notes

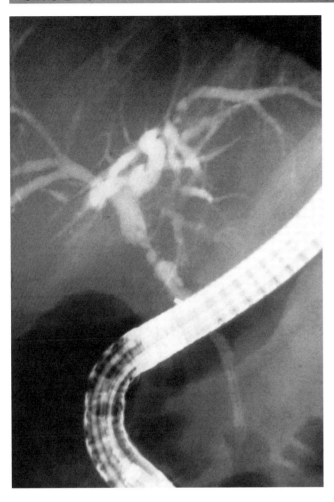

History: A 53-year-old man who had recently undergone cholecystectomy; operative cholangiogram found abnormal bile ducts.

1. Which of the following should be included in the differential diagnosis of the imaging finding shown in the figure? (Choose all that apply.)
   A. Mirizzi's syndrome
   B. Cholangiocarcinoma
   C. Primary biliary cirrhosis
   D. Primary sclerosing cholangitis
   E. Recurrent biliary tract infection

2. What is the most common disease associated with sclerosing cholangitis?
   A. Retroperitoneal fibrosis
   B. Mediastinal fibrosis
   C. Crohn's disease
   D. Ulcerative colitis

3. What is the most common cause of recurrent biliary tract infection worldwide?
   A. AIDS
   B. Bacterial cholangitis
   C. Clonorchis sinensis
   D. Ascaris lumbricoides

4. Which of the following statements regarding malignancy and sclerosing cholangitis is true?
   A. Patients are at risk of developing hepatocellular carcinoma.
   B. Patients are at risk of developing cholangiocarcinoma.
   C. About 50% of patients develop malignant complications.
   D. There is no malignant association.

Sclerosing Cholangitis

1. B, D, and E

2. D

3. D

4. B

References

Chapman R, Fevery J, Kalloo A, et al. Diagnosis and management of primary sclerosing cholangitis. *Hepatology* 2010;51:660-678.

MacCarthy RL: Inflammatory disorders of the biliary tract. In Gore RM, Levine MS, editors: *Textbook of Gastrointestinal Radiology*, 2nd ed. Philadelphia: WB Saunders, 2000, pp 1375-1394.

Cross-Reference

Gastrointestinal Imaging: *THE REQUISITES,* 3rd ed, p 228.

Comment

Primary sclerosing cholangitis is a chronic biliary disease of unknown etiology. The majority (70% or more) of cases are related to underlying inflammatory bowel disease, particularly ulcerative colitis. It is estimated that anywhere from 3% to 10% of patients with ulcerative colitis will develop sclerosing cholangitis. It is a disease of young people (third and fourth decades), with male predominance. Pathologically the condition is caused by multifocal areas of periductal fibrosis, which produce the narrowing, with intervening normal areas developing ductal ectasia (see figure).

Similar radiologic changes are apparent in patients with recurrent biliary tract infections. The groups that typically develop this condition are postoperative patients with complications and the AIDS population. Worldwide, the most likely cause is intestinal parasites, particularly *Ascaris lumbricoides.* This roundworm migrates into the ducts from the small bowel and causes recurrent cholangitis. The usual course of disease is one of secondary biliary cirrhosis, recurrent sepsis, and eventual hepatic failure. The time between the appearance of the initial symptoms and death is usually 5 to 10 years. Total colectomy (in cases of ulcerative colitis) sometimes halts or diminishes the course of the disease.

Approximately 10% to 20% of patients with sclerosing cholangitis secondary to ulcerative colitis develop cholangiocarcinoma. Interestingly this condition does not develop in patients with Crohn's disease. Sometimes, total colectomy arrests the liver disease, but this effect is not predictable. If the disease progresses, the only treatment is liver transplantation.

Notes

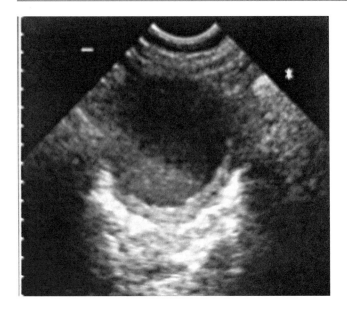

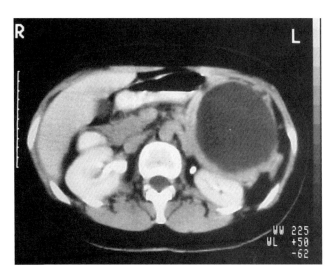

History: A 39-year-old woman presents with 3 months of pain in the left hypochondrium. On examination, a mass is easily palpable in the left upper quadrant.

1. Which of the following should be included in the differential diagnosis of the imaging finding shown in the figures? (Choose all that apply.)
   A. Abscess
   B. Hydatid cyst
   C. Pseudocyst
   D. Pseudoaneurysm
   E. Cystic pancreatic tumor

2. Which statement concerning mucinous cystadenoma of the pancreas is true?
   A. They most often occur in the pancreatic head.
   B. They have no malignant potential.
   C. Calcification is very rare.
   D. Average age of patients is 50 years.
   E. Typically there are multiple cysts.

3. Which of the following statements regarding pancreatic microcystic adenomas is true?
   A. This tumor is similar on imaging to mucinous tumors.
   B. On CT, the solid component of the tumor is nonenhancing.
   C. Calcification contributes to a well-defined surrounding capsule.
   D. The tumor is associated with von Hippel–Lindau disease.

4. Which is the most common of these pancreatic tumors?
   A. Cystic teratoma
   B. Microcystic adenoma
   C. Mucinous cystadenoma
   D. Papillary epithelial tumor

Cystic Tumor of the Pancreas

1. A, B, C, and E

2. D

3. D

4. C

References

Lundstedt C, Dawiskiba S: Serous and mucinous cystadenoma/cystadenocarcinoma of the pancreas. *Abdom Imaging* 2000;25:201-206.

Sahani DV, Kadavigere R, Saokar A, et al: Cystic pancreatic lesions: a simple imaging-based classification system for guiding management. *Radiographics* 2005;25:1471-1484.

Cross-Reference

Gastrointestinal Imaging: THE REQUISITES, 3rd ed, p 166.

Comment

Several neoplasms of the pancreas manifest as cystic lesions, although all are fairly rare compared with ductal adenocarcinoma, which almost never has a cystic component. Central necrosis is usually easily distinguishable from a cystic component.

The term *mucinous cystic neoplasms* describes what has been termed mucinous cystadenoma and mucinous cystadenocarcinoma. These tumors are difficult to distinguish, and because cystadenomas have malignant potential, they are now classified together and all are considered malignant or potentially malignant. Often the cyst is unilocular, resembling a pseudocyst, or cysts can be large, with multiple distinct septations. These tumors are hypovascular, and if they calcify, they do so in a peripheral location.

Another cystic tumor is microcystic adenoma, which has multiple small cysts of varying size. If the cysts are too numerous to count, the diagnosis should be considered microcystic adenoma. This condition occurs in older patients, mostly female. This tumor is associated with von Hippel–Lindau disease. It is a hypervascular tumor that develops central necrosis and scarring, often with calcification.

Another tumor that can resemble a mucinous cystic neoplasm is a cystic teratoma, although this tumor is rare. This tumor also has multiple large cysts and dystrophic calcification. Papillary epithelial neoplasms can be cystic. The cyst is usually thick walled, with mural tumor projections. This tumor occurs in young women and is considered a low-grade malignancy. Also, islet cell tumors that undergo necrosis can show cystic changes.

Notes

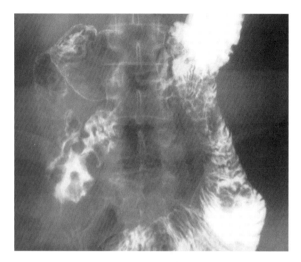

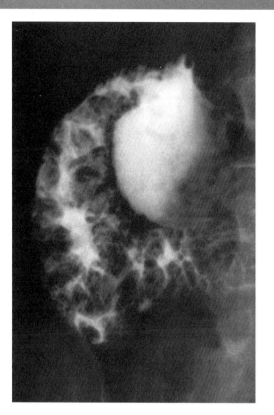

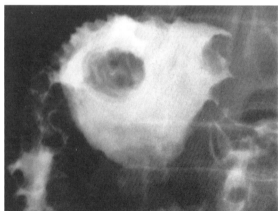

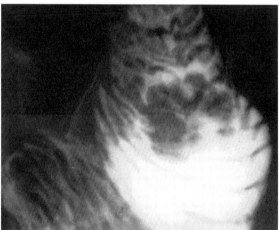

History: A 68-year-old woman presents with abnormal liver function tests.

1. Which of the following should be included in the differential diagnosis of the imaging finding shown in the figures? (Choose all that apply.)
   A. Varices
   B. Polyposis
   C. Pancreatitis
   D. Wilkie's syndrome
   E. Zollinger-Ellison syndrome

2. Histologically, of what tissue type are most duodenal polyps?
   A. Adenomatous polyps
   B. Hyperplastic polyps
   C. Brunner's gland tumors
   D. Hamartomatous polyps

3. What is the most common cause of polypoid-like filling defects at the base of the duodenal bulb?
   A. Duodenal adenoma
   B. Brunner's gland hyperplasia
   C. Prolapse of gastric mucosa
   D. Hyperplastic polyps

4. With which polyposis syndrome is small bowel and duodenal polyps most commonly associated?
   A. Cowden's disease
   B. Familial polyposis coli
   C. Peutz-Jeghers syndrome
   D. Cronkhite-Canada syndrome

Villous Adenomas of the Duodenum

1. A, B, C, and E

2. A

3. C

4. B

References

Dahnert W: *Radiology Review Manual*, 6th ed. Philadelphia: Lippincott Williams & Wilkins, 2007, p 774.

Witteman BJ, Janssens AR, Griffioen G, Lamers CB: Villous tumours of the duodenum. An analysis of the literature with emphasis on malignant transformation. *Neth J Med* 1993;42:5-11.

Cross-Reference

Gastrointestinal Imaging: *THE REQUISITES,* 3rd ed, p 94.

Comment

Once thought to be rare, in recent decades the occurrence of solitary polyps in the duodenum has been found to be more common than once thought. In contrast to the stomach, where most polyps are hyperplastic, in the duodenum, solitary polyps are most often adenomas and dangerous. Hyperplastic polyps of the duodenum are rare, despite the inflammatory changes that occur there. As is true of colonic polyps, the larger the adenoma, the more likely it is to be malignant. However, unlike the colon, any adenomatous polyp in the duodenum has a greater risk for malignancy.

The location of the polyp may be a helpful distinguishing feature. A polypoid filling defect in the bulb may be a gastric polyp, prolapsing through the pylorus along with gastric mucosa, a Brunner's gland adenoma (not a true adenomatous polyp), another type of tumor (e.g., gastrointestinal stromal tumor [GIST], metastasis), an adenoma, or an ectopic pancreatic rest. The more distal the polyp is in the duodenum, the more likely it is to be an adenoma or villous adenoma. Villous adenomas are particularly common in the periampullary region and can result in biliary and pancreatic duct obstruction. GIST tumors and ectopic pancreatic rests can occur anywhere but are more common in the proximal half of the duodenum. As a general rule, the more distal the lesion is in the duodenum, the more likely it is to be clinically important.

Duodenal polyps are more common in the patient with virtually any of the polyposis syndromes (see figures). In the patient with familial polyposis coli, the growths may be either adenomas or hyperplastic polyps. Patients with Gardner's syndrome or familial polyposis coli have a high incidence of periampullary malignancies, particularly those with Gardner's syndrome.

Notes

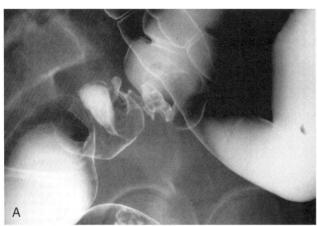

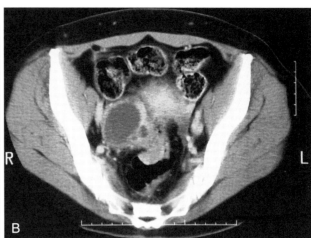

History: A 40-year-old woman presents with intermittent rectal bleeding.

1. Which of the following should be included in the differential diagnosis of the imaging finding shown in Figure A? (Choose all that apply.)
   A. Primary colon carcinoma
   B. Peritoneal metastatic cancer
   C. Primary gynecologic malignancy
   D. Pelvic inflammatory disease
   E. Pelvic congestion syndrome

2. If this patient's symptoms were monthly cyclical, what would be a likely diagnosis?
   A. Hydrosalpinx
   B. Endometriosis
   C. Uterine leiomyoma
   D. Polycystic ovary syndrome

3. What imaging modalities would be most helpful if endometriosis is suspected?
   A. CT
   B. MRI
   C. Ultrasound
   D. Hysterosalpingography

4. What is the anatomic space anterior to the superior rectum?
   A. Glisson's capsule
   B. Space of Retzius
   C. Morison's pouch
   D. Pouch of Douglas

Endometriosis Involving the Rectum

1. A, B, C, and D

2. B

3. B

4. D

References

Jeong YY, Outwater EK, Kang HK: Imaging evaluation of ovarian masses. *Radiographics* 2000;20:1445-1470.

Woodward PJ, Sohaey R, Mezzetti TP: Endometriosis: radiologic-pathologic correlation. *Radiographics* 2001;21:193-216.

Cross-Reference

Gastrointestinal Imaging: *THE REQUISITES,* 3rd ed, p 307.

Comment

The anterior wall of the rectum abuts some major structures and can be involved by disease processes arising from these organs. Most important, however, the lowermost portion of the peritoneal cavity, the cul-de-sac, overlies the anterior portion of the upper rectum. Typically this abuts the rectum above the first or second valve of Houston. In this location, any peritoneal process can reside and secondarily involve the rectum.

Inflammatory processes or bleeding from above can result in fluid or pus in the pouch of Douglas (cul-de-sac), but malignancy is the most important factor, and any abdominal tumor can seed the peritoneal cavity with metastatic disease involving the cul-de-sac and the contiguous rectal wall. The most important consideration in a female patient is ovarian carcinoma. Endometrial carcinoma is another possibility. In both sexes, gastric, pancreatic, or colon cancer can produce peritoneal metastases. The appearance of all these tumors is identical.

Inflammatory processes include appendicitis, diverticulitis, and pelvic inflammatory disease. Because the region is the most dependent portion of the peritoneum, all pelvic inflammatory processes can spread to it either before or after surgery.

Endometriosis is a condition produced when there are extrauterine deposits of endometrial tissue. The etiology is uncertain. When endometrial tissue becomes implanted on intra-abdominal structures, it is typically on the ovaries (chocolate cysts) or the serosal surface of the bowel. The tissue is able to maintain viability, and it also responds to the monthly hormonal cycles. The tissue undergoes its normal cyclic changes, including proliferation and then desquamation, just as if it were in the uterine cavity. It is this recurrent shedding of tissue that can lead to complications, including fibrosis. The changes apparent on barium enema relate to fibrotic changes occurring in the wall of the bowel, with some mass effect produced by the tissue (see figures). In addition to the anterior rectum, the sigmoid colon, distal small bowel, cecum, appendix, and other pelvic structures may be involved. Very rarely the condition spreads to the upper abdominal cavity.

Notes

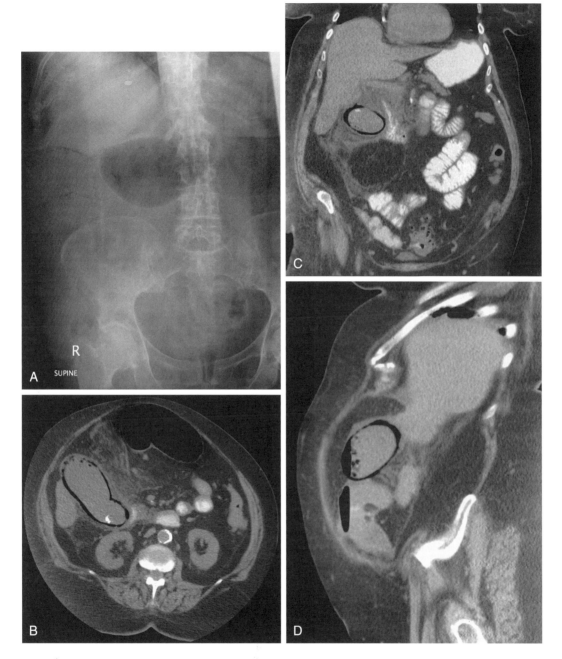

History: A 78-year-old woman presents feeling very unwell and with abdominal pain.

1. Which of the following should be included in the differential diagnosis of the imaging finding shown in Figure A? (Choose all that apply.)
   A. Hepatic abscess
   B. Pneumatosis coli
   C. Pneumatosis intestinalis
   D. Emphysematous cholecystitis
   E. Emphysematous pyelonephritis

2. What organism typically produces the process shown in these images of the right upper quadrant?
   A. *Escherichia coli*
   B. Cytomegalovirus

C. Coliform species
D. *Clostridium* species

3. What underlying condition does this patient probably have?
   A. AIDS
   B. Emphysema
   C. Atherosclerosis
   D. Diabetes mellitus

4. What is the major complication leading to a high mortality rate?
   A. Perforation
   B. Pancreatitis
   C. Cystic duct obstruction
   D. Common bile duct obstruction

CASE 68

Emphysematous Cholecystitis

1. A, B, C, and D

2. D

3. D

4. A

References

Gill KS, Chapman AH, Weston MJ: The changing face of emphysematous cholecystitis. *Br J Radiol* 1997;70:986-991.

Grand D, Horton KM, Fishman E: CT of the gallbladder: spectrum of disease. *Am J Roentgenol* 2004;183:163-170.

Cross-Reference

Gastrointestinal Imaging: *THE REQUISITES,* 3rd ed, p 255.

Comment

The appearance of gas in the lumen or the wall of the gallbladder is diagnostic of a condition known as emphysematous cholecystitis. The gas is the result of the gas-forming organism that is causing the cholecystitis. Most commonly, clostridial organisms are to blame. Patients who develop this condition are typically diabetic; rarely does emphysematous cholecystitis occur in persons without diabetes as an underlying condition. Often the patient is older and has had diabetes for many years, resulting in vascular insufficiency to the gallbladder, which is probably a major underlying cause for the development of emphysematous cholecystitis. Usually, cystic duct obstruction is also present. Although gas is present in the gallbladder lumen, gas is rarely encountered in the rest of the biliary system. The risk of perforation in patients with emphysematous cholecystitis is five times higher than that in patients with ordinary acute cholecystitis.

Emphysematous cholecystitis is one of the few diagnoses that can be readily made based on conventional radiographs (see figures). When the patient is experiencing severe abdominal pain and there is gas in the gallbladder lumen, particularly if the patient is diabetic, the diagnosis of emphysematous cholecystitis must be a primary consideration. Many conditions can result in the accumulation of gas in the lumen of the gallbladder, but there is usually an abnormal connection of the biliary tract to the bowel lumen allowing this to occur. Also, in some instances gas is visible in the wall of the gallbladder, indicating necrosis of the gallbladder wall. On CT the abnormalities are shown quite well and pericholecystic complications of inflammation and abscess are demonstrated (see figures). This condition might not be readily diagnosed on ultrasound, however, because the gas can mimic gallstones and produce acoustic shadowing.

Notes

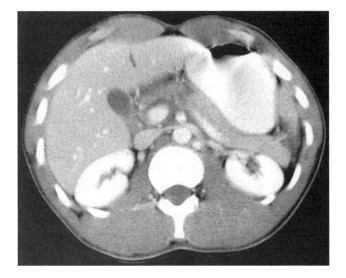

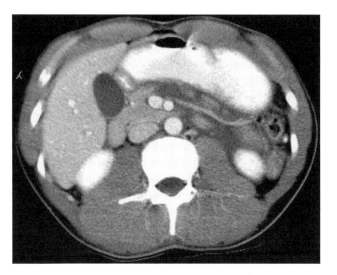

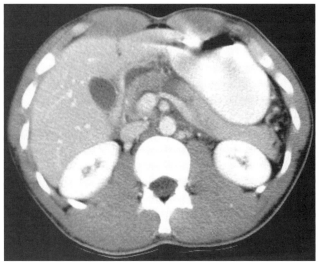

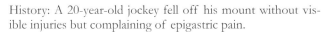

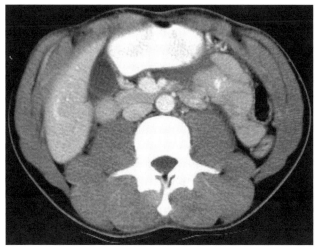

History: A 20-year-old jockey fell off his mount without visible injuries but complaining of epigastric pain.

1. Which of the following should be included in the differential diagnosis of the imaging finding shown in the figures? (Choose all that apply.)
   A. Pancreatic hematoma
   B. Pancreatic pseudocyst
   C. Pancreatic cystic tumor
   D. Splenic vein thrombosis
   E. Splenic artery pseudoaneurysm

2. What is the most common cause of pancreatic injury in adults?
   A. Sports injury
   B. Abuse or assault
   C. Penetrating injury
   D. Motor vehicle accident

3. What structure must be assessed to determine definitive treatment of pancreatic trauma?
   A. Splenic vein
   B. Splenic artery
   C. Mesenteric root
   D. Pancreatic duct

4. What is the most common treatment for this condition?
   A. Laparotomy and resection
   B. Antibiotics and conservative management
   C. Percutaneous drainage of any fluid collections
   D. Endoscopic pancreatography and pancreatic duct stenting

Pancreatic Trauma

1. A, B, and C

2. D

3. D

4. A

References

Gupta A, Stuhlfaut JW, Fleming KW, et al: Blunt trauma of the pancreas and biliary tract: a multimodality imaging approach to diagnosis. *Radiographics* 2004;24:1381-1395.

Sivit CJ, Eichelberger MR, Taylor GA, et al: Blunt pancreatic trauma in children: CT diagnosis. *Am J Roentgenol* 1992;158:1097-1100.

Cross-Reference

Gastrointestinal Imaging: THE REQUISITES, 3rd ed, p 174.

Comment

The pancreas is not often injured by blunt abdominal trauma. (It is injured in less than 12% of cases of blunt abdominal trauma.) The spleen and liver are much more commonly injured. However, the pancreas extends rather far anteriorly in the abdomen and crosses the spine, and both factors contribute to its risk of injury during blunt trauma. Motor vehicle accidents and deceleration injuries are the leading causes of pancreatic injury in adults, whereas child abuse or sports-related or bicycle injuries more typically produce the damage in children. Penetrating trauma is another common cause of pancreatic injury.

When pancreatic injury occurs, there is a high incidence of associated injuries to the bowel, spleen, liver, and blood vessels. The mortality rate for this injury approaches 20% because of both the pancreatic injury and all the other associated injuries. Patients with pancreatic injury have pain, leukocytosis, and elevated amylase levels. The injury may be just a contusion, a laceration, or a complete transection. The integrity of the pancreatic duct is important; if the duct is compromised or transected, surgical resection is required. For this type of injury, CT is the imaging modality of choice (see figures).

The appearance of the injury can be quite variable. Sometimes little or nothing can be seen. Changes related to pancreatitis, involving fluid, inflammation, or both, can be evident in the region. A contusion can produce a low-density area in the parenchyma or an area of higher density if there is hemorrhage. The actual laceration or tear of the pancreatic tissue may be evident, particularly on high-resolution scans through the pancreas. Surgery is often indicated for patients with this injury to at least drain the peripancreatic tissues of fluid that can accumulate. If the pancreatic duct is injured, the treatment usually requires surgical resection of the pancreas proximal to the injury. Ductal patency might have to be determined by endoscopic retrograde cholangiopancreatography.

Notes

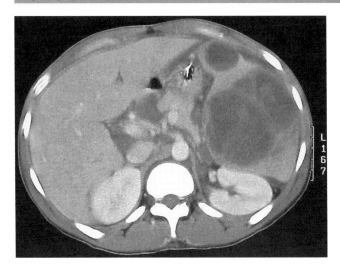

History: A 30-year-old man presents with fever and abdominal pain.

1. Which of the following should be included in the differential diagnosis of the imaging finding shown in the figure? (Choose all that apply.)
   A. Abscesses
   B. Hematomas
   C. Cysts
   D. Infarcts
   E. Lymphoma

2. What clinical condition is a major predisposing factor to the development of splenic abscesses?
   A. Polycythemia
   B. Thrombocytopenia
   C. Immunosuppression
   D. Pneumococcal infection

3. What is the most common source of septic emboli that can result in splenic abscesses?
   A. Kidney
   B. Gallbladder
   C. Heart
   D. Colon

4. What local condition is most commonly associated with the development of a splenic abscess?
   A. Pyelonephritis
   B. Diverticulitis
   C. Pancreatitis
   D. Empyema

Splenic Abscess

1. A, B, and E

2. C

3. C

4. C

References

Kamaya A, Weinstein S, Desser TS: Multiple lesions of the spleen: differential diagnosis of cystic and solid lesions. *Semin Ultrasound CT MRI* 2006;27:389-403.

Warshauer DM, Hall HL: Solitary splenic lesions. *Semin Ultrasound CT MRI* 2006;27:370-388.

Cross-Reference

Gastrointestinal Imaging: THE REQUISITES, 3rd ed, p 218.

Comment

Splenic abscesses are being encountered more commonly as a result of better diagnostic studies, such as CT (see figure) and ultrasound, and the increased number of patients with immunosuppression (e.g., patients with AIDS, transplant recipients, and those undergoing chemotherapy). Splenic abscesses can develop in several ways, including as a result of metastatic infection from septic emboli (endocarditis), as a result of contiguous infection (pyelonephritis or pancreatitis), as a sequela of an infarct or trauma with secondary infection, and as a result of generalized immunosuppression with sepsis. A small fraction of splenic abscesses develop in the absence of any underlying condition. Most infectious organisms, such as staphylococci, streptococci, and *Escherichia coli,* are aerobic. There is often a high incidence of fungal abscesses, no doubt because many of these patients are immunosuppressed.

The most common finding on plain radiography is a left pleural effusion. CT is the best modality for detecting splenic abscesses, although they also may be demonstrated by ultrasound or even MRI. The problem with CT is that many other conditions have an appearance similar to that of an abscess, and from an imaging perspective it might be impossible to differentiate an epithelial or a posttraumatic splenic cyst from an abscess. Clinical history is as important to the radiologist as it is to the clinician. Those who do not understand this have a poor grasp of the role of imaging in patient care.

Abscesses are areas of low density caused by necrotic or infected tissue. Gas is rarely demonstrated but is pathognomonic of an abscess if present. A hematoma or an infarct can appear like an abscess, as would a neoplastic process, such as lymphoma. The wall of an abscess is usually thick and somewhat irregular, which can help to differentiate it from a splenic cyst. The rim of a splenic cyst enhances only when a well-defined capsule develops about the edge of the cyst, which occurs only later in the inflammatory process. Nuclear imaging may be helpful if there is concern about the nature of a splenic mass. Gallium scans and labeled white blood cell studies are active in areas of an abscess; however, lymphoma is also gallium positive. Labeled leukocyte studies always show splenic activity and can obscure an abscess.

Notes

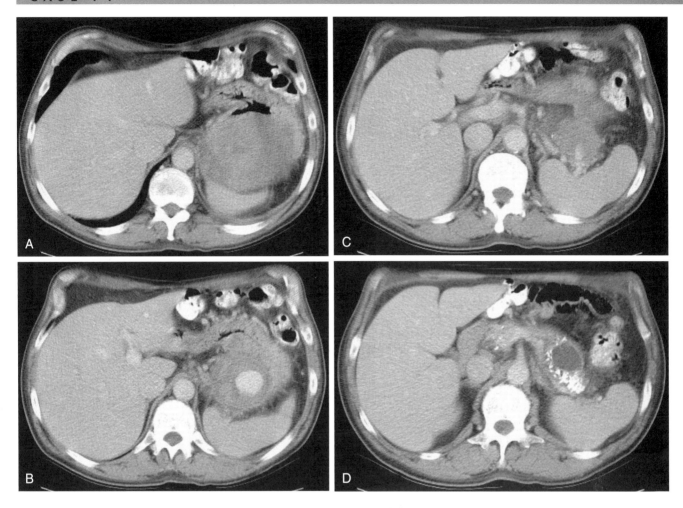

History: A 53-year-old man presents with hematemesis. Upper gastrointestinal endoscopy identified an extramucosal mass distorting the greater curvature of the stomach.

1. Which of the following should be included in the differential diagnosis of the imaging finding shown in Figures A to C? (Choose all that apply.)
   A. Intramural gastric tumor
   B. Splenic vein thrombosis
   C. Retroperitoneal hematoma
   D. Splenic artery pseudoaneurysm
   E. Communicating peripancreatic fluid collection

2. The pancreas is a small organ. Several of its anatomic features allow acute pancreatitis to have a widespread impact. Which of the following is *not* one of these contributing features?
   A. Capsule
   B. Location
   C. Exocrine function
   D. Endocrine function

3. What is the condition in acute pancreatitis called when significant bleeding occurs?
   A. Gastric varices
   B. Pancreatic necrosis
   C. Hemorrhagic pancreatitis
   D. Disseminated intravascular coagulopathy

4. What is the major cause of acute pancreatitis?
   A. Alcoholism
   B. Biliary disease
   C. Hypercalcemia
   D. Viral infection

Hemorrhagic Pancreatitis

1. A, C, D, and E

2. D

3. C

4. A

References

Agrawal GA, Johnson PT, Fishman EK: Splenic artery aneurysms and pseudoaneurysms: clinical distinctions and CT appearances. *Am J Roentgenol* 2007;188:992-999.

Balthazar EJ, Robinson DL, Megibow AJ, Ranson JH: Acute pancreatitis: value of CT in establishing prognosis. *Radiology* 1990;174:331-336.

Cross-Reference

Gastrointestinal Imaging: *THE REQUISITES,* 3rd ed, p 155.

Comment

Pancreatitis is a relatively common inflammatory condition in which, for various reasons, autodigestion of the gland occurs, resulting in edema and fluid around the gland, swelling and loss of the normal planes around the gland, and, in the acute phase, almost invariably, changes at the left lung base secondary to diminished diaphragmatic excursion, hypoventilation, and resultant atelectasis and effusion. If a vessel is eroded, significant bleeding can occur, such as in this case. The incidence ranges from 20 to 30 cases per 100,000 population. The usual presentation is epigastric pain, sometimes radiating to the back, nausea, tachycardia, tachypnea, and often fever. Occasionally the patient is hypotensive, especially in severe hemorrhagic pancreatitis. The swollen head of the gland can impress the common bile duct, causing some degree of biliary obstruction.

The most common cause is alcohol abuse. However, other causes include endoscopic retrograde cholangiopancreatography (ERCP), trauma, gallstones, certain medications, penetrating peptic ulcers, and pancreatic divisum. One of the more interesting complications is splenic artery pseudoaneurysm (see figures). These pseudoaneurysms develop as a result of inflammation and enzymatic activity weakening a point in the splenic artery wall. Although this complication is unusual, if found it constitutes a danger to the patient of sudden life-threatening bleeding.

Notes

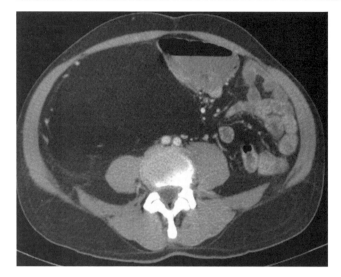

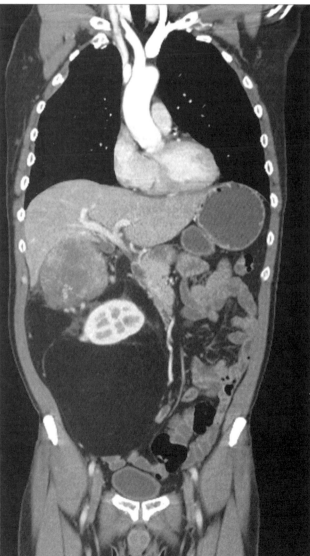

History: A 42-year-old man presents with diffuse, gradual abdominal enlargement and abdominal pain.

1. Which of the following should be included in the differential diagnosis of the imaging finding shown? (Choose all that apply.)
   A. Angiomyolipoma
   B. Leiomyosarcoma
   C. Liposarcoma
   D. Teratoma
   E. Desmoid

2. Which of the following statements regarding liposarcoma is true?
   A. Liposarcoma typically occurs in children.
   B. Liposarcoma usually arises from a pre-existing lipoma.
   C. Liposarcoma is appropriately treated with radiotherapy.
   D. Liposarcoma is encapsulated and therefore easily resected.

3. In adults, what is the most common retroperitoneal soft tissue sarcoma?
   A. Liposarcoma
   B. Mesothelioma
   C. Leiomyosarcoma
   D. Malignant fibrous histiocytoma

4. Which of the following statements relevant to imaging of liposarcomas is true?
   A. The most common location is the retroperitoneum.
   B. A retroperitoneal fatty tumor is most likely a liposarcoma.
   C. Liposarcoma usually invades the adjacent kidney and ureter.
   D. The most common intra-abdominal location is the anterior perirenal space.

Liposarcoma of the Abdomen

1. A, C, D, and E

2. C

3. A

4. B

References

Kim T, Murakami T, Oi H, et al: CT and MR imaging of abdominal liposarcoma. *Am J Roentgenol* 1996;166:829-833.

Liles JS, Tzeng CW, Short JJ, et al: Retroperitoneal and intra-abdominal sarcoma. *Curr Probl Surg* 2009;46:445-503.

Cross-Reference

Gastrointestinal Imaging: *THE REQUISITES,* 3rd ed, p 279.

Comment

Liposarcomas are relatively uncommon lesions seen in approximately 5000 patients in the United States annually. They are lipogenic tumors that can become widespread in the abdomen and extremely difficult to remove surgically. They are seen more commonly in adults, as opposed to the small, well-contained lipomas of the gut seen in children and young adults. Liposarcomas are rare in children. They can be mostly lipomatous with some soft tissue component, such as in this case, or almost purely lipomatous. They occur slightly more in male patients, and the less well differentiated the lesion, the poorer the outlook. Most patients have few or no symptoms until the tumor reaches a very large size. Eventually the patients become aware of swelling or pain and consult a physician. The imaging modality of choice is CT, in which the size, nature, and extent of involvement can be well described. CT diagnosis is usually quite accurate (see figures). Plain film can be helpful in determining the presence of a mass.

Notes

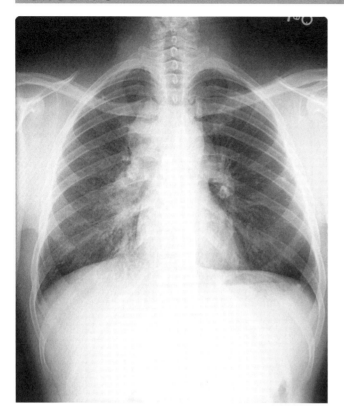

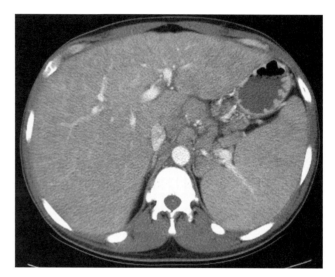

History: A 43-year-old woman presents with a rash.

1. Which of the following should be included in the
   differential diagnosis of the imaging finding shown in the
   figures? (Choose all that apply.)
   A. AIDS
   B. Lymphoma
   C. Sarcoidosis
   D. Metastatic cancer
   E. Whipple's disease

2. What is the most common intra-abdominal site of
   involvement by sarcoidosis?
   A. Liver
   B. Spleen
   C. Pancreas
   D. Peritoneum

3. Which of the following statements about abdominal
   sarcoid is true?
   A. Sarcoid is typically a thoracic disease. Abdominal dis-
      ease occurs when pulmonary disease is advanced.
   B. The most common imaging abnormality in abdominal
      sarcoidosis is extensive lymphadenopathy.
   C. Hepatic involvement by sarcoid usually leads gradually
      but progressively to portal hypertension.
   D. Biliary involvement by sarcoidosis results in strictures
      of the extrahepatic bile ducts.

4. Less than 10% of patients with sarcoidosis have
   gastrointestinal tract involvement. What places in the gut
   are most commonly involved?
   A. Stomach
   B. Small bowel
   C. Appendix
   D. Rectum

Sarcoidosis with Hepatosplenomegaly

1. A, B, C, and D

2. A

3. D

4. A

References

Farman J, Ramirez G, Rybak B, et al: Gastric sarcoidosis. *Abdom Imaging* 1997;22:248-252.

Warshauer DM, Lee JK: Imaging manifestations of abdominal sarcoidosis. *Am J Roentgenol* 2004;182:15-28.

Cross-Reference

Gastrointestinal Imaging: THE REQUISITES, 3rd ed, p 61.

Comment

Sarcoidosis is a disease generally seen involving the thorax, skin, or eyes, but it is also seen, on occasion, involving both solid and hollow viscera of the abdomen (see figures). The disease is of unknown etiology; at times correlation with some microorganism has been suggested but never proved. It is a noncaseating granulomatous disease. Most involvement of the liver is not a serious issue and usually goes unnoticed. However, about a third of patients with liver involvement have some abnormalities of liver enzymes. Most of these patients show no clinical symptoms. However, in a very small subset of that third (less than 2%) sarcoid involvement of the liver can lead to significant and serious hepatic disease. Clinically this includes jaundice and pruritus as a result of chronic progressive disease. Hepatic enlargement may be seen radiologically. In some patients there might be diffuse involvement with the spleen. Most sarcoid involvement of the spleen does not result in splenomegaly, but infrequently it is seen, such as in this patient. Patients with diffuse severe involvement of both spleen and liver can develop portal hypertension.

Notes

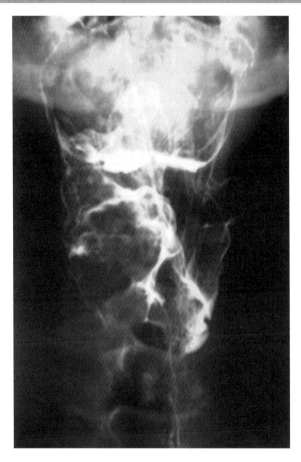

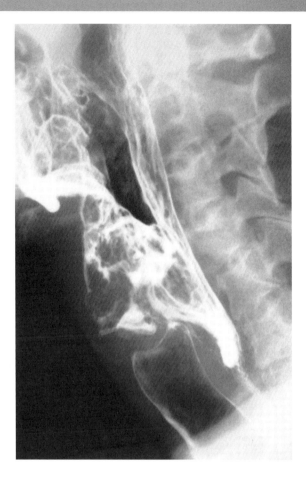

History: A 50-year-old man presents with right neck swelling but no dysphagia or dysphonia.

1. Which of the following should be included in the differential diagnosis of the imaging finding shown in the figures? (Choose all that apply.)
   A. Lymphoma
   B. Kaposi's sarcoma
   C. Metastatic melanoma
   D. Squamous cell carcinoma
   E. Gastrointestinal stromal tumor

2. What is the most common tumor of the pharynx?
   A. Lymphoma
   B. Kaposi's sarcoma
   C. Metastatic melanoma
   D. Squamous cell carcinoma

3. What is the most common risk factor for the development of pharyngeal cancer?
   A. Tobacco
   B. Betel nut
   C. Epstein-Barr virus
   D. Human papillomavirus

4. Which of the following statements relevant to imaging of pharyngeal cancers is true?
   A. Pharyngeal cancers usually manifest early.
   B. In staging pharyngeal tumors, T2 describes primary tumor between 2 and 4 cm in diameter.
   C. In staging pharyngeal tumors, N2 describes lymph nodes between 2 and 4 cm in diameter.
   D. A second primary tumor is found in 15% of patients, and 75% of these are found at the time of diagnosis (synchronous).

Squamous Carcinoma of the Pharynx

1. A, B, C, and D

2. D

3. A

4. B

References

Dammann F, Horger M, Mueller-Berg M, et al: Rational diagnosis of squamous cell carcinoma of the head and neck region: comparative evaluation of CT, MRI, and [18]FDG PET. *Am J Roentgenol* 2005;184:1326-1331.
Schmalfuss IM: Imaging of the hypopharynx and cervical esophagus. *Neuroimag Clin North Am* 2004;14:647-662.

Cross-Reference

Gastrointestinal Imaging: THE REQUISITES, 3rd ed, p 5.

Comment

The majority of tumors involving the pharynx are squamous in origin. These tumors are seen radiologically as small nodules or masses or sometimes as a thickening or obliteration of the normal structures. Laryngoscopy is the method of choice for identification, but with the increase in swallowing studies being performed to diagnose conditions causing dysphagia, the radiologist may be the first to encounter these tumors.

The pharynx and hypopharynx are repositories of a substantial amount of lymph tissue. Thus it is to be expected that patients with lymphoma might develop neoplastic infiltration of these structures. In patients with lymphoma and dysphagia, the hypopharynx must be studied closely. Squamous tumors of the hypopharynx typically arise in the vallecula, piriform sinuses, or epiglottis.

Lymphomas more commonly involve the posterior or lateral wall and may be submucosal, producing subtle changes. If a tumor is substantially posterior, lymphoma must be strongly considered. Potentially, all tumors can metastasize to this region. However, it is a rare event, given the number of patients with malignancies. Two common cancers—breast and lung—are known to metastasize to the pharynx on occasion. Also, cancers of the skin, such as melanoma and Kaposi's sarcoma, seem to metastasize to the hypopharynx relatively commonly.

Patients with Plummer-Vinson syndrome have anemia associated with cervical esophageal webs. Although it is controversial, some authors believe that the syndrome is a premalignant condition and that affected patients have a higher incidence of pharyngeal and esophageal carcinoma.

Notes

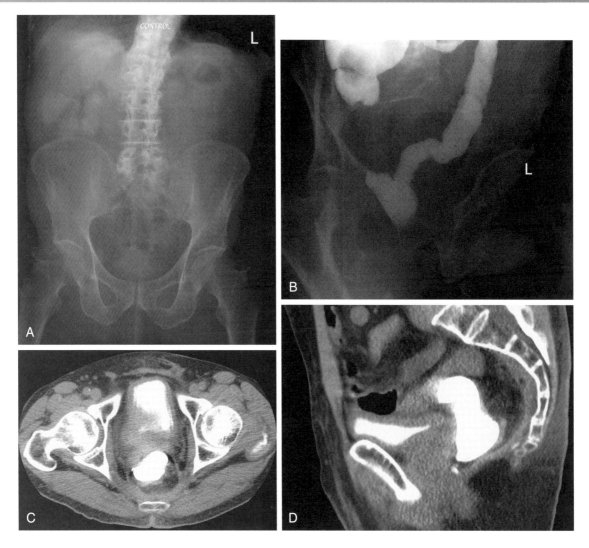

History: A 68-year-old man underwent ultra-low anterior resection 6 months ago. He had recovered well from his surgery. Earlier today he underwent a Gastrografin enema. He is now undergoing a CT scan without intravenous contrast.

1. There is high-density material in the urinary bladder. Which of the following should be included in the differential diagnosis of this imaging finding as shown in Figures C and D? (Choose all that apply.)
   A. Colovesical fistula
   B. Hemorrhagic cystitis
   C. Renal excretion of iodinated contrast administered intravascularly in the last few days
   D. Vicarious renal excretion of iodinated contrast absorbed from the lumen of the intact colon
   E. Renal excretion of iodinated contrast absorbed from the peritoneal cavity after extravasation from the perforated colon

2. Several contributing factors that might increase the incidence of absorption of iodinated contrast from the colonic lumen have been recognized. Which of the following is *not* such a factor?
   A. Ischemic colitis
   B. Radiation colitis
   C. Irritable bowel syndrome
   D. Inflammatory bowel disease

3. Apart from the diagnostic confusion, what other complication might the patient suffer from the absorption of iodinated contrast from the colonic lumen?
   A. Anaphylaxis
   B. Nephrotoxicity
   C. Colonic impaction
   D. Nephrogenic fibrosis

4. What is the most common finding on Gastrografin enema following resection for colorectal cancer with creation of diverting ileostomy?
   A. Leak
   B. Fistula
   C. Stricture
   D. Normal

Vicarious Excretion

1. A, C, D, and E

2. C

3. A

4. D

References

Low VHS, Chu BK: Diagnostic error due to vicarious excretion of rectal iodinated contrast. *Austral Radiol* 2006;50:369-372.

Sohn KM, Lee SY, Kwon OH: Renal excretion of ingested Gastrografin. *Am J Roentgenol* 2002;178:1129-1132.

Cross-Reference

Gastrointestinal Imaging: *THE REQUISITES,* 3rd ed, p 267.

Comment

The use of iodinated water-soluble contrast agent is common in radiologic practice. Occasionally vicarious excretion, usually following an enema study, can be seen in the kidneys (see figures). It is important in these studies to ensure that the contrast agent was not present before the examination. Vicarious excretion has also been reported following endoscopic retrograde cholangiopancreatography (ERCP). When iodinated water-soluble contrast agent is used in imaging the colon, vicarious excretion has been seen in as many as 20% of normal subjects in one study. Thus, its appearance in the kidneys does not necessarily indicate diseased colon. However, it is very likely that inflamed or ischemic bowel mucosa can allow the contrast agent to cross the mucosal barrier at such a rate that it may be detected in the kidneys. Indeed, the main function of the colon, apart from storage, is water absorption, which it does quite efficiently under normal circumstances.

Notes

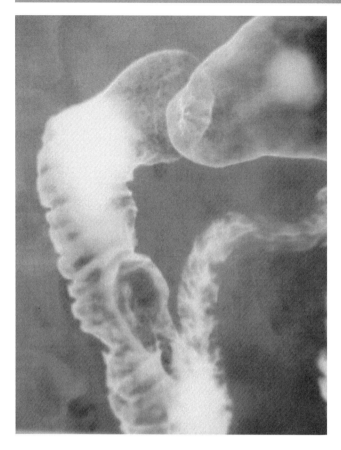

History: A 52-year-old man presents with nausea.

1. Which of the following should be included in the differential diagnosis of the imaging finding shown in the figure? (Choose all that apply.)
   A. Normal
   B. Carcinoma
   C. Pancreatitis
   D. Choledochocele
   E. Villous adenoma

2. What is the most common pathologic cause of enlargement of the papilla?
   A. Carcinoma
   B. Pancreatitis
   C. Choledochocele
   D. Choledocholithiasis

3. Pancreatitis can result in enlargement of papillae due to edema and swelling. What is the name of this sign?
   A. Oddi's sign
   B. Vater's sign
   C. Poppel's sign
   D. Brunner's sign

4. With which polyposis syndrome are tumors of the papilla most commonly associated?
   A. Cowden's disease
   B. Familial polyposis coli
   C. Peutz-Jeghers syndrome
   D. Cronkhite-Canada syndrome

Enlarged Papilla of the Duodenum

1. A, B, C, and D

2. D

3. C

4. B

Reference

Dahnert W: *Radiology Review Manual*, 6th ed. Philadelphia: Lippincott Williams & Wilkins, 2007, p 774.

Cross-Reference

Gastrointestinal Imaging: *THE REQUISITES,* 3rd ed, p 98.

Comment

On normal upper gastrointestinal tract examinations the papilla and associated structures may be identified along the medial wall of the second portion of the duodenum (see figure). The papilla is an elevated mound of tissue that is typically smaller than 1 cm. It is considered abnormal when larger than 1.5 cm, although healthy patients have been known to have papillae enlarged up to 3 cm. Inferior to the papilla, folds may be visible, extending up to 3 cm in length.

The papilla is usually enlarged as a result of benign disease. The most common cause of edema of the papilla is the presence of stones in the distal common bile duct. Other causes include pancreatitis (either short term or long term), which can produce swelling (Poppel's sign). Typically the enlargement of the papilla with edema produces a smooth and symmetrical enlargement. Rarely, acute duodenal ulcer disease produces papillary enlargement but is usually associated with duodenal fold thickening. A choledochocele, an abnormal enlargement of the most distal end of the common bile duct and ampullary region, also causes enlargement of the papilla.

Tumors arising in or about the papilla are called perivaterian malignancies. Carcinoma of the papilla is the most common tumor. Polyps or mesenchymal tumors, such as leiomyoma, can also arise in the region and produce enlargement. Certain polyposis syndromes—familial polyposis coli and the associated Gardner's syndrome—predispose patients to tumor development in the perivaterian region. Such a patient can require routine screening of the upper gastrointestinal tract throughout his or her life because of this association.

Notes

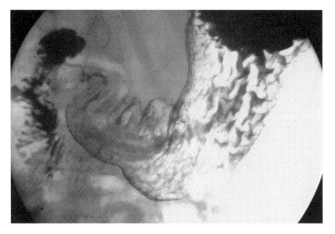

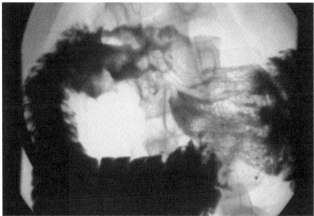

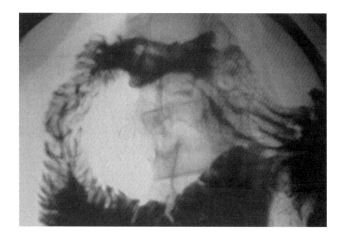

History: A 41-year-old woman presents with recurrent dyspepsia despite H2 blocker treatment.

1. Which of the following should be included in the differential diagnosis of the imaging finding shown in the figures? (Choose all that apply.)
   A. Normal
   B. Lymphoma
   C. Carcinoma
   D. NSAID gastritis
   E. *Helicobacter* gastritis

2. What is the leading cause of gastroduodenal ulcer disease in industrialized societies?
   A. Recreational drugs
   B. Therapeutic drugs
   C. Hypergastrinemia
   D. *Helicobacter pylori*

3. What substance does the breath test for gastric *H. pylori* infection in the upper gastrointestinal tract detect?
   A. Nitric oxide
   B. Hydrogen
   C. Xylose
   D. Urease

4. What is the treatment of choice for this infection?
   A. Antacids
   B. Antibiotics
   C. Triple therapy
   D. Histamine (H2) blockers

Helicobacter Gastritis

1. B, C, D, and E

2. D

3. D

4. C

References

Levine MS: Inflammatory conditions of the stomach and duodenum. In Gore RM, Levine MS (eds): *Textbook of Gastrointestinal Radiology,* 2nd ed. Philadelphia: WB Saunders, 2000, pp 546-574.

Nadgir RN, Levine MS: Update on *Helicobacter pylori. Appl Radiol* 1999;28: 10-14.

Cross-Reference

Gastrointestinal Imaging: *THE REQUISITES,* 3rd ed, p 66.

Comment

The presence of *H. pylori* in the upper gastrointestinal tract is now believed to be the major cause of peptic ulcer disease among persons who live in industrialized countries. The majority of gastric ulcers also are attributed to this organism, which is considered a major cause of chronic gastritis as well. Almost all duodenal ulcer patients also have *H. pylori* infection.

The radiologic abnormalities in these patients can be quite variable, and many patients have normal radiologic studies. By far the most common radiologic abnormality seen in patients with *H. pylori* infection is thickened gastric folds (see figures). The abnormality can vary from mild thickening of the folds in either the proximal stomach or antral region to bizarrely nodular folds involving a large portion of the stomach. These folds can become so thickened that they resemble a neoplastic process, such as lymphoma. Often these fold abnormalities can be detected on CT examination. Polyps of varying sizes also have been described. Typically these are small hyperplastic polyps, although rarely a large focal polypoid mass is encountered. In many of these patients, endoscopy is necessary to exclude malignancy. Of course, ulcers and erosions can be identified in the stomach, but this finding is less common than are the fold abnormalities. Enlarged areae gastricae also have been described, although this finding is subtle. In the duodenum, radiologic findings include ulcers, thickened folds, and narrowing or deformity.

Noninvasive techniques for detecting *H. pylori* include a breath test that detects urease activity within the upper gastrointestinal tract. Serologic tests can detect antibodies to the *H. pylori* antigen. Endoscopic studies are considered the mainstay for detection because the bacteria can be identified on biopsy specimens. However, the infection itself is patchy, and multiple biopsies are often necessary to detect the organism.

Treatment includes antibiotic therapy, usually involving a combination of agents, including metronidazole, tetracycline, or amoxicillin. Oral bismuth therapy is also recommended, and histamine blockers or proton-pump inhibitors are given to reduce acid levels.

Notes

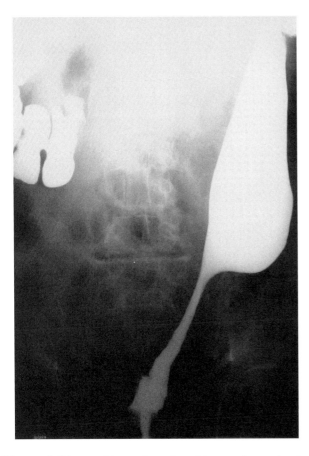 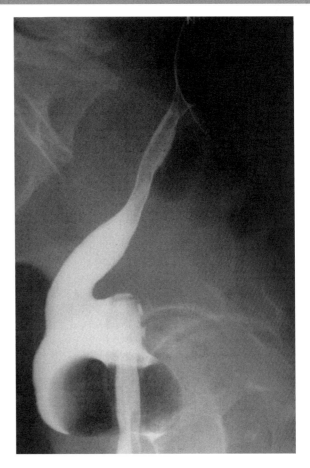

History: A 27-year-old man has a long history of constipation dating back to his infancy.

1. Which of the following should be included in the differential diagnosis of the imaging finding shown in the figures? (Choose all that apply.)
   A. Pelvic mass
   B. Colon carcinoma
   C. Radiation stricture
   D. Hirschsprung's disease
   E. Postinflammatory stricture

2. What is the pathologic basis of Hirschsprung's disease?
   A. A segment of colonic aperistalsis
   B. A segment of submucosal fibrosis
   C. A segment of persistent contraction of intramural smooth muscle
   D. A segment of congenitally absent ganglion cells in the distal colon

3. What other conditions is most commonly seen with Hirschsprung's disease?
   A. Cardiac malformations
   B. Imperforate anus
   C. Meconium ileus
   D. Trisomy 21

4. Which of the following statements about Hirschsprung's disease is *true*?
   A. The disease is more common in girls than boys.
   B. In about 5% of cases, the entire colon is involved.
   C. Treatment of choice is dilatation of the narrow segment.
   D. Barium enema and rectal manometry are the optimal diagnostic tools.

Adult Hirschsprung's Disease

1. A, C, D, and E

2. D

3. D

4. B

References

Crocker NL, Messmer JM: Adult Hirschsprung's disease. *Clin Radiol* 1991;44:257-259.

Fernbach SK: Neonatal gastrointestinal radiology. In Gore RM, Levine MS, editors: *Textbook of Gastrointestinal Radiology*, 2nd ed. Philadelphia: WB Saunders, 2000, pp 2042-2073.

Cross-Reference

Gastrointestinal Imaging: THE REQUISITES, 3rd ed, p 304.

Comment

Hirschsprung's disease is named after Harald Hirschsprung, the Danish physician who described the disease in 1888. It is a congenital disorder of the gut characterized by a segment of absent ganglion cells in the distal colon. The degree of involvement can vary, but most cases are diagnosed in the neonatal stage with the failure to pass meconium. However, lesser degrees of aganglionosis can result in a delayed diagnosis. The massive enlargement of the colon is obvious. The aganglionic segment is also visible in the rectum. The disease is more common in boys and has no racial predilection. Patients who have delayed diagnosis are much affected by the disease. They suffer from chronic severe debilitating constipation, abdominal distention, some with encopresis and an overall life-altering health state.

Plain films are suggestive in most cases. CT may be diagnostic, showing the classic features recognized by barium enema of a narrowed distal colon with proximal dilation (see figures). Barium enema has the benefit of acquiring a 24-hour-delayed radiograph that will show retention of the contrast. Rectal biopsy is the definitive diagnostic procedure. Surgery aimed at the removal of the aganglionic segment and some excess colon is usually the treatment of choice. Laparoscopic surgery for Hirschsprung's disease in newborns has been reported with some initial success.

Notes

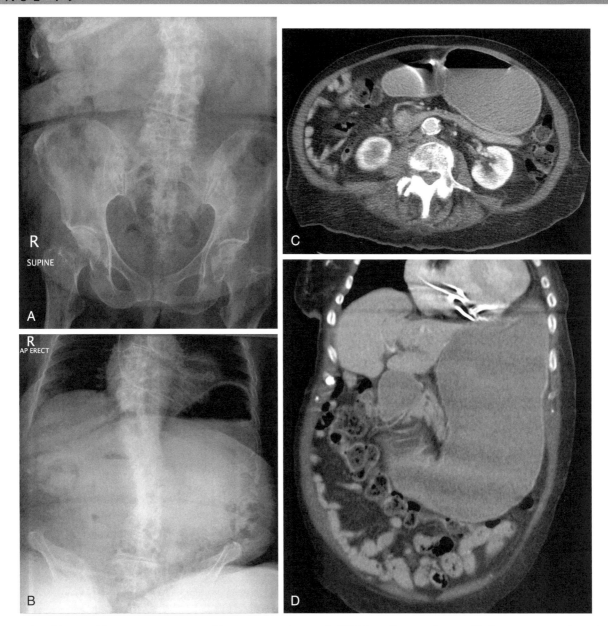

History: An 86-year-old woman presents with nausea and vomiting for 2 weeks.

1. Which of the following should be included in the differential diagnosis of the imaging finding shown in Figure A? (Choose all that apply.)
   A. Gastroparesis
   B. Pyloric spasm
   C. Portal gastropathy
   D. Gastric antral malignancy
   E. Proximal duodenal scarring

2. What is the most common cause of gastric outlet obstruction?
   A. Malignancy
   B. Pancreatitis
   C. Crohn's disease
   D. Peptic ulcer disease

3. Which malignancy is most likely to cause gastric outlet obstruction?
   A. Gastric adenocarcinoma
   B. Duodenal carcinoma
   C. Pancreatic cancer
   D. Lymphoma

4. Which of the following statements about gastric outlet obstruction is *false*?
   A. A short history of symptoms is suspicious for malignancy.
   B. The organoaxial type of gastric volvulus is more likely to cause gastric outlet obstruction.
   C. Gastric outlet obstruction is the most common complication of gastroduodenal tuberculosis.
   D. Gastric outlet obstruction can occur as a complication of percutaneous gastrostomy tube migration

Gastric Outlet Obstruction

1. A, B, D, and E

2. D

3. C

4. B

Reference

Eisenberg RL, Levine MS: Miscellaneous abnormalities of the stomach and duodenum. In Gore RM, Levine MS (eds): *Textbook of Gastrointestinal Radiology*, 2nd ed. Philadelphia: WB Saunders, 2000, pp 659-681.

Cross-Reference

Gastrointestinal Imaging: THE REQUISITES, 3rd ed, p 49.

Comment

With newer and more-effective medications inhibiting acid secretion, gastric outlet obstruction is not as common as it was 20 years ago. However, peptic ulcer disease (PUD) is still the most common cause. Malignancy is becoming a larger and more dangerous issue as a cause for gastric outlet obstruction in the 21st century. Patients who have a long history of PUD and who have ineffective treatment or do not comply with the medication regimen (e.g., alcoholics) and who present with pain and gastric distention probably have ulceration and inflammation as the cause of their obstruction. Alternatively, severe pancreatitis that causes inflammation and spasm of the second portion of the duodenum can also obstruct the gastric outlet. In patients who have little or no history of PUD and who present with gastric outlet obstruction, the possibilities are more ominous, such as carcinoma of the distal antrum or pylorus, as well as pancreatic carcinoma invading and obstructing the duodenum. In this case, pancreatic cancer with duodenal invasion was the cause of the outlet obstruction (see figures).

Notes

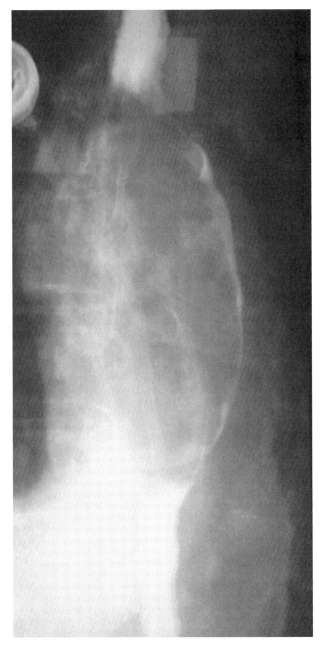

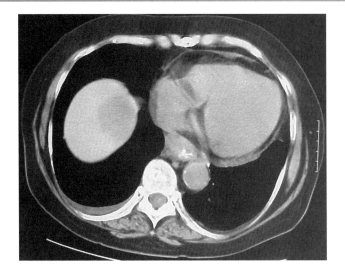

History: A 64-year-old woman presents with dysphagia and hematemesis.

1. Which of the following should be included in the differential diagnosis of the imaging finding shown in the figures? (Choose all that apply.)
   A. Achalasia
   B. Bolus impaction
   C. Spindle cell carcinoma
   D. Inverted diverticulum
   E. Intussusception

2. What tumor most often invades the esophagus through direct extension?
   A. Lymphoma
   B. Bronchogenic tumor
   C. Gastric cardia
   D. Pharyngeal

3. What is the most common cause of hematogenous metastases to the esophagus?
   A. Breast cancer
   B. Bronchogenic
   C. Colorectal
   D. Melanoma

4. Which of the following statements regarding metastatic disease to the esophagus is *true*?
   A. Odynophagia is the most common symptom.
   B. Metastatic spread to the esophagus usually occurs late in the disease.
   C. Secondary achalasia from malignant infiltration is most commonly the result of breast cancer.
   D. Mediastinal lymphadenopathy involving the esophagus usually results in a lobulated ulcerated stricture.

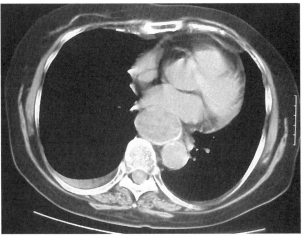

CASE 80

Metastatic Disease to the Esophagus

1. A, B, and C

2. C

3. A

4. B

Reference

Levine MS: Other malignant tumors of the esophagus. In Gore RM, Levine MS (eds): *Textbook of Gastrointestinal Radiology*, 2nd ed. Philadelphia: WB Saunders, 2000, pp 435-451.

Cross-Reference

Gastrointestinal Imaging: *THE REQUISITES*, 3rd ed, p 11.

Comment

Metastases to the esophagus are not uncommon findings on autopsy studies. However, it is somewhat more rare for them to be encountered in radiologic practice. The most common cause of secondary tumor involvement of the esophagus is direct invasion or extension of an adjacent neoplasm. The most likely of these neoplasms is gastric carcinoma, which extends into the distal esophagus. However, with new knowledge about Barrett's metaplasia and its progression toward adenocarcinoma of the distal esophagus and gastroesophageal junction, direct spread from stomach to esophagus is much less common than previously thought. Carcinoma of the lung also involves the esophagus either by direct extension or by secondary involvement of the mediastinal adenopathy. Breast cancer is the most likely distant tumor to secondarily involve the esophagus. It usually involves the esophagus by first spreading to mediastinal lymph nodes and then invading into the esophagus. However, it is also the most common cancer to have direct hematogenous metastases to the esophagus, as was the primary site and situation in this case (see figures). Hematogenous metastases are quite rare. Although all tumors can metastasize to the esophagus, the hematogenous metastases are more commonly associated with breast cancer, Kaposi's sarcoma, melanoma, and renal cell carcinoma.

Notes

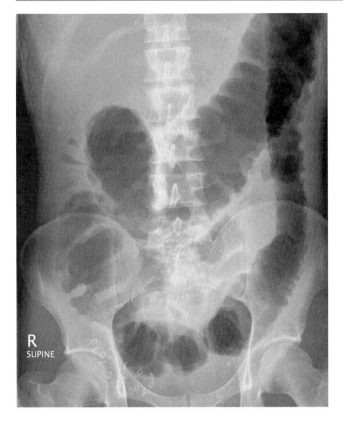
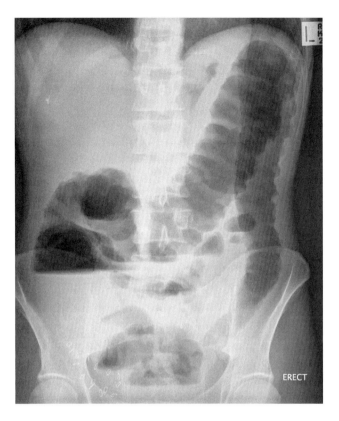

History: A 34-year-old man with chronic diarrhea presents acutely unwell with abdominal distention, fever, rectal bleeding, and passage of clots.

1. Which of the following should be included in the differential diagnosis of the imaging finding shown in the figures? (Choose all that apply.)
   A. Ischemia
   B. Infectious colitis
   C. Irritable bowel syndrome
   D. Pseudomembranous colitis
   E. Inflammatory bowel disease

2. What measurement is used to indicate the seriousness of toxic megacolon?
   A. Hypoalbuminemia
   B. Hemoglobin
   C. Colonic diameter
   D. None

3. What is the pathogenesis for the development of toxic megacolon?
   A. Severe electrolyte imbalance
   B. Failure of cholinergic neurotransmission
   C. Transmural inflammation damaging the ganglion cells
   D. Dilation due to mechanical failure of downstream passage of colonic contents

4. Which of the following correctly describes the thumbprinting sign?
   A. Reticular mucosal pattern similar to the fine lines of a thumbprint or fingerprint
   B. Thickened valvulae resembling fingers or thumbs standing close together
   C. Lobules of edematous mucosa separated by lines of ulceration
   D. Lobulated thickening of haustral folds

Toxic Megacolon

1. A, B, D, and E

2. D

3. C

4. D

References

Imbriaco M, Balthazar EJ: Toxic megacolon: role of CT in evaluation and detection of complications. *Clin Imaging* 2001;25(5):349-354.

Sheikh RA, Yasmeen S, Prindiville T: Toxic megacolon: a review. *JK Practitioner* 2003;10:176-178.

Cross-Reference

Gastrointestinal Imaging: *THE REQUISITES,* 3rd ed, p 312.

Comment

Toxic megacolon is a relatively uncommon complication of colitis but is one of the most life-threatening. Its incidence varies, but it probably affects less than 10% of ulcerative colitis patients. It has also been described in Crohn's disease, pseudo-membranous colitis, ischemia, and infectious colitis (particularly in AIDS patients).

Toxic megacolon occurs when there is severe transmural inflammation extending into the muscularis propria. There is accompanying vasculitis of the arterioles and destruction of the ganglion cells in the myenteric plexuses. Inflammation can extend all the way to the serosa, producing peritoneal inflammation and clinical changes of peritonitis, even without perforation. The bowel wall becomes quite thin because the mucosa and submucosa are often sloughed as a result of the inflammation. An associated loss of muscle tone is caused by the inflammation of the muscle layers and the destruction of ganglion cells. Adding to this problem are the effects of the narcotic drugs and steroids that may be given to the patient for treatment, as well as possible electrolyte disturbances. These problems all lead to an atony of the bowel, with subsequent dilation.

Some authors have stated that a transverse colon exceeding 8 cm is an indication of impending megacolon. The transverse colon usually dilates the most because it is in the least dependent portion of the colon, and air accumulates in it. However, other parts of the colon may be involved as well. It may be better to disregard measurements because a large colon may be present without severe disease, and perforation can occur without significant dilation.

Perforation is the most serious complication, with an associated high mortality rate. Often it is clinically occult because the high-dose steroids used to treat toxic megacolon mask the symptoms of peritonitis, which accompanies the perforation. The diagnosis can be made only on plain abdominal radiographs or CT scans (see figures). Patients who are successfully medically treated for toxic megacolon still do poorly in the future and are often at risk for recurrence or require colectomy at a later date.

Notes

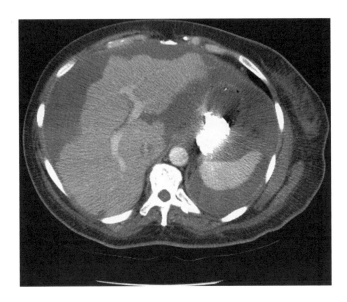

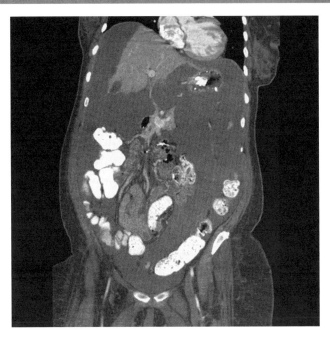

History: A 54-year-old woman presents with abdominal distention.

1. Which of the following should be included in the differential diagnosis of the imaging finding shown in the figures? (Choose all that apply.)
   A. Loculated ascites
   B. Peritoneal tuberculosis
   C. Pseudomyxoma peritonei
   D. Traumatic hemoperitoneum
   E. Subphrenic abscesses

2. What is the original tumor described to cause pseudomyxoma peritonei?
   A. Mucinous gastric tumor
   B. Mucinous ovarian tumor
   C. Mucinous pancreatic tumor
   D. Mucinous appendiceal tumor

3. Which of the following statements regarding pseudomyxoma peritonei is true?
   A. The disease has equal sex distribution.
   B. The most common presentation in women is increasing abdominal girth.
   C. The most common presentation in men is the development of an inguinal hernia.
   D. Disease tends to involve the peritoneal surfaces of the bowel.

4. What is the definitive treatment for pseudomyxoma peritonei?
   A. Chemotherapy
   B. Radiation therapy
   C. Surgical resection
   D. No definitive treatment

Pseudomyxoma Peritonei

1. A, B, and C

2. D

3. B

4. D

References

Levy AD, Shaw JC, Sobin LH: Secondary tumors and tumorlike lesions of the peritoneal cavity: imaging features with pathologic correlation. *Radiographics* 2009;29:347-373.

Yeh HC, Shafir MK, Slater G, et al: Ultrasonography and computed tomography in pseudomyxoma peritonei. *Radiology* 1984;153:507-510.

Cross-Reference

Gastrointestinal Imaging: *THE REQUISITES*, 3rd ed, p 138.

Comment

These CT images demonstrate large collections of low-density material throughout the abdominal cavity, resembling ascites. However, in this instance the material appears loculated or cystic in the lower abdominal cavity. Scalloping of the liver edge also is present. Finally, areas of fine calcification are evident within the peritoneal cavity on some of the images. All these findings make this case atypical for conventional ascites and suggest the possibility of pseudomyxoma peritonei.

Pseudomyxoma peritonei is the presence of gelatinous or mucinous material in the peritoneal cavity. It is produced by the rupture of a mucin-producing neoplasm into the peritoneal cavity. It can be either a malignant process, such as a mucinous adenocarcinoma, or a benign process, such as a mucocele of the appendix. Once the tumor ruptures, the cellular debris continues to produce mucin within the peritoneum, and the process tends to be progressive whether it is the result of a benign or a malignant cause.

In women by far the most common cause of pseudomyxoma peritonei is a mucinous neoplasm of the ovary, typically mucinous cystadenocarcinoma. In men the usual origin of the process is an appendiceal tumor, such as a mucocele of the appendix or a mucinous cystadenocarcinoma. Mucinous cystic tumors of the pancreas also can cause this condition. Mucinous tumors of the stomach, intestines, or bile ducts are even more rare. In this patient the scalloping of the liver and the calcification favor the diagnosis of a malignant mucinous process. Treatment is typically supportive because the material cannot be successfully removed surgically, and the remaining cells within the peritoneum will continue to produce the material.

Notes

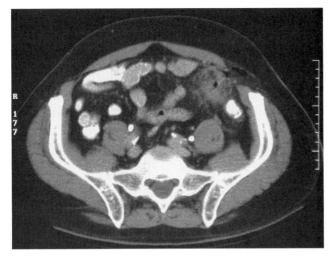

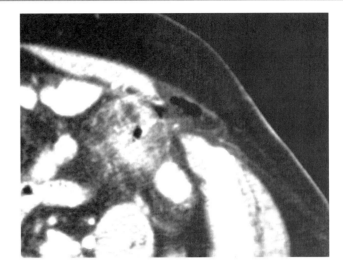

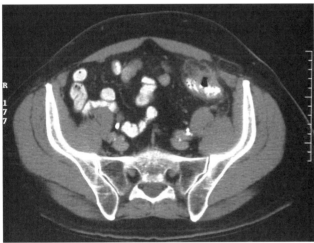

History: A 66-year-old man presents with left flank pain.

1. Which of the following should be included in the differential diagnosis of the imaging finding shown in the figures? (Choose all that apply.)
   A. Spontaneous perforation
   B. Iatrogenic perforation
   C. Pneumatosis coli
   D. Gunshot injury
   E. Stab injury

2. What is the examination of choice in a patient with an abdominal stab injury?
   A. Erect abdominal radiograph
   B. Peritoneal lavage
   C. CT scan
   D. Laparotomy

3. Which of the following statements about abdominal stab injuries is true?
   A. The colon is often involved in stab injuries.
   B. The most commonly injured viscus is the spleen.
   C. Stab injuries are less common than gunshot injuries.
   D. The liver and spleen protect the diaphragm from stab injury.

4. Which of the following statements about abdominal gunshot injuries is true?
   A. The most commonly injured viscus is the spleen.
   B. Gunshot wounds are responsible for most of the fatalities of penetrating abdominal injuries.
   C. Upper abdominal wounds are difficult to evaluate owing to the subtlety of injury to the pancreas.
   D. Flank wounds are difficult to evaluate owing to the subtlety of injury to the ascending and descending colon.

Colonic Trauma: Stab Wound

1. A, B, D, and E

2. C

3. A

4. B

References

Goodman CS, Hur JY, Adajar MA, Coulam CH: How well does CT predict the need for laparotomy in hemodynamically stable patients with penetrating abdominal injury? A review and meta-analysis. *Am J Roentgenol* 2009;193:432-437.

Shanmuganathan K, Mirvis SE, Chiu WC, et al: Penetrating torso trauma: triple-contrast helical CT in peritoneal violation and organ injury—a prospective study in 200 patients. *Radiology* 2004;231:775-784.

Cross-Reference

Gastrointestinal Imaging: *THE REQUISITES,* 3rd ed, p 300.

Comment

CT imaging, especially multidetector CT imaging, is the examination of choice in penetrating abdominal trauma when the patient is hemodynamically stable (see figures). Penetrating wounds are mostly stab wounds and bullet wounds. When the hollow viscus is penetrated, not only blood can be spilled into the peritoneal cavity but also the content of the hollow viscus. Small collections of air or bubbles must be accounted for. If it is determined that the air collections or bubbles are outside the bowel, and there has been no other cause for such a finding (recent surgery or peritoneal lavage), then a breeching injury of the bowel must be presumed. It is possible for bowel to be injured but not necessarily penetrated. This is usually seen as blood in the bowel wall. Some small amount of bleeding into the peritoneal cavity can occur even in this situation. Penetration of the colon will lead to widespread peritonitis, sepsis, and death within a few days. The morbidity and mortality rates for stab wounds depend entirely on how early diagnosis and surgical intervention occur. Penetrating trauma to the abdomen accounts for about 30% of patients in urban trauma centers and less than half that in suburban centers.

Notes

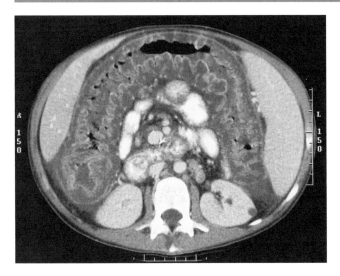 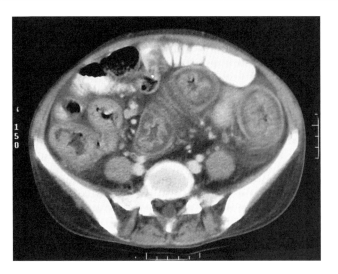

History: A 20-year-old woman presents with several days of watery diarrhea and cramping abdominal pain.

1. Which of the following should be included in the differential diagnosis of the imaging finding shown in the figures? (Choose all that apply.)
   A. Pseudomembranous colitis
   B. Ulcerative colitis
   C. Crohn's disease
   D. Diverticulitis
   E. Viral colitis

2. What is the predisposing factor for the development of pseudomembranous colitis?
   A. Antibiotics
   B. Vasculopathy
   C. Immunocompromise
   D. Recent abdominal surgery

3. What is the treatment for pseudomembranous colitis?
   A. *Clostridium botulinum* antitoxin
   B. Change the antibiotic regimen
   C. Corticosteroids
   D. Colectomy

4. Which of the following statements about the pseudomembranous colitis is true?
   A. The colitis is due to a toxin produced by *Clostridium perfringens*.
   B. 20% or more of patients carry *Clostridium* species without symptoms.
   C. The disease causes a pancolitis from cecum to rectum.
   D. The disease does not extend to the small bowel.

Pseudomembranous Colitis

1. A, B, C, and E

2. A

3. B

4. B

References

Kawamoto S, Horton KM, Fishman EK: Pseudomembranous colitis: spectrum of imaging findings with clinical and pathologic correlation. *Radiographics* 1999;19:887-897.

Ramachandran I, Sinha R, Rodgers P: Pseudomembranous colitis revisited: spectrum of imaging findings. *Clin Radiol* 2006;61:535-544.

Cross-Reference

Gastrointestinal Imaging: THE REQUISITES, 3rd ed, p 313.

Comment

Pseudomembranous colitis is commonly encountered. It actually represents an infection with the bacillus *Clostridium difficile,* although the relationship is variable. *C. difficile* can be found in many healthy patients (20% of the population), in whom it does not produce extensive colonization. Under certain circumstances (e.g., during the course of antibiotic therapy or chemotherapy), an overgrowth of this bacterium can develop, which is why this condition is often called antibiotic-associated colitis. However, many episodes of diarrhea associated with antibiotic use are not caused by *C. difficile* infection; probably only the most severe cases are caused by this bacterium. The relationship is even more difficult to establish in that the onset of symptoms can occur anywhere from a few days to 8 weeks after antibiotics have been initiated, although typically it takes less than 2 weeks.

C. difficile produces several endotoxins, some of which are detectable with laboratory assays. These toxins produce an inflammatory and necrotic change in the mucosa, with subsequent loss of fluid through the wall of the bowel. On sigmoidoscopy there are small raised yellowish plaques, cellular debris, and mucus, hence the term pseudomembranous colitis. The inflammatory process can involve the whole colon, but in a substantial number of patients the rectum is spared or only segments of the colon are involved.

Radiologically, in severe cases the abnormalities may be apparent on plain abdominal images. The findings include thickening of the haustral folds, thickening of the bowel wall, and a shaggy appearance of the mucosa. The changes can mimic ischemia. Barium studies are usually not indicated but show the thickened folds and irregular margins to the barium. Toxic megacolon can occur in patients with this condition. CT is probably the best modality for evaluating severe cases because the thickened bowel is readily apparent and the study does not precipitate any complications (see figures). Treatment is discontinuation of the antibiotics, sometimes use of vancomycin, and supportive therapy.

Notes

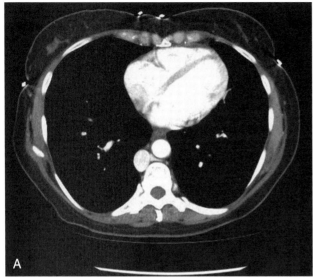

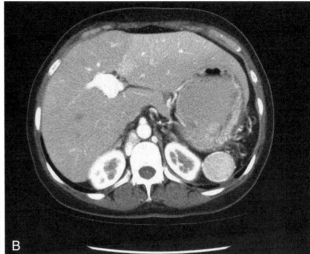

History: A 32-year-old man with an abnormality noted on a routine chest x-ray.

1. Which of the following should be included in the differential diagnosis of the imaging finding shown in Figure A? (Choose all that apply.)
   A. Azygous continuation of the inferior vena cava (IVC)
   B. Congestive heart failure
   C. Obstruction of the IVC
   D. Obstruction of the superior vena cava
   E. Lymphadenopathy

2. What is the physical cause of azygous continuation?
   A. Portal hypertension
   B. Fistula from an artery
   C. Lateral course of the azygous vein in a pleural septum
   D. Occlusion, or failure of development of the IVC

3. Which of the following statements regarding azygous continuation is true?
   A. The diagnosis is recognized on the frontal chest radiograph by the absence of the shadow of the IVC.
   B. Because of the absence of the hepatic segment of the IVC, the hepatic veins drain through collaterals.
   C. Müller's maneuver would cause the enlarged azygous vein to decrease in size.
   D. This can be a congenital anomaly.

4. Which of the following is *not* a clinical significance of azygous continuation?
   A. It may be mistaken for a mediastinal mass.
   B. The patient is at risk for paradoxical embolism.
   C. It is relevant in being able to undertake vascular procedures.
   D. It alerts to the presence of other significant congenital disorders.

Azygous Continuation

1. A, B, C, and D

2. D

3. D

4. B

References

Bass JE, Redwine MD, Kramer LA, et al: Spectrum of congenital anomalies of the inferior vena cava: cross-sectional imaging findings. *Radiographics* 2000;20:639-652.

Kellman GM, Alpern MB, Sandler MA, Craig BM: Computed tomography of vena caval anomalies with embryologic correlation. *Radiology* 1990;8:533-555.

Cross-Reference

Gastrointestinal Imaging: *THE REQUISITES,* 3rd ed, p 183.

Comment

Azygous continuation can be seen in a variety of settings. It can be a congenital failure of the development of the inferior vena cava or it can be chronic disease that slowly occludes the hepatic vein or the IVC over time. Any condition that results in hepatic venous occlusion can result in hepatomegaly and, if chronic, distention of the azygous-hemiazygous system as an alternative collateral route to return venous blood from the lower body to the heart. Such conditions include hepatoma and other indolent neoplasms as well as blood dyscrasias, such as sickle cell anemia and leukemia. In this case, the reason for the unusually large size of the azygous vein is failure of development of the IVC (see figures). Hepatic veins are visible but no IVC is identifiable (see figures). The finding was incidental. Other incidental CT findings in this vein would include duplication of the IVC, persistent cardinal vein, and commonly retroaortic left renal vein.

Notes

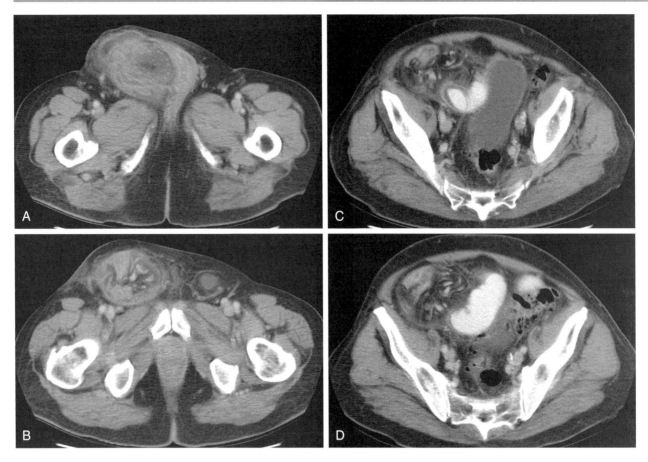

History: A 77-year-old man presents with abdominal pain and distention and vomiting.

1. Which of the following should be included in the differential diagnosis of the imaging finding shown in Figure A? (Choose all that apply.)
   A. Hematoma
   B. Inguinal hernia
   C. Femoral hernia
   D. Scrotal abscess
   E. Testicular tumor

2. Which of the following statements about inguinal herniation is true?
   A. The most common tumor of the inguinal canal is a lipoma.
   B. Littre's hernia is an inguinal hernia containing the vermiform appendix.

C. Inguinal herniation of the ovary typically occurs in post-menopausal women.
D. The most common primary site of metastases to the inguinal canal is melanoma from the skin.

3. What is the most common cause of small bowel obstruction?
   A. Body wall hernia
   B. Colon carcinoma
   C. Small bowel tumor
   D. Fibrous adhesions

4. What is the optimal method for demonstrating mechanical small bowel obstruction?
   A. Plain radiograph
   B. Barium study
   C. Ultrasound
   D. CT

Inguinal Hernia

1. A, B, D, and E

2. A

3. D

4. D

References

Aguirre DA, Santosa AC, Casola G, Sirlin CB: Abdominal wall hernias: imaging features, complications, and diagnostic pitfalls at multi-detector row CT. *Radiographics* 2005;25:1501-1520.

Bhosale PR, Patnana M, Viswanathan C, Szklaruk J: The inguinal canal: anatomy and imaging features of common and uncommon masses. *Radiographics* 2008;28:819-835.

Cross-Reference

Gastrointestinal Imaging: *THE REQUISITES,* 3rd ed, p 314.

Comment

Although the main cause of small bowel obstruction is surgical adhesions, hernias are another important cause, either in the abdominal wall or internally. Inguinal hernias are very common. Only ventral hernias are seen with more frequency. Both can lead to obstructive pathology, with inguinal hernia being more likely to incarcerate and obstruct as well as threaten the bowel's blood supply (strangulated bowel).

For decades, contrast examination of the small bowel, along with plain film radiography, has been the standard for evaluating the patient with suspected obstruction. Enteroclysis or a dedicated small bowel follow-through have been shown to be of benefit, but they are often impractical for the postoperative patient, are time consuming, and are very uncomfortable for patients. Most now advocate the use of CT, which can assess the site of obstruction and possible underlying causes of the problem. It is as sensitive as the other modalities and can be quite specific for determining the cause of the problem, which is most helpful for clinicians (see figures).

Notes

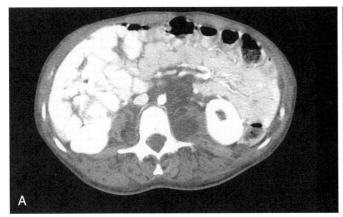

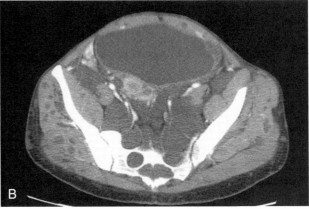

History: A 35-year-old woman with 6 months of vague abdominal discomfort.

1. Which of the following should be included in the differential diagnosis of the imaging finding shown in Figure A? (Choose all that apply.)
   A. Multiple endocrine neoplasia (MEN)
   B. Melanoma metastases
   C. Proteus syndrome
   D. Neurofibromatosis
   E. Polycystic disease

2. What is the hereditary description of neurofibromatosis?
   A. Autosomal dominant
   B. Spontaneous mutation
   C. Autosomal recessive
   D. X-linked

3. What part of the body does neurofibromatosis most commonly affect?
   A. Skin
   B. Gastrointestinal tract
   C. Central nervous system
   D. Musculoskeletal system

4. Which of the following statements regarding neurofibromatosis is true?
   A. Hypertension developing in a patient with neurofibromatosis is usually due to a pheochromocytoma.
   B. Abdominal lesions in neurofibromatosis usually arise in the mesentery.
   C. Most abdominal tumors in neurofibromatosis are leiomyomas.
   D. Barium small bowel series can show malabsorption.

Neurofibromatosis of the Abdomen

1. B, C, and D

2. A

3. A

4. D

References

Hartley N, Rajesh A, Verma R, et al: Abdominal manifestations of neurofibromatosis. *J Comput Assist Tomogr* 2008;32:4-8.

Levy AD, Patel N, Dow N, et al: Abdominal neoplasms in patients with neurofibromatosis type 1: radiologic-pathologic correlation. *Radiographics* 2005;25:455-480.

Cross-Reference

Gastrointestinal Imaging: THE REQUISITES, 3rd ed, p 131.

Comment

Neurofibromatosis is an autosomal dominant disease that can affect multiple organ systems. The best-known area affected is the skin. However, the process can be much more far ranging and dangerous. The disease has been divided into two types, neurofibromatosis type 1 (von Recklinghausen's disease), which accounts for almost 90% of cases, and type 2, which involves the acoustic nerves. Neurofibromatosis type 1 is one of the more common autosomal hereditary disorders (1 in 4000). Involvement of the abdomen and GI tract can be extensive, as seen in this patient (see figures). Tumors may be found within the liver or mesentery as well as in the bowel itself. It can result in GI bleeding, obstruction, or intussusception, chronic abdominal pain, and distention. There is thought to be an increased incidence of adenocarcinoma of the small bowel when the gut is involved.

Notes

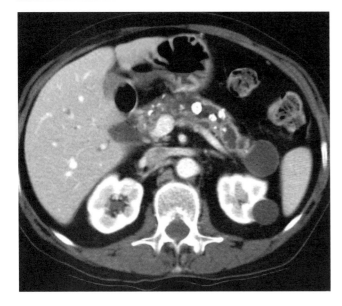

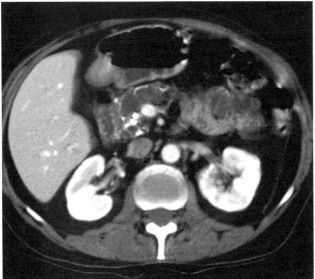

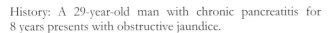

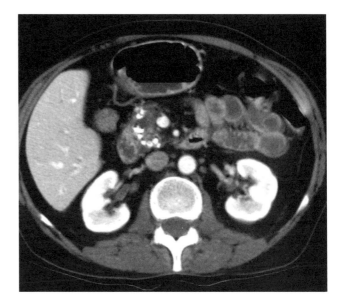

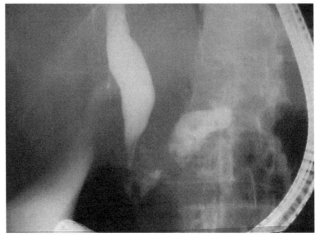

History: A 29-year-old man with chronic pancreatitis for 8 years presents with obstructive jaundice.

1. Which of the following should be included in the differential diagnosis of the imaging finding shown in the figures? (Choose all that apply.)
   A. Choledochal cyst type 1
   B. Chronic pancreatitis stricture
   C. Cancer of the pancreatic head
   D. Calculus impacted at the ampulla
   E. Intraductal papillary mucinous tumor

2. Which of the following statements regarding complications of chronic pancreatitis is true?
   A. The cardinal symptom is abdominal pain.
   B. Malabsorption occurs early in the course of the disease.
   C. Endocrine insufficiency is usually mild, manifesting as non–insulin-dependent diabetes.
   D. With chronic pancreatitis, the significant loss of viable active tissue prevents the recurrence of acute pancreatitis.

3. Which of the following statements regarding investigation of chronic pancreatitis is true?
   A. Glandular calcification is radiographically visible in about 5% of patients.
   B. Serum amylase and lipase levels are in a constant state of mild elevation.
   C. MRI shows generalized increase in glandular signal owing to fatty replacement.
   D. Endoscopic retrograde cholangiopancreatography (ERCP) allows demonstration of diagnostic features and provides access for biliary and pancreatic duct intervention

4. What is the double duct sign?
   A. Dilation of the common bile and pancreatic ducts
   B. Double pancreatic duct due to ectopic pancreatic rest
   C. Endoscopic observation of double ducts draining the pancreas
   D. Sonographic appearance of paired tubular anechoic structures in the liver

Benign Stricture of Chronic Pancreatitis

1. B, C, and D

2. A

3. D

4. A

References

Remer EM, Baker ME: Imaging of chronic pancreatitis. *Radiol Clin North Am* 2002;40:1229-1242.

Robinson PJ, Sheridan MB: Pancreatitis: computed tomography and magnetic resonance imaging. *Eur Radiol* 2000;10:401-440.

Cross-Reference

Gastrointestinal Imaging: *THE REQUISITES,* 3rd ed, p 227.

Comment

Unlike stone formation in the bile duct, pancreatic stones (which usually form in the pancreatic ductal system rather than the acinar tissue) are not a major factor in pancreatic duct obstruction. In cases of benign stricture of the pancreas, the cause is usually chronic pancreatitis (see figures). When the stricture is located directly over the spine and there has been a prior history of blunt trauma to the abdomen, trauma should be included in the etiologic considerations.

Pancreatic strictures present a difficult therapeutic problem. The surgical approach, which includes the Puestow procedure (longitudinal pancreaticojejunostomy) and the Whipple procedure, involves long and highly invasive surgery, especially if there is no demonstrable mass on imaging. In recent years, placement of stents across a benign pancreatic duct has become more common, but there are problems associated with this as well. Although there have been reports of pain relief with stent placement, there is a question of whether a chronically dilated pancreatic duct can provide intrinsic drainage despite surgical intervention or stent placement. Moreover, pancreatic duct stents have an increased incidence of occlusion and are suspected by many investigators of causing chronic pancreatitis by their presence.

Notes

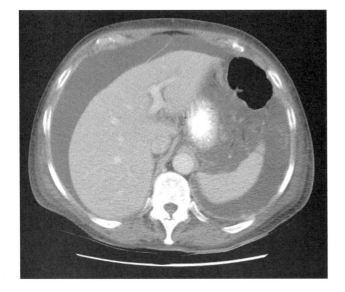

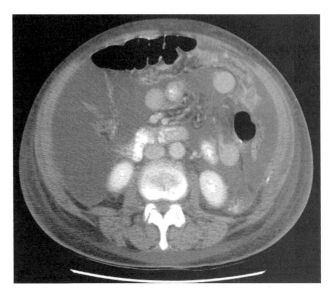

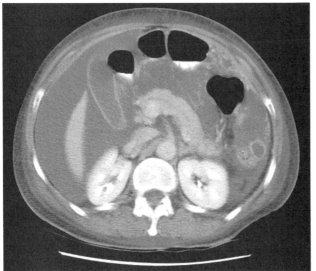

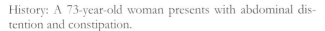

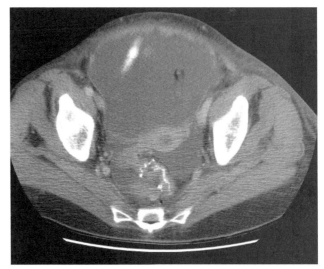

History: A 73-year-old woman presents with abdominal distention and constipation.

1. Which of the following should be included in the differential diagnosis of the imaging finding shown in the figures? (Choose all that apply.)
   A. Pneumoperitoneum
   B. Hemoperitoneum
   C. Carcinomatosis
   D. Dialysis
   E. Ascites

2. What is the most common cause of ascites?
   A. Cirrhosis and severe liver disease
   B. Carcinomatosis peritonei
   C. Cardiac failure
   D. Trauma

3. In the supine patient, what is the lowest, most dependent part of the abdomen?
   A. Rectouterine pouch (pouch of Douglas)
   B. Hepatorenal recess (Morison's pouch)
   C. Subphrenic spaces
   D. Paracolic gutters

4. What is the dog ears imaging sign of ascites?
   A. Ovoid or triangular densities just above and lateral to the urinary bladder on supine abdominal radiography
   B. Medial displacement of the lateral liver edge from the thoracoabdominal wall
   C. Small bowel loops lined up in a polycyclic or arcuate arrangement
   D. Diaphragmatic crus displaced laterally on CT

Mass Effect Displacing Bowel

1. B, C, D, and E

2. A

3. A

4. A

References

Gore RM, Gore MD: Ascites and peritoneal fluid collections. In Gore RM, Levine MS (eds): *Textbook of Gastrointestinal Radiology*, 2nd ed. Philadelphia: WB Saunders, 2000, pp 1969-1979.

Thoeni RF: The role of imaging in patients with ascites. *Am J Roentgenol* 1995;165:16-18.

Cross-Reference

Gastrointestinal Imaging: *THE REQUISITES,* 3rd ed, p 132.

Comment

Bowel can be displaced by a number of processes in the abdomen. Fluid in the peritoneal cavity, ascites, and blood can displace bowel. Large amounts cause air-filled loops of bowel to rise as the fluid level increases (see figures). Because the abdomen is dome-shaped in most of us, when the bowel reaches the top of the dome, it will appear as if the bowel (with air in it) has collected in a circle in the middle of the abdomen. This is called *centralization of bowel loops* and is a wonderful sign for a large amount of fluid in the abdomen on plain films of the abdomen. Lesser degrees of fluid in the abdomen may be suspected when there is separation (more than 2 cm) of the properitoneal fat stripe from air in the ascending or descending colon. A less-specific sign is loss of the inferior margin of the liver. This is usually a fat–soft tissue interface. However, when fluid occupies the Morrison pouch it becomes a soft tissue–soft tissue interface, which is an invisible interface on plain film. This sign does require the patient to have some intraperitoneal fat, and the extremely thin patient may be an exception. Another sign of fluid in the abdomen is fluid in the lateral pelvic recesses, giving the dog ears sign. This is also a soft sign and can be reproduced by fluid in bowel and even loops of collapsed bowel. Mass effect owing to massive enlargement of viscera (e.g., hepatosplenomegaly) or large tumors can also displace bowel loops.

Notes

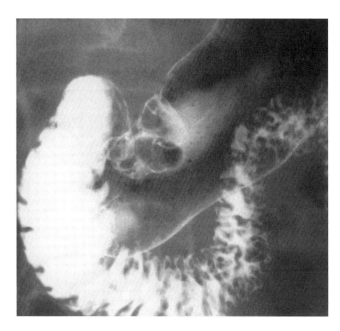 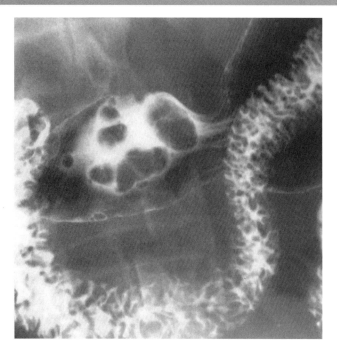

History: A 74-year-old man presents after noticeable darkening of his feces.

1. Which of the following should be included in the differential diagnosis of the imaging finding shown in the figures? (Choose all that apply.)
   A. Hyperplastic polyps
   B. Polyposis syndrome
   C. Metastases
   D. Erosions
   E. Artifact

2. What is the most common type of multiple gastric polyps?
   A. Adenomatous polyps
   B. Hyperplastic polyps
   C. Hamartomas
   D. Metastases

3. With which polyposis syndrome is gastric adenomas associated?
   A. Cowden's
   B. Gardner's
   C. Peutz-Jeghers
   D. Cronkhite-Canada

4. A patient with multiple gastric polyps also manifests circumoral papillomatosis and skeletal malformations. What polyposis syndrome does the patient have?
   A. Cowden's
   B. Gardner's
   C. Peutz-Jeghers
   D. Cronkhite-Canada

Multiple Gastric Polyps

1. A, B, and C

2. B

3. B

4. A

References

Buck JL, Harned RK: Polyposis syndromes. In Gore RM, Levine MS (eds): *Textbook of Gastrointestinal Radiology*, 2nd ed. Philadelphia: WB Saunders, 2000, pp 44-65, 1075-1088.

Feczko PJ, Halpert RD, Ackerman LV: Gastric polyps: radiological evaluation and clinical significance. *Radiology* 1985;155:581-584.

Cross-Reference

Gastrointestinal Imaging: THE REQUISITES, 3rd ed, p 72.

Comment

With the increased use of biphasic upper gastrointestinal examination, it is not uncommon to encounter multiple small polyps within the gastric lumen. These growths are often found throughout the body and in the proximal stomach. For the most part these small polyps are the sequelae of previous inflammation of the stomach and histologically are hyperplastic or inflammatory polyps (see figures). On occasion, they are due to metastases, and rarely they indicate the presence of a polyposis syndrome of the gastrointestinal tract.

Almost all polyposis syndromes can cause polyps to develop in the stomach. Patients with familial polyposis (or Gardner's syndrome) have a high incidence of gastric polyps. Unlike their adenomatous counterparts in the colon, gastric polyps can be either adenomatous or hyperplastic. Patients with Peutz-Jeghers syndrome develop hamartomatous lesions in the stomach with no malignant potential. Juvenile polyps also are hamartomas and can occur sporadically or as part of a diffuse juvenile polyposis syndrome.

Cronkhite-Canada syndrome is a nonfamilial polyposis syndrome. It is associated with a group of skin abnormalities, including alopecia, onychodystrophy, and hyperpigmentation. Clinically these patients also have weight loss and depletion of protein and electrolytes. It is this last group of symptoms that may be life threatening. The condition usually occurs in middle-aged patients and sometimes in the elderly. Patients with Peutz-Jeghers syndrome develop hamartomatous lesions in the stomach with no malignant potential. Juvenile polyps also are hamartomas and can occur sporadically or as part of a diffuse juvenile polyposis syndrome. The polyps are inflammatory or hamartomatous and have no malignant potential. Typically the growths are quite small. Cowden's disease is a rare cause of hamartomatous polyps in the stomach; this disorder is hereditary and results in formation of diffuse hamartomatous and ectodermal abnormalities throughout the body.

Occasionally one encounters what appear to be multiple small beadlike polyps lined up on folds in the body and antrum of the stomach. Erosions occurring in the stomach evoke an edematous response around the erosions that are sometimes mistaken for multiple small polyps. Careful barium coating of the stomach often shows the erosion (a tiny barium collection) on a raised edematous mound.

Notes

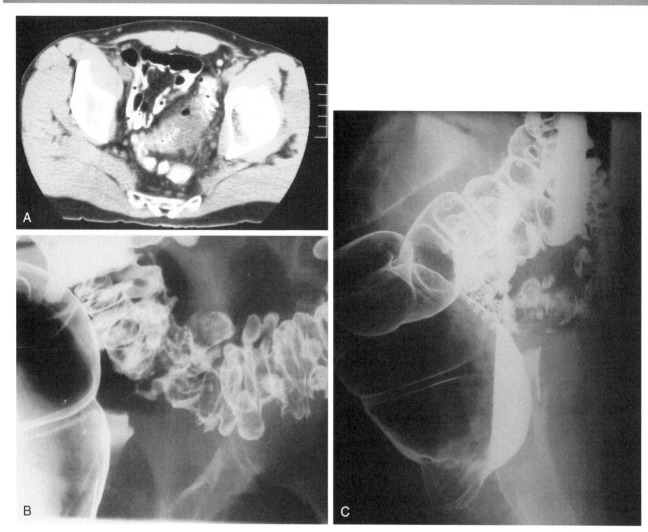

History: A 63-year-old woman presents with perineal soiling.

1. Which of the following should be included in the differential diagnosis of the imaging finding shown in Figure A? (Choose all that apply.)
   A. Colonic mass
   B. Diverticular disease
   C. Extrinsic mass
   D. Inflammatory bowel disease
   E. Within normal limits

2. Where is the fistula shown in figures 2 and 3 extending to?
   A. Small bowel
   B. Peritoneum
   C. Nowhere
   D. Bladder
   E. Vagina

3. Which statement about colonic fistulas to the urogenital tract is true?
   A. The most common fistula site is colovaginal.
   B. The fistula is usually directly visualized on CT.
   C. Sigmoidoscopy usually shows the fistula.
   D. The most common cause is colonic diverticulitis.
   E. Colovesical fistulas occur more commonly in female patients.

4. What is the worldwide most common cause of rectovaginal fistulas?
   A. Trauma
   B. Surgery
   C. Infection
   D. Radiotherapy
   E. Crohn's disease

Colovaginal Fistula

1. A, B, and D

2. E

3. D

4. A

References

Cho KC, Morehouse HT, Alterman DD, Thornhill BA: Sigmoid diverticulitis: diagnostic role of CT. Comparison with barium enema studies. *Radiology* 1990;176:111-115.

Pickhardt PJ, Bhalla S, Balfe DM: Acquired gastrointestinal fistulae: classification, etiologies, and imaging evaluation. *Radiology* 2002;224:9-23.

Cross-Reference

Gastrointestinal Imaging: *THE REQUISITES,* 3rd ed, p 303.

Comment

A fistula is defined as an abnormal tract extending from one mucosa-lined organ into the mucosal surface of another organ. The possible types include enteroenteric (between two loops of bowel), enterovesical (bowel to bladder), enterovaginal, and enterocutaneous, among others. A sinus is also a tract communicating with bowel, but it ends blindly or in a cavity that is not normally lined with mucosa.

In the colon, diverticulitis is the most common cause of fistulas in industrialized society, such as seen in this case; figures 2 and 3 show a tract developing from inflamed sigmoid colon directing toward the vagina. Other inflammatory conditions also lead to the formation of numerous fistulas. Crohn's disease is a relatively common and well-known cause of fistula formation in the gastrointestinal tract. Fistula formation occurs between adjacent loops of bowel, as well as with other structures. Some infections that can produce fistulas are tuberculosis and actinomycosis. This chronic inflammatory process ulcerates and produces a variety of unusual fistulas. Fistulas can form as a complication of surgery, typically at an anastomotic site that dehisces. Malignancy can also result in fistulous formation, especially if it is fairly extensive or is already being treated (leading to necrosis) before the fistula occurs. Radiation is a well-known cause of fistula development; this complication results from microvascular ischemic changes and fibrosis and matting together of organs.

Fluoroscopic studies (cystogram, contrast enema, small bowel study, even vaginogram) are valuable for confirming and defining the anomalous communication. Evaluation of fistulas can be quite difficult. Often, contrast material travels in only one direction through a fistula. Also, the fistula must be open at the time of the study, or it cannot be demonstrated. CT and MRI are good modalities for revealing the presence of the underlying condition leading to the fistula (see figures).

Notes

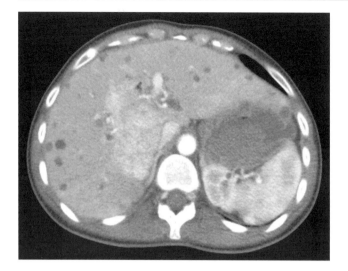

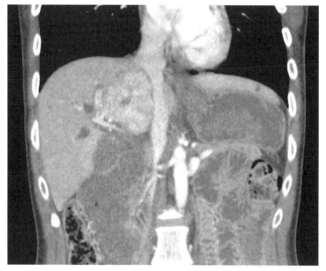

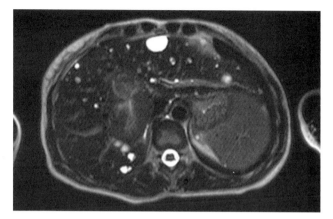

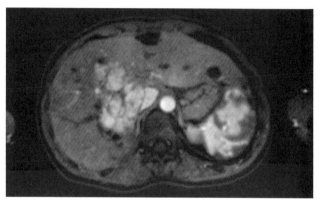

History: A 32-year-old woman presents with chest pain.

1. Which of the following should be included in the differential diagnosis of the imaging finding shown in the figures? (Choose all that apply.)
   A. Hepatoma
   B. Hemangioma
   C. Hydatid abscess
   D. Hepatic adenoma
   E. Focal nodular hyperplasia

2. Why do focal nodular hyperplasia (FNH) lesions take up sulfur colloid?
   A. The lesion contains hepatocytes.
   B. The lesion contains Kupffer cells.
   C. The lesion contains blood pools.
   D. The lesion is hypervascular.

3. In what demographic group is FNH most commonly seen?
   A. Children
   B. Young women
   C. Middle-aged men
   D. Chronic liver disease

4. What is the vascular supply usually serving FNH?
   A. Peripheral
   B. Central
   C. Portal
   D. None

Focal Nodular Hyperplasia

1. A, B, D, and E

2. B

3. B

4. B

References

Brancatelli G, Federle MP, Grazioli L, et al: Focal nodular hyperplasia: CT findings with emphasis on multiphasic helical CT in 78 patients. *Radiology* 2001;219:61-68.

Silva AC, Evans JM, McCullough AE, et al: MR imaging of hyper-vascular liver masses: a review of current techniques. *Radiographics* 2009;29:385-402.

Cross-Reference

Gastrointestinal Imaging: *THE REQUISITES,* 3rd ed, p 198.

Comment

Focal nodular hyperplasia (FNH) of the liver is the second most common benign tumor of the liver after hemangiomas. The tumor is a hyperplasia of normal, non-neoplastic liver tissue that has an abnormal arrangement and is similar to a hamartomatous type of lesion. It is believed to develop as some type of response to a congenital vascular abnormality in the region, and there is a slight association between hemangiomas and FNH. Histologically, the liver tissue is arranged in small nodules, with septa in between. Arterial vessels feed the nodules from a centrally located artery that is often within a central scar or septum. They do not have a portal venous supply. FNH contains Kupffer cells in most instances.

Adenomas and FNH are similar in that they both occur in young women, although FNH also occurs in children and older patients. Unlike adenomas, FNH is not associated with use of oral contraceptives. This tumor is rarely found in men. FNH must be differentiated from other hepatic tumors, such as adenomas, fibrolamellar hepatomas, and giant cavernous hemangiomas. All these tumors are large vascular tumors that affect young women and often have a central scar.

Focal nodular hyperplasia is sometimes detected on ultrasound as a well-defined lesion with echogenicity different from that of the normal liver. A large central vessel may be detectable on Doppler scanning. On CT scanning, the lesion's density may be similar to that of the liver and therefore may be difficult to distinguish from the normal liver parenchyma (see figures). A central scar or low-density area may be visible (see figures).

Because of the functional reticuloendothelial cells, FNH may be detectable on sulfur colloid scanning as an area of increased uptake. On MRI, FNH is only slightly hyperintense on T2-weighted images, but the central scar may be markedly hyperintense (see figures).

Notes

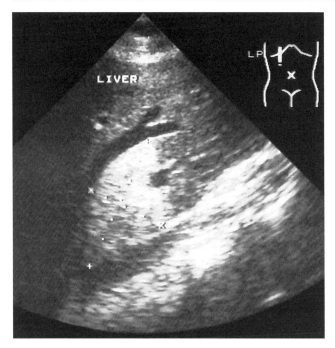

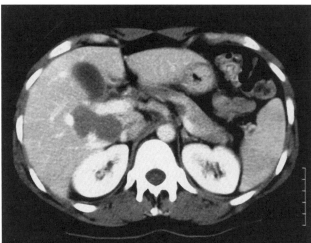

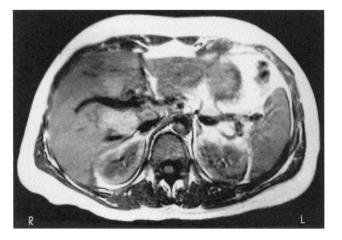

History: A 36-year-old woman presents with 8-month history of nocturnal upper abdominal pain.

1. Which of the following should be included in the differential diagnosis of the imaging finding shown in the figures? (Choose all that apply.)
   A. Hepatic adenoma
   B. Hydatid abscess
   C. Hemangioma
   D. Hepatic cyst
   E. Lipoma

2. Which of the following predisposes to the development of hepatic adenoma?
   A. Hepatic cirrhosis
   B. Iron storage disorder
   C. Use of catabolic steroids
   D. Use of oral contraceptives

3. How does a hepatic adenoma appear on a sulfur colloid liver scan?
   A. Cold photopenic defect
   B. Hot spot, increased uptake
   C. Isointense uptake to normal liver
   D. Uptake with gallbladder accumulation

4. What is the most common clinical presentation of a hepatic adenoma?
   A. Incidental imaging finding
   B. Abdominal pain
   C. Acute abdomen
   D. Palpable mass

Hepatic Adenoma

1. A, B, C, and E

2. D

3. A

4. B

References

Grazioli L, Federle MP, Brancatelli G, et al: Hepatic adenomas: imaging and pathologic findings. *Radiographics* 2001;21:877-892.
Silva AC, Evans JM, McCullough AE, et al: MR imaging of hyper-vascular liver masses: a review of current techniques. *Radiographics* 2009;29:385-402.

Cross-Reference

Gastrointestinal Imaging: *THE REQUISITES*, 3rd ed, p 196.

Comment

Hepatic adenomas are composed of hepatocytes that are loosely arranged, have no portal tracts, and have poorly formed hepatic veins. They form bile to a slight extent. These tumors tend to be large and solitary, often exceeding 10 cm in diameter. They are also quite vascular and because of their poorly developed venous system have a propensity for spontaneous hemorrhage, which is the major clinical presentation. Usually the hemorrhage is internal within the adenoma, and liver produces pain by hepatic capsular distention, such as in this case, but if the hemorrhage spreads into the peritoneal cavity, it could be fatal.

Adenomas occur predominantly in women, usually younger women. They are believed to be estrogen-associated tumors, and their incidence is increased in women taking oral contraceptives. Cessation of oral contraceptive use causes the tumors to shrink. Rarely the tumor occurs spontaneously in men. Men taking anabolic steroids are at increased risk for developing a tumor that is similar to both an adenoma and a hepatocellular carcinoma. Patients with glycogen storage disease also are at greater risk for developing adenomas.

Hepatic adenomas are usually easily identifiable on cross-sectional imaging, but their differentiation from other hepatic tumors is the major concern. Ultrasound typically reveals a large hyperechoic lesion (see figure), which can have central areas of low density caused by hemorrhage or necrosis. On CT the lesion may be hypodense because of glycogen, which is often within the tumor (see figure). After contrast material is injected, the tumor enhances and can become isodense. At the periphery of the tumor are large vessels, which are feeding vessels for the tumor. This finding is apparent on angiography; large peripheral arteries can be seen draped around the tumor and feeding into the center of the mass. Adenomas are visible as cold defects on sulfur colloid scans; this point is important in differentiating the tumor from focal nodular hyperplasia, which appears "hot" on sulfur colloid scan. On MRI, adenomas may be hyperintense on T1-weighted images because of the presence of glycogen and fat in the tumors (see figure).

Notes

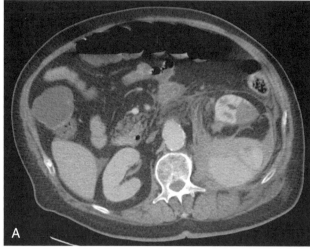

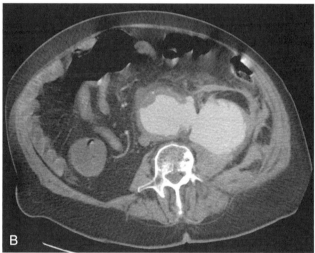

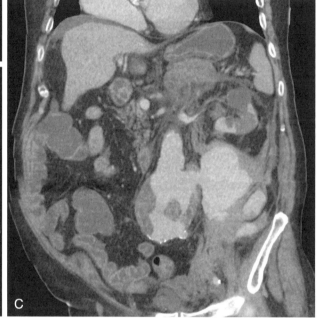

History: A 76-year-old man presents with left flank pain.

1. Which of the following should be included in the differential diagnosis of the imaging finding shown in Figure A? (Choose all that apply.)
   A. Abscess
   B. Hemorrhage
   C. Pseudocyst
   D. Neoplasia
   E. Urinoma

2. Which of the following statements regarding aortic aneurysm is true?
   A. Male and female patients are equally affected.
   B. It is most commonly located just above the bifurcation.
   C. Smoking is the major risk factor for aneurysm formation.
   D. Aneurysm is defined as aortic dilation more than 2 cm diameter.

3. What is the most common clinical presentation of a patient with an abdominal aortic aneurysm?
   A. Imaging finding
   B. Back pain
   C. Collapse
   D. Mass

4. What is the preferred imaging modality for screening for aortic aneurysm?
   A. Plain radiography
   B. Ultrasound
   C. MRI
   D. CT

CASE 94

Abdominal Aortic Aneurysm

1. A, B, and D

2. C

3. A

4. B

References

LaRoy LL, Cormier PJ, Matalon TA, et al: Imaging of abdominal aortic aneurysms. *Am J Roentgenol* 1989;152:785-792.

Sparks AR, Johnson PL, Meyer MC: Imaging of abdominal aortic aneurysms. *Am Fam Physician* 2002;65(8):1565-1570.

Cross-Reference

Gastrointestinal Imaging: THE REQUISITES, 3rd ed, p 138.

Comment

Abdominal aneurysms are relatively common in elderly patients. Whites are more likely to have it and men are affected seven times more often than women. The aorta comprises three layers: intima, media, and adventitia. Abdominal aortic aneurysms (AAAs) occur over long periods of time during which medial degeneration takes place, resulting in a gradual dilation of the vessel.

However, not all AAAs are caused by degenerative disease. In a small percentage of cases (3% to 5%), the mycotic aneurysm results from the hematogenous spread of bacteria. Most AAAs are fusiform in shape and are located below the renal arteries and the bifurcation. Some extend into the iliac vessels.

Most AAAs are asymptomatic until they suddenly expand, leak, rupture, or compromise renal or enteric vessels. Almost two thirds of patients with sudden rupture die from rapid cardiovascular collapse before reaching the hospital. CT usually reveals a large dilated abdominal aorta with varying degrees of intramural thrombus. Care should be taken to evaluate for dissection, blood leakage, and quality of kidney and bowel perfusion. Pain associated with AAA can be misdiagnosed, because the classic presentation of tachycardia, hypotension, and a pulsatile mass on physical diagnosis is, as most classical presentations, not the most common. Often these patients present with flank pain and kidney stones. multidetector CT protocols are performed looking for the offending calculi. In the event of an elderly patient presenting with flank pain with no obvious urologic source, with or without an AAA, the possibility of dissection should not be overlooked.

Uncommon causes of AAA include Marfan's syndrome and Ehlers-Danlos disease.

Notes

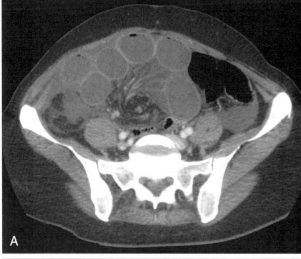

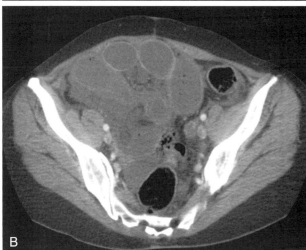

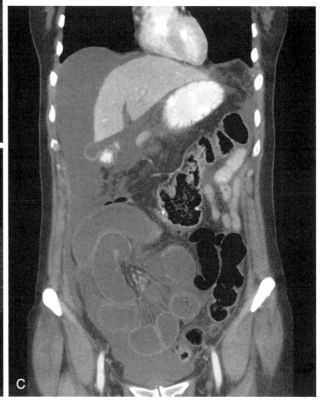

History: A 60-year-old woman presents with 6 hours of abdominal pain. History includes bowel resection for angiodysplasia and more recent laparotomy for division of adhesions.

1. Which of the following should be included in the differential diagnosis of the imaging finding shown in Figure A? (Choose all that apply.)
   A. Large bowel obstruction
   B. Small bowel obstruction
   C. Adynamic ileus
   D. Gastroparesis
   E. Enteritis

2. What is the origin of the gas in dilated bowel in a patient with obstruction?
   A. Swallowed air
   B. Bacterial production
   C. Outgassing of dissolved gases
   D. By-product of digestion of food

3. Strangulation is closed-loop obstruction with intestinal ischemia. Which finding on CT is most diagnostic of this complication?
   A. Ascites
   B. Halo sign
   C. Whirl sign
   D. Abnormal enhancement

4. What is the optimal modality for investigating acute small bowel dilatation?
   A. Plain radiography
   B. Enteroclysis
   C. Ultrasound
   D. CT

Dilated Small Bowel

1. A, B, and C

2. A

3. D

4. D

References

Maglinte DD, Kelvin FM, Rowe MG, et al: Small bowel obstruction: optimizing radiologic investigation and nonsurgical management. *Radiology* 2001;218:39-46.

Silva AC, Pimenta M, Guimaraes LS: Small bowel obstruction: what to look for. *Radiographics* 2009;29:423-439.

Cross-Reference

Gastrointestinal Imaging: *THE REQUISITES,* 3rd ed, p 106.

Comment

One of the problems most commonly evaluated by the radiologist (and surgeon) is dilated loops of small bowel. This evaluation is particularly difficult in the patient who develops distention after a surgical procedure. The main differential diagnostic concern is whether a true mechanical obstruction has developed or whether the bowel dilation is secondary to an adynamic ileus.

Most mechanical obstructions occur as the result of fibrous adhesions, which develop within days after surgery. However, mechanical obstruction within the first few days after abdominal surgery is quite rare. Usually it takes months or years before obstructions from adhesions become symptomatic (if they become symptomatic). When they are symptomatic, most are treated successfully with nasogastric decompression. The CT images in this case show high-grade small bowel obstruction (see figures). At surgery, a closed-loop obstruction of the distal and terminal ileum was found, including a 20-cm segment of ischemic nonviable bowel.

In the postoperative patient, the radiologist should be wary of diagnosing a mechanical obstruction when the colon is dilated up to the level of the anatomic splenic flexure (the point where the descending colon passes behind the phrenicocolic ligament and becomes retroperitoneal). Spasm at that site is relatively common in patients immediately following abdominal surgery, and the radiologist should consider this before deciding it is a mechanical obstruction.

Other causes of grossly dilated small bowel include hernias, either in the abdominal wall or internally. Fibrous bands also can lead to volvulus or closed-loop obstructions. For decades, contrast examination of the small bowel, along with plain film radiography, had been the standard for evaluation of the patient with suspected obstruction. Enteroclysis has been shown to be of somewhat greater benefit but is impractical for the postoperative patient. Today the use of CT has become standard. This modality can assess the site of obstruction and possible underlying causes of the problem. It is as sensitive as the other modalities and can be quite specific for determining the cause of the problem and identifying complications, which is most helpful for clinicians.

Notes

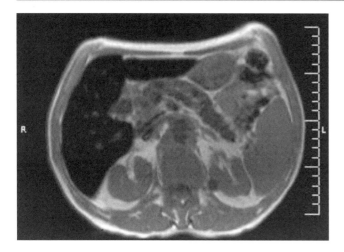

History: A 46-year-old man is undergoing investigations for an abnormal heartbeat.

1. Which of the following should be included in the differential diagnosis of the imaging finding shown in the figure? (Choose all that apply.)
   A. Amiodarone
   B. Wilson's disease
   C. Hemosiderosis
   D. Hemochromatosis
   E. Therapeutic gold

2. Which of the following statements regarding primary hemochromatosis is true?
   A. Disease more commonly affects male patients.
   B. Inheritance is X-linked recessive.
   C. Iron deposition is visible on imaging in the liver and spleen.
   D. Severity of diabetes is related to the severity of pancreatic iron deposition and therefore signal loss.

3. What is the gold standard for the measurement of the iron deposition in the liver?
   A. Serum ferritin
   B. Biopsy
   C. CT density
   D. MR signal

4. What is the most serious complication of hemochromatosis?
   A. Arthropathy
   B. Hormonal changes
   C. Cirrhosis
   D. Diabetes

Hemochromatosis

1. C and D

2. A

3. B

4. C

References

Gandon Y, Guyader D, Heautot JF, et al: Hemochromatosis: diagnosis and quantification of liver iron with gradient-echo MR imaging. *Radiology* 1994;193:533-538.

Queiroz-Andrade M, Blasbalg R, Ortega CD, et al: MR imaging findings of iron overload. *Radiographics* 2009;29:1575-1589.

Cross-Reference

Gastrointestinal Imaging: THE REQUISITES, 3rd ed, p 207.

Comment

Hemochromatosis is an inherited disorder of increased iron absorption from dietary food sources, which over time leads to overload of iron deposition in different sites within the body. This iron deposition leads to cirrhosis, insulin-dependent diabetes, arthropathy, and cardiac problems. In hereditary or primary hemochromatosis, the liver is the main organ of iron deposition initially. Hemosiderosis or secondary hemochromatosis can develop in patients who receive multiple blood transfusions over time. Other causes of increased iron body stores can be from thalassemia with increased demand for iron in the bone marrow secondary to ineffective erythropoiesis and also hemolytic anemias.

Bantu siderosis is a condition found in parts of Africa resulting from abnormal iron deposition in the liver. It is most commonly found in those with an increased predisposition for iron absorption and a thirst for homemade beer. This beer, brewed locally, contains a large amount of iron.

Iron deposition can be detected and quantified by MRI. Iron results in signal loss, particularly on T2-weighted sequences (long TE), including gradient echoes, which are the best sequence for assessing iron (see figure).

Hemochromatosis and hemosiderosis cause the liver to increase in density owing to the accumulation and metabolism of iron in the liver. Hemochromatosis is a primary disorder of iron metabolism. Hemosiderosis occurs in a patient who has received multiple blood transfusions or has had a high turnover of blood, such as with hemolytic anemia.

Relative density on an unenhanced CT scan of the liver should raise the question of the use of the antiarrhythmic drug amiodarone. This drug causes the liver to increase in density owing to its accumulation and metabolism in the liver and the fact that amiodarone contains iodine. Increased liver density may be common inpatients taking this useful medication, but actual hepatotoxicity is uncommon.

Other considerations for a high-density liver include Wilson's disease, a disease of copper metabolism; malfunction is rare but can result in a dense liver. Older patients who received Thorotrast in the 1960s and who are still alive (there are very few today) have increased density of liver and spleen. Patients treated with intramuscular gold for rheumatoid arthritis might have such a finding as well as those with some of the glycogen storage diseases.

Notes

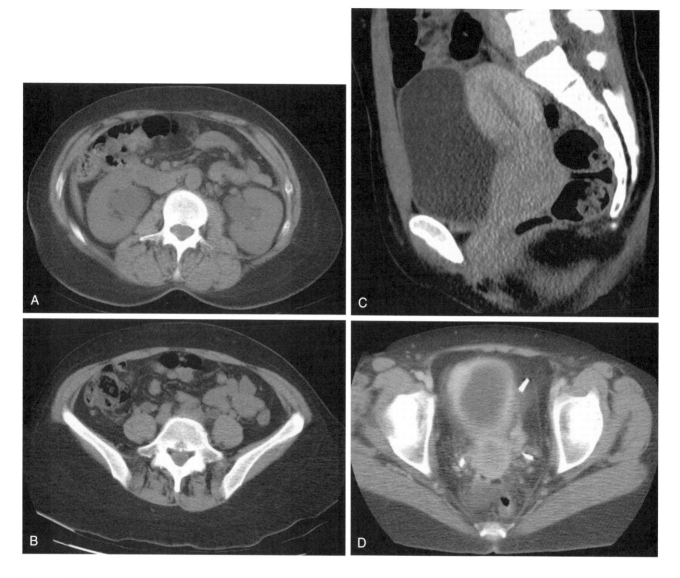

History: A 54-year-old woman presents with lower abdominal pain.

1. Which of the following should be included in the differential diagnosis of the imaging finding shown in Figures A and B? (Choose all that apply.)
   A. Pelvic tumor
   B. Bladder tumor
   C. Prostatomegaly
   D. Vesicoureteric reflux
   E. Retroperitoneal fibrosis

2. Which of the following statements regarding clinical aspects of cervical carcinoma is true?
   A. It is a disease of postmenopausal women.
   B. Papillomavirus exposure is a risk factor.
   C. Common symptoms are abdominal distention and constipation.
   D. It commonly involves the adjacent bladder, producing urinary symptoms.

3. Which of the following statements about the spread of cervical carcinoma is true?
   A. The close relationship of the rectum allows invasion from cervical cancer early in the disease.
   B. Early spread of cervical carcinoma is usually anterior to the bladder.
   C. Hematogenous spread usually occurs first to the vertebral column.
   D. Lymph node status is the most important prognostic factor.

4. What is the optimal imaging modality for the local evaluation of cervical carcinoma?
   A. Hysterosalpingography
   B. Ultrasound
   C. CT
   D. MRI

CASE 97

Cervical Carcinoma with Ureteral Obstruction

1. A, B, D, and E

2. B

3. D

4. D

References

Dahnert W. *Radiology Review Manual*, 6th ed. Philadelphia: Lippincott Williams & Wilkins, 2007, pp 1031-1033.

Fielding JR: MR imaging of the female pelvis. *Radiol Clin North Am* 2003;41:179-192.

Cross-Reference

Genitourinary Radiology: *THE REQUISITES,* 2nd ed, pp 305-309.

Comment

Cervical carcinoma is a disease of younger women compared with ovarian carcinoma, which usually affects middle-aged and older women. The most important risk factor is exposure to specific subtypes of the human papillomavirus (HPV). Other risk factors include early age at first intercourse, multiple sexual partners, high-risk male sexual partners, and low socioeconomic status.

Cervical carcinoma usually extends by contiguous spread laterally to the parametrium and to the vagina. Fascial planes delay its spread to adjacent gut (rectum) or bladder; these occur late in the course of the disease. Lymph node assessment is an important role of staging imaging because the state of the lymph nodes is a major prognostic factor. The 5-year survival rates are estimated to be 90% for node-negative disease and 55% for node-positive disease.

Endovaginal and endorectal ultrasonography play a limited role in the imaging of cervical cancer. Cervical cancer is isoechoic to normal cervical tissue; cervical enlargement may be the only sign of the presence of malignancy. Ultrasound can demonstrate uterine or urinary obstruction. CT lacks the contrast resolution to stage low-volume disease. CT is preferred for advanced disease. The superior contrast resolution of MRI makes it an ideal modality for evaluating cervical carcinoma. Cervical carcinoma is identified as a high signal intensity mass on T2-weighted images. This is in stark contrast to the low signal of normal cervical stroma.

Notes

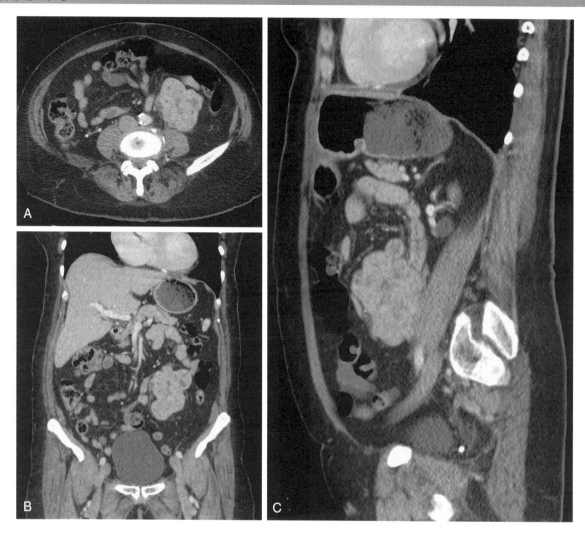

History: An 82-year-old woman presents with right flank pain and suspected renal colic.

1. Which of the following should be included in the differential diagnosis of the imaging finding shown in Figure A? (Choose all that apply.)
   A. Internal hernia
   B. Small bowel tumor
   C. Retroperitoneal cyst
   D. Asymptomatic and can be ignored
   E. Retroperitoneal or mesenteric mass

2. What is the most common incidental finding of *moderate* importance on CT?
   A. Renal cyst
   B. Gallstones
   C. Hiatal hernia
   D. Lymphadenopathy

3. In which viscus is the finding of an incidental lesion containing fat most commonly found?
   A. Colon
   B. Ovary
   C. Kidney
   D. Adrenal

4. Which of the following incidental findings should *not* be ignored?
   A. Bosniak 3 renal cyst
   B. Adrenal nodule with washout
   C. Liver lesion with nodular enhancement
   D. Vertebral body lucency with polka-dot sclerotic foci

Incidental Finding

1. A, B, and E

2. B

3. D

4. A

References

Berland LL, Silverman SG, Gore RM, et al: Managing incidental findings on abdominal CT: white paper of the ACR incidental findings committee. *J Am Coll Radiol* 2010;7:754-773.

Hellstrom M, Svensson MH, Lasson A: Extracolonic and incidental findings on CT colonography (virtual colonoscopy). *Am J Roentgenol* 2004;182:631-638.

Cross-Reference

Gastrointestinal Imaging: *THE REQUISITES,* 3rd ed, p 138.

Comment

This patient presented with symptoms suggesting right renal colic. A low-dose CT scan without contrast enhancement was performed to evaluate for renal tract calculi and obstruction. An unusual appearance was observed by the radiologist on the left asymptomatic side. This then led to the standard contrast-enhanced CT scan presented here (see figures). The patient eventually went to surgery for resection of the mass, which was diagnosed histologically as a retroperitoneal leiomyosarcoma.

Improvements in imaging, especially CT, have seen an increase in the incidence of detecting incidental findings. Sometimes given the name *incidentalomas,* they are defined as findings that are unrelated to the clinical indication for the imaging examination performed. Most of these incidental findings are benign and have little or no clinical significance, but a small but significant proportion are serious. A careful decision needs to be made between performing appropriate further investigation and follow-up versus considered reassurance. Subjecting a patient with an incidentaloma to unnecessary testing and treatment can result in a potentially injurious and expensive cascade of tests and procedures.

Notes

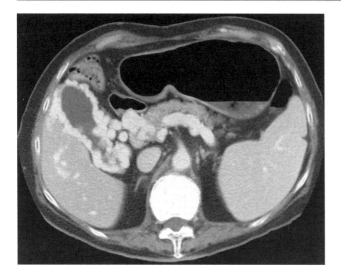

History: A 38-year-old man presents with abdominal distention.

1. Which of the following should be included in the differential diagnosis of the imaging finding shown in the figure? (Choose all that apply.)
   A. Adherent calculi
   B. Biliary sludge
   C. Porcelain gallbladder
   D. Gallbladder varices
   E. Emphysematous cholecystitis

2. What is the most likely underlying condition resulting in this abnormality?
   A. Alcoholic cirrhosis
   B. Schistosomiasis
   C. Chronic viral hepatitis
   D. Congenital hepatic fibrosis

3. Why is this finding important for future reference?
   A. Surgery
   B. Cholecystitis
   C. Carcinoma
   D. Perforation

4. What is the name given to a chronically occluded portal vein?
   A. Cavernous transformation
   B. Caput medusa
   C. Coronary vein
   D. Uphill varices

Gallbladder Varices

1. A, C, and D

2. A

3. A

4. A

References

Chawla Y, Dilawari JB, Katariya S: Gallbladder varices in portal vein thrombosis. *Am J Roentgenol* 1994;162:643-645.
West MS, Garra BS, Horii SC, et al: Gallbladder varices: imaging findings in patients with portal hypertension. *Radiology* 1991;179:179-182.

Cross-Reference

Gastrointestinal Imaging: *THE REQUISITES,* 3rd ed, p 211.

Comment

Gallbladder varices are a rare finding in patients with portal hypertension. In the West, the most common cause of portal hypertension is alcoholic cirrhosis of the liver. Fewer patients develop cirrhosis and portal hypertension as a result of portal or splenic vein thrombosis, parasitic infection involving the portal system (schistosomiasis), chronic hepatitis or liver injury secondary to hypervitaminosis A, congenital diseases such as congenital absence of portal vein or congenital hepatic fibrosis, and a host of relatively uncommon prehepatic, hepatic, and posthepatic causes. All these conditions can result in either occlusion or increased pressures in the portal vein, causing collateralization of veins in the splenic circulation. Although the incidence of varices in portal hypertension secondary to hepatic cirrhosis is high (up to 75% to 80%), the most common manifestation is distention of the coronary veins that ascend to the gastroesophageal junction and give rise to uphill varices. Other manifestations of varices are dilated veins in the abdominal wall around the umbilicus (caput medusa sign) and splenorenal shunting. Duplex Doppler ultrasound can gauge the flow in the portal vein, collateralization, and the texture of the liver. CT in patients who are able to have IV contrast material is an excellent way to demonstrate collateralizations without flow quantification, such as obtained in ultrasound, and to evaluate the liver (see figure).

Notes

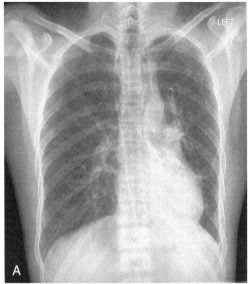

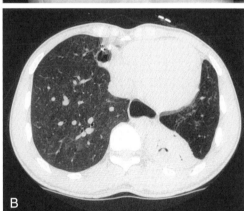

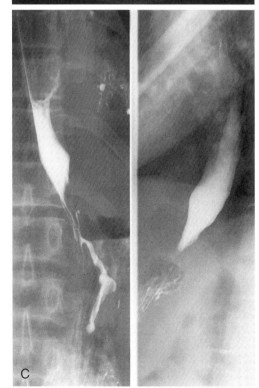

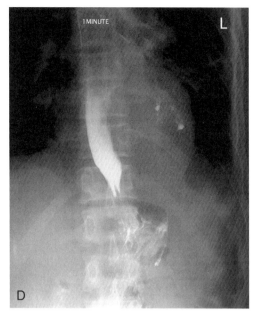

History: A 24-year-old man presents with recurrent episodes of pneumonia.

1. Which of the following should be included in the differential diagnosis of the imaging finding shown in Figures A and B? (Choose all that apply.)
   A. Epidermolysis bullosa dystrophica
   B. Gastroesophageal reflux disease
   C. Distal esophageal obstruction
   D. Esophageal motility disorder
   E. Esophageal varices

2. What is the etiologic basis for primary achalasia?
   A. Cancer
   B. Infection
   C. Idiopathic
   D. Connective tissue disease

3. What radiographic finding on barium swallow is most commonly seen and useful to differentiate secondary achalasia due to malignancy from primary achalasia?
   A. Narrowed segment nodularity
   B. Narrowed segment length
   C. Proximal shouldering
   D. Gastric cardia mass

4. What is the most common etiology of secondary achalasia?
   A. Cancer
   B. Infection
   C. Idiopathic
   D. Connective tissue disease

C A S E 1 0 0

Achalasia

1. B, C, and D

2. C

3. B

4. A

References

Ott DJ. Motility disorders of the esophagus:In Gore RM, Levine MS, (eds): *Textbook of Gastrointestinal Radiology*, 2nd ed. Philadelphia: WB Saunders, 2000, pp 316-328.

Woodfield CA, Levine MS, Rubesin SE, et al: Diagnosis of primary versus secondary achalasia: reassessment of clinical and radiographic criteria. *Am J Roentgenol* 2000;175:727-731.

Cross-Reference

Gastrointestinal Imaging: THE REQUISITES, 3rd ed, pp 21-23.

Comment

Achalasia is a fairly common but poorly understood disorder of the myenteric plexuses of the esophagus resulting in dilation, absence of peristaltic activity, and spasm at the gastroesophageal junction. It is more common in men and is usually seen in the third or fourth decade of life. In the images accompanying this case, a barium esophagogram demonstrates the classic area of tapered narrowing and spasm in the distal esophagus at the gastroesophageal junction (see figures). With chronic achalasia, the esophagus will over time become grossly dilated, with a sigmoid configuration. This may be confused with the appearance of esophageal resection and gastric pull-up or colonic interposition.

Other conditions, such as scleroderma and other collagen vascular disorders, can mimic achalasia. They are described as secondary achalasia. In these patients, the underlying condition is usually of long standing and well known to the patient. There have been reports of patients with diffuse esophageal spasm with dilated esophagus, minimal peristaltic activity, and spasm at the gastroesophageal junction. In fact, some investigators feel that achalasia and diffuse esophageal spasm may be part of the same spectrum of diseases. Although this is occasionally seen, it is not the usual pattern of presentation seen in most cases of achalasia. Primary and secondary achalasia may be identical in imaging appearance and presentation.

An important and common cause of secondary achalasia occurs where the underlying condition is esophageal or gastric cardiac carcinoma, which has infiltrated the wall of the lower esophagus or gastroesophageal junction and destroyed the myenteric plexuses. This is usually seen in an older age group, with a short history of dysphagia and weight loss. The differentiating feature on a barium swallow may be some mucosal irregularity at the site of spasm, proximal shouldering, or a mass at the gastric cardia. The length of the segment narrowing is a key differentiating feature, with malignant achalasia having a narrow segment greater than 3.5 cm. Endoscopic ultrasound and, in many cases, CT are more sensitive methods for making the diagnosis of secondary achalasia. Some authors refer to this etiology for secondary achalasia as pseudo-achalasia, recognizing that unlike the other secondary causes where the etiology is known, the patient and clinician might not be aware of the underlying malignancy when the patient presents with dysphagia.

Notes

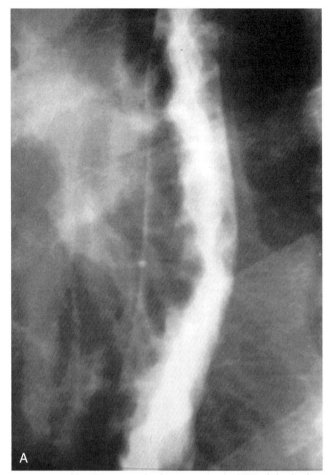

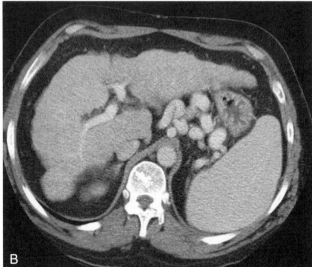

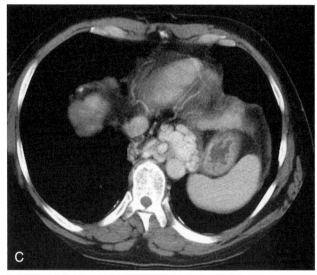

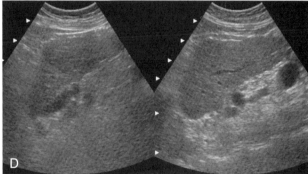

C. Varices
D. Stricture
E. Esophagitis

2. What is the usual physiologic basis for the development of uphill varices?
   A. Portal hypertension
   B. Occlusion of the splenic vein
   C. Incompetent perforators
   D. Superior obstruction of the vena cava

3. What is the most common cause of upper gastrointestinal bleeding?
   A. Varices
   B. Carcinoma
   C. Peptic ulcers
   D. Esophageal tears

4. Where do downhill varices occur?
   A. Stomach
   B. Umbilicus
   C. Distal esophagus
   D. Proximal esophagus

History: A 48-year-old man presents with chronic hepatitis C and cirrhosis.

1. Which of the following should be included in the differential diagnosis of the imaging finding shown in Figure A? (Choose all that apply.)
   A. Webs
   B. Cancer

Esophageal Varices

1. B, C, and E

2. A

3. C

4. D

References

Kim SH, Kim YJ, Lee JM, et al: Esophageal varices in patients with cirrhosis: multidetector CT esophagography—comparison with endoscopy. *Radiology* 2007;242:759-768.

Mazzeo S, Caramella D, Gennai A, et al: Multidetector CT and virtual endoscopy in the evaluation of the esophagus. *Abdom Imaging* 2004;29:2-8.

Cross-Reference

Gastrointestinal Imaging: *THE REQUISITES,* 3rd ed, p 9.

Comment

In Western society the most common cause of portal hypertension and the formation of esophageal varices is hepatic cirrhosis (see figures). This is usually the result of chronic alcoholism. However, many other causes can lead to liver cirrhosis, especially chronic hepatocellular disease (such as hepatitis), chronic portal vein occlusion by thrombus, or parasitic infection. Chronic portal vein occlusion can also result in cavernous transformation of the portal vein, in which collateralization along the entire route of the former portal vein is seen. This results in less-evident esophageal varices, and indeed, the patient may be asymptomatic. Cavernous transformation in portal hypertension related to liver cirrhosis is uncommon. Esophageal varices can bleed. This most alarming complication of the condition carries a high morbidity rate.

At the other end of the esophagus, obstruction of the superior vena cava can result in downhill varices seen in the upper esophagus and representing prominent collateralization of the venous system in an attempt to bypass an occluded superior vena cava, usually secondary to marked adenopathy resulting from adjacent malignancy, most commonly small cell carcinoma of the lung. Lymphoma can also be the underlying condition. The diagnosis is usually not difficult from the patient's physical appearance of congested facial features and engorged neck veins.

Notes

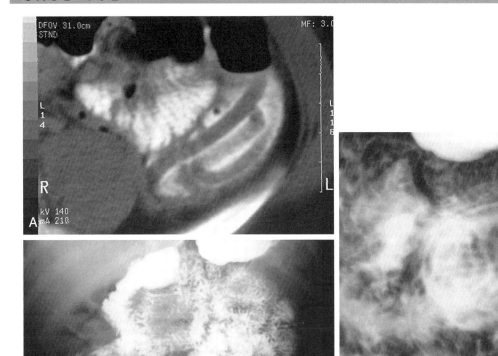

History: A 16-year-old boy presents with abdominal discomfort, nausea, and weight loss.

1. Which of the following should be included in the differential diagnosis of the imaging finding shown in Figure A? (Choose all that apply.)
   A. Filiform polyposis
   B. Worm infestation
   C. Ingested foreign bodies
   D. Trichobezoar fragments
   E. Intramural hemorrhage

2. Which of the following statements regarding ascariasis is true?
   A. The majority of sufferers come from Africa.
   B. It is the most common intestinal parasitic infection.
   C. The disease spreads most easily during the dry season.
   D. The disease is transmitted through dogs as the animal reservoir.

3. What is the most common abdominal visceral complication of this infestation?
   A. Renal
   B. Biliary
   C. Splenic
   D. Lymphatic

4. Which of the following is *not* a recognized manifestation of pulmonary involvement by this organism?
   A. Bronchospasm
   B. Eosinophilia
   C. Cavitation
   D. Infiltrates

Ascariasis of the Small Bowel

1. B, C, and D

2. B

3. B

4. C

References

Herlinger H, Ekberg TO: Other inflammatory conditions of the small bowel. In Gore RM, Levine MS (eds): *Textbook of Gastrointestinal Radiology*, 2nd ed. Philadelphia: WB Saunders; 2000, pp 746-758.

Reeder MM: The radiological and ultrasound evaluation of ascariasis of the gastrointestinal, biliary, and respiratory tracts. *Semin Roentgenol* 1998;33:57-58.

Cross-Reference

Gastrointestinal Imaging: *THE REQUISITES,* 3rd ed, p 135.

Comment

One of the most common parasitic infections is produced by the nematode *Ascaris lumbricoides*. It infects a major proportion of the world's population. With the ease of worldwide travel, as well as immigration, this parasite is encountered in all areas of the world. The pathway of infection is quite complicated. The eggs of this parasite are ingested when infected water or food is consumed. In the gastrointestinal tract (small bowel) the larvae hatch and burrow through the intestinal wall. From there, they reach the portal venous system and travel to the liver and the lungs. The larvae then reach the bronchial system, where they can be found in the sputum, and reach the intestines by being swallowed in the sputum. Once they again reach the intestines, they grow into adult worms, which can be quite large.

The parasite produces diseases in many ways. The larvae may produce a local hypersensitivity reaction, which is particularly evident when they are in the lungs. When they are in the intestines, the worms cause nutritional deficiencies. As the worms grow, the large mass of the worms can produce obstruction and even appendicitis. Perforation of the intestines with peritonitis can even occur. Often the patient's symptoms are quite vague, with occasional pain and diarrhea. The worms can also migrate into the biliary system, where they can produce cholangitis or pancreatitis because of their size as well as a local inflammatory response.

Radiologically the worms are visible on barium studies because they are so large (see figures). There may be a single worm, or they can occur in large masses. A hallmark of these worms is that they ingest the barium during the examination, and then barium outlines the intestinal tract of the worms, as is evident in this case (see figures).

Notes

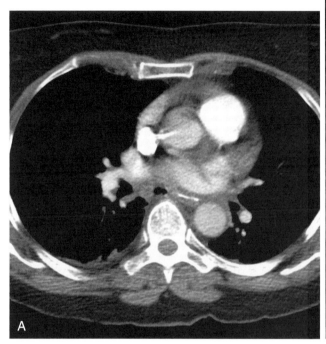

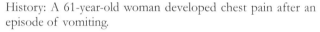

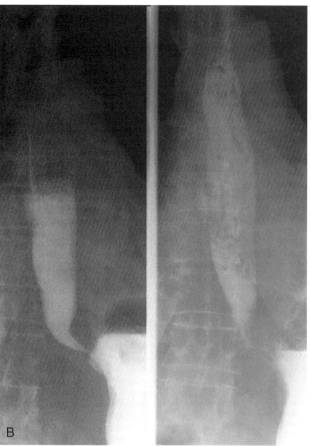

History: A 61-year-old woman developed chest pain after an episode of vomiting.

1. Which of the following should be included in the differential diagnosis of the imaging finding shown in Figure A? (Choose all that apply.)
   A. Esophageal tear
   B. Esophageal duplication
   C. Esophageal perforation
   D. Esophageal diverticulum
   E. Esophageal pseudodiverticulosis

2. This patient has developed a distal esophageal mucosal tear and intramural dissection after forceful retching. What is this syndrome?
   A. Paterson-Kelly
   B. Mallory-Weiss
   C. Boerhaave's
   D. Barrett's

3. Which of the following statements regarding Mallory-Weiss tears is true?
   A. They are usually multiple.
   B. They are caused by vomiting or retching.
   C. They are usually associated with alcohol abuse.
   D. Left untreated, they usually progress to perforation.

4. Which of the following statements regarding Boerhaave's syndrome is true?
   A. It usually resolves spontaneously.
   B. Endoscopy is the investigation of choice.
   C. It is most commonly due to vomiting or straining.
   D. The treatment of choice in all cases is surgical.

Esophageal Tear

1. A, C, and D

2. B

3. C

4. C

References

de Lutio di Castelguidone E, Merola S, Pinto A, et al: Esophageal injuries: spectrum of multidetector row CT findings. *Eur J Radiol* 2006;59:344-348.

Fadoo F, Ruiz DE, Dawn SK, et al: Helical CT esophagography for the evaluation of suspected esophageal perforation or rupture. *Am J Roentgenol* 2004;182:1177-1179.

Cross-Reference

Gastrointestinal Imaging: *THE REQUISITES*, 3rd ed, p 19.

Comment

Air in the esophageal wall is an uncommon finding. It is extremely difficult to see on plain film or even on barium esophagograms. However, the finding is easily identified on CT (see figures). The Mallory-Weiss patient can have air in the esophageal wall if an open mucosal tear exists (see figures). These patients usually are alcoholics (but not always). The condition has also been described in a few patients with severe hiccups. They present with blood-tinged vomiting and chest pain. The tears are almost always treated conservatively, and about 95% spontaneously heal. Patients with portal hypertension and a Mallory-Weiss tear are a more serious problem. A full-thickness tear of the distal esophagus (Boerhaave syndrome) is a surgical emergency and requires immediate intervention. The morbidity rate is high. Endoscopic instrumentation occasionally is the cause of mucosal tears. However, the risk of iatrogenic injury to the mucosa will probably increase as newer methods of endoscopic ablation of Barrett's metaplasia are being tried with varying degrees of success and associated complications (including pneumatosis). Some of these procedures include photodynamic therapy, laser therapy, electrocoagulation, argon plasma coagulation therapy, and mucosal surface resection. In addition, radiofrequency and cryotherapy are being evaluated.

Notes

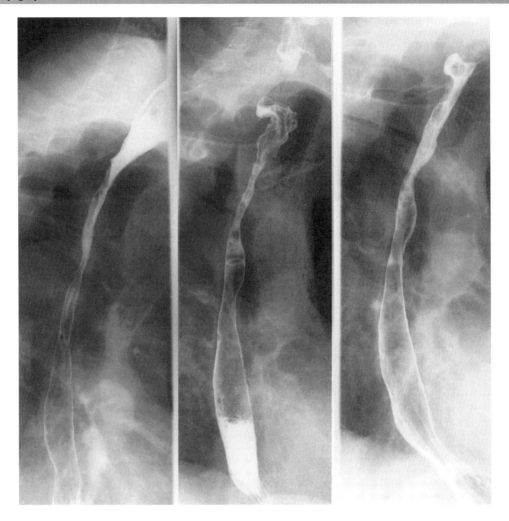

History: A 53-year-old man presents with dysphagia since childhood.

1. Which of the following should be included in the differential diagnosis of the imaging finding shown in the figures? (Choose all that apply.)
   A. Cervical web
   B. Radiation therapy
   C. Caustic ingestion
   D. Nasogastric intubation
   E. Squamous cell carcinoma

2. Ingestion of which of these caustic agents produces the worst outcomes?
   A. Acid
   B. Alkali
   C. Bleach
   D. Batteries

3. What is the potentially fatal complication of esophageal corrosive injury?
   A. Adenocarcinoma
   B. Barrett's esophagus
   C. Squamous cell carcinoma
   D. Tracheoesophageal fistula

4. Which of the following obstructive lesions of the esophagus is usually not found in the proximal or mid esophagus?
   A. Achalasia
   B. Barrett's esophagus
   C. Cricopharyngeal incoordination
   D. Drug (medication) ingestion

CASE 104

Esophageal Strictures from Ingestion of a Caustic Substance

1. B and C

2. A

3. C

4. A

Reference

Luedtke P, Levine MS, Rubesin SE, et al: Radiologic diagnosis of benign esophageal strictures: a pattern approach. *Radiographics* 2003;23:897-909.

Cross-Reference

Gastrointestinal Imaging: THE REQUISITES, 3rd ed, p 17.

Comment

Ingestion of alkaline (lye) or acid substances may be either intentional or, in rare cases, accidental. Many household cleaners contain alkali or caustic substances. The degree of injury that occurs in the gastrointestinal tract is related to both the concentration and the volume of the ingested substances. The immediacy of treatment also has a significant impact regarding the sequelae of this injury. Alkaline substances produce coagulative necrosis and tend to cause a more deeply penetrating injury to the bowel.

Radiologic studies may be performed (but are not recommended in known cases of caustic ingestion) as long as there are no signs of perforation, such as a widened mediastinum, soft tissue emphysema, or intraperitoneal air. Initial radiologic assessment may be performed before endoscopy is attempted and should be done with water-soluble contrast agent followed by thin barium. In the early stages (less than 12 hours after the ingestion) the only apparent problem may be a motility disorder, ranging from spasm to atony and even dilation. If there has been a severe caustic burn, superficial ulceration may be apparent in the mucosa. Over the ensuing days, the damaged mucosa sloughs and becomes edematous, with the most severe changes subsiding after several days. Radiologic examination typically is not performed during this time unless there is suspected perforation. A water-soluble study can show the location and size of the leak. The final phase of scarring, fibrosis, and stricture formation takes several weeks to months to develop. Not all patients develop esophageal stricturing, but it is more common in patients who ingested lye than in those who ingested acid. The strictures that are apparent can be either long and diffuse or weblike areas of narrowing (see figure). A significant number of these patients have developed, over time, squamous cell carcinoma of the esophagus, a well-known complication of lye ingestion.

Ingestion of alkaline and acid substances can involve the stomach, usually in the distal antrum along the greater curvature, which is where the ingested substance often comes to rest when the patient is upright. The degree of gastric injury is usually worse with ingestion of acids. The appearance looks almost identical to a malignancy: a large ulcerated mass on the greater curve of the stomach. Alkaline substances may be neutralized by the gastric acidity. However, up to 20% of patients who ingested lye develop gastric injury.

Notes

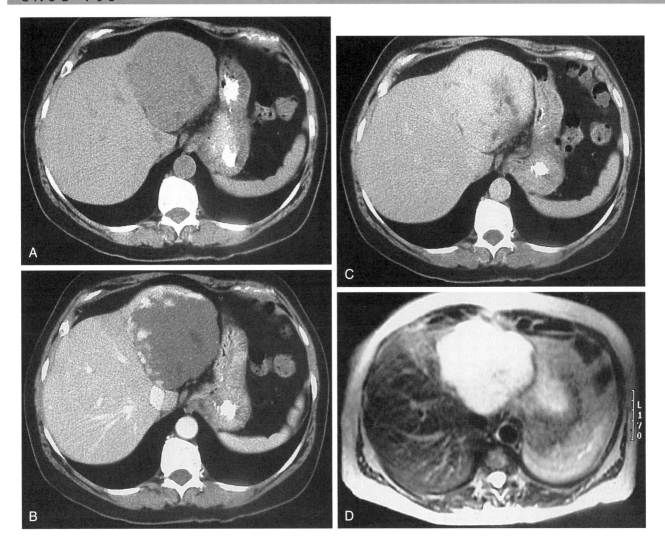

History: A 34-year-old woman presents with right upper quadrant discomfort.

1. Which of the following should be included in the differential diagnosis of the imaging finding shown in Figures A to C? (Choose all that apply.)
   A. Adenoma
   B. Hepatoma
   C. Giant cyst
   D. Metastasis
   E. Hemangioma

2. Which of the following statements regarding clinical features of hepatic hemangiomas is true?
   A. They are usually solitary.
   B. There is equal sex incidence.
   C. They are found with increasing incidence with age.
   D. The most common symptom is right upper quadrant discomfort.

3. Which of the following imaging descriptions suggest hepatic hemangioma?
   A. On ultrasound, they are usually hypoechoic with slight distal acoustic enhancement.
   B. On CT, centrifugal progressive enhancement is diagnostic.
   C. On MRI, marked hyperintensity on T1-weighted images is characteristic.
   D. On nuclear scintigraphy scans with tagged red blood cells, there is early phase defect with delayed fill in.

4. Hemangiomas are usually asymptomatic. What is the rare syndrome with associated thrombocytopenia?
   A. Klippel-Trenaunay-Weber syndrome
   B. Osler-Rendu-Weber syndrome
   C. Kasabach-Merritt syndrome
   D. Von Hippel–Lindau disease

Hepatic Hemangioma

1. A, B, D, and E

2. A

3. D

4. C

References

Ros PR, Taylor HM: Benign tumors of the liver. In Gore RM, Levine MS (eds): *Textbook of Gastrointestinal Radiology*, 2nd ed. Philadelphia: WB Saunders, 2000, pp 1487-1522.

Vilgrain V, Boulus L, Villuerme MP, et al: Imaging of atypical hemangiomas of the liver with pathologic correlation. *Radiographics* 2000;20:379-397.

Cross-Reference

Gastrointestinal Imaging: *THE REQUISITES,* 3rd ed, p 186.

Comment

Hemangiomas of the liver, unlike those of the rest of the gastrointestinal tract, are a common finding. In the rest of the gastrointestinal tract, they are rare lesions. There is no malignant potential associated with this lesion. The problem is one of attempting to distinguish the harmless hemangioma from other lesions such hepatic metastatic disease. There are two different types of hemangiomas to consider: simple hemangioma (by far the most common) and cavernous hemangioma, such as is seen in this case. Hemangiomas of the liver are the most common benign neoplastic tumors of the liver. It is thought that these tumors affect at least 2% to 5% of the population. They are more common in women and occur most commonly in the right lobe of the liver. Multiple hemangiomas occur in 10% to 15% of these patients. By themselves, hemangiomas are rarely symptomatic and are of no consequence to the patient. Their importance lies more in the fact that their appearance can mimic that of more sinister conditions of the liver, such as metastases or malignant tumors.

Most discussions regarding hemangiomas concern the diagnostic tests that can help distinguish them from other lesions. Dynamic scanning of the liver by CT is quite helpful. In this case, initial CT scans show the hemangioma to be a low-attenuation lesion in the liver. Delayed images of the lesion over the next several minutes demonstrate increasing opacification of the hemangioma from the periphery toward the center, the *centripetal opacification*. However, not all cavernous hemangiomas show the classic findings, and often other studies are required. Ultrasound often shows a well-defined echogenic lesion, although the findings are not always pathognomonic. MRI is often useful because hemangiomas have a high signal intensity on T2-weighted images, but cysts and even some metastatic lesions can have a similar appearance. Radionuclide scanning is quite helpful for evaluating the liver hemangioma. On tagged red blood cell studies the hemangioma typically appears as a cold defect during the early scans, but in later images the lesion fills in and actually has increased activity on delayed images. With all these imaging studies, the greatest difficulty is encountered when the hemangioma has a central area of necrosis or fibrosis (see figures), which can mimic other lesions.

Notes

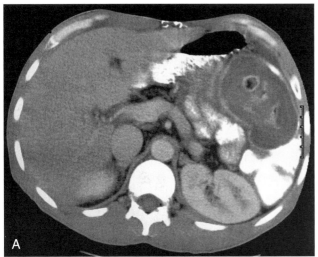

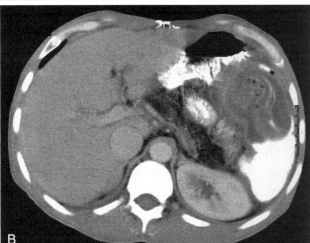

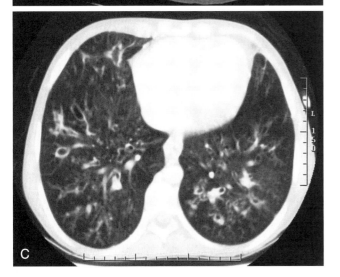

History: A 25-year-old man has been under lifelong medical care for recurrent chest infections.

1. Which of the following should be included in the differential diagnosis of the imaging finding shown in Figure A? (Choose all that apply.)
   A. Cystic fibrosis
   B. Diabetes mellitus
   C. Hemochromatosis
   D. Chronic pancreatitis
   E. Shwachman's syndrome

2. Which is the most common of the following abdominal complications of cystic fibrosis?
   A. Infertility
   B. Meconium ileus
   C. Rectal prolapse
   D. Pancreatic exocrine insufficiency

3. What is the definitive treatment for cystic fibrosis?
   A. Lung transplantation
   B. Pancreas transplantation
   C. Prenatal genetic testing
   D. There is no definitive (curative) treatment

4. Cystic fibrosis affects the pancreas in a variety of ways. Which of the following is *not* a pancreatic complication of cystic fibrosis?
   A. Cancer
   B. Pancreatitis
   C. Diabetes mellitus
   D. Pancreatic exocrine insufficiency

CASE 106

Cystic Fibrosis and Atrophy of the Pancreas

1. A, C, D, and E

2. A

3. D

4. A

References

Agrons GA, Corse WR, Markowitz RI, et al: Gastrointestinal manifestations of cystic fibrosis: radiologic-pathologic correlation. *Radiographics* 1996;16:871-893.

Fields TM, Michel SJ, Butler CL, et al: Abdominal manifestations of cystic fibrosis in older children and adults. *Am J Roentgenol* 2006;187:1199-1203.

Robertson MB, Choe KA, Joseph PM: Review of the abdominal manifestations of cystic fibrosis in the adult patient. *Radiographics* 2006;26:679-690.

Cross-Reference

Gastrointestinal Imaging: *THE REQUISITES,* 3rd ed, p 158.

Comment

Cystic fibrosis is a recessive genetic disorder caused by the malfunction of a single gene on chromosome 7. The gene, cystic fibrous transmembrane conductance regulator (CFTR), has to do with transport of chloride and, to a lesser extent, sodium ions from within the cell to outside the cell. There can be a variety of mutations of this gene, all resulting in the production of excessive, thick mucus within the cells of the glandular structures. This, in part, accounts for the salty skin of patients with CF. The thick mucus has its most deadly effect on the lungs, where it provides a near-perfect medium for chronic bacterial infections, which over time, distort and destroy the lung and bronchial architecture and further decrease respiratory capability.

Pancreatic involvement resulting in marked pancreatic atrophy and deficiency (such as in this case: note the absence of pancreatic tissue in its expected anatomic location) is extremely common. Supplementation with pancreatic enzymes is the common treatment along with a careful diet. With the use of CT over the years, we have come to recognize pancreatic atrophy as a common finding in older patients, with fatty infiltration of the pancreas. It seems to be a senile atrophy of the pancreas. However, the pancreatic atrophy of CF is seen in younger patients and is striking in its absence of pancreatic tissue.

Notes

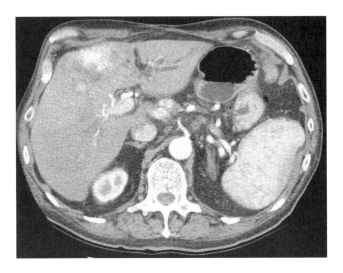 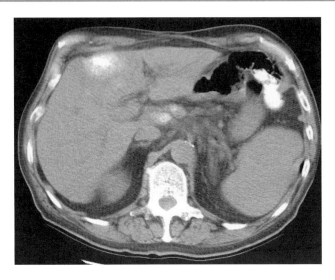

History: A 70-year-old man presents for surveillance CT to follow up previously resected colorectal carcinoma.

1. Which of the following should be included in the differential diagnosis of the imaging finding shown in the figures? (Choose all that apply.)
   A. Hematoma
   B. Primary liver tumor
   C. Choledocholithiasis
   D. Granulomatous disease
   E. Metastatic cancer deposits

2. What is the most common metastatic lesion to the liver to calcify?
   A. Ovarian cancer
   B. Breast carcinoma
   C. Colorectal carcinoma
   D. Osteogenic sarcoma

3. What is the most common cause of calcified liver lesions in children?
   A. Hemangioendothelioma
   B. Hepatoblastoma
   C. Neuroblastoma
   D. Hamartoma

4. Infection of the liver by many organisms results in calcified lesions. Which of these organisms would you *not* expect to see with calcification?
   A. *Candida albicans*
   B. *Pneumocystis jiroveci*
   C. *Schistosoma mansoni*
   D. *Echinococcus multilocularis*

Calcified Hepatic Metastatic Disease

1. A, B, D, and E

2. C

3. C

4. C

References

Paley MR, Ros PR: Hepatic calcification. *Radiol Clin North Am* 1998;36:391-398.
Stoupis C, Taylor HM, Paley MR, et al: The rocky liver: radiologic-pathologic correlation of calcified hepatic masses. *Radiographics* 1998;18:675-685.

Cross-Reference

Gastrointestinal Imaging: *THE REQUISITES,* 3rd ed, p 206.

Comment

The CT image demonstrates calcified liver and lymph nodes lesions (see figures). Primary liver tumors may calcify and typically are solitary. Infectious processes that have involved the liver, such as granulomatous infections, also can produce liver calcifications. Parasitic diseases, such as echinococcal cysts, can cause calcification. However, the illustrated case shows multiple lesions that are either partially or completely calcified, which is strongly suggestive of metastatic disease.

Metastases to the liver rarely calcify. In the adult population, calcification of liver metastases is typically the result of a mucinous adenocarcinoma, which produces a psammomatous type of calcification that is detectable on CT scans. Most often, mucinous adenocarcinoma is found in the colon. Other sites of mucinous carcinoma include the pancreas, stomach, and ovaries. Tumors such as osteogenic sarcoma and chondrosarcoma can produce calcification or ossification, and their metastases could have this appearance as well. In children the most likely cause is neuroblastoma; up to 25% of neuroblastoma metastases calcify. Tumors outside the abdominal cavity rarely produce calcified liver metastases, but lung tumors, breast tumors, melanomas, and testicular tumors produce these lesions on rare occasion. Tumors that have been treated with chemotherapy or radiation also can calcify, although admittedly this presentation is rare. Calcification has been reported in various treated tumors and in treated lymphoma of the liver.

Notes

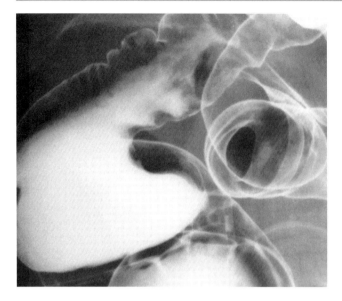

History: A 38-year-old woman presents with chronic constipation and recent rectal bleeding.

1. Which of the following should be included in the differential diagnosis of the imaging finding shown in the figure? (Choose all that apply.)
   A. Hemorrhoids
   B. Endometriosis
   C. Peritoneal metastases
   D. Colitis cystica profunda
   E. Rectal adenocarcinoma

2. On defecography, what finding may be evident in this patient?
   A. Rectocele
   B. Enterocele
   C. Pelvic floor prolapse
   D. Internal rectal prolapse

3. Which of the following statements regarding clinical aspects of solitary rectal ulcer syndrome is true?
   A. It is mainly a disease of women.
   B. A quarter of patients may be asymptomatic.
   C. Patients usually present within 3 months of onset of symptoms.
   D. The most common presentation is a feeling of incomplete evacuation.

4. In patients with solitary rectal ulcer syndrome, what is the most common finding on barium enema?
   A. Mucosal granularity
   B. Thickened folds
   C. Stricture
   D. Normal

CASE 108

Colitis Cystica Profunda

1. B, C, D, and E

2. D

3. B

4. D

References

Goei R, Baeten C, Arends JW: Solitary rectal ulcer syndrome: findings at barium enema study and defecography. *Radiology* 1988;168:303-306.

Ledesma-Medina J, Reid BS, Girdany BR: Colitis cystic profunda. *Am J Roentgenol* 1978;131:529-530.

Cross-Reference

Gastrointestinal Imaging: THE REQUISITES, ed 3, p 300.

Comment

The anterior wall of the rectum is a relatively common location for pathologic findings. Probably the most common abnormalities in this area are external diseases of the cul-de-sac, including endometriosis and numerous abdominal tumors (ovarian, gastric, pancreatic, and intestinal) that produce peritoneal seeding or drop metastases to this region. All these processes have a similar appearance on barium enema. Primary tumors of the colon, mainly adenocarcinoma, can also develop in this region.

However, the anterior mucosal wall of the rectum also is a location for abnormalities that occur as the sequelae of anorectal defecation disorders. Patients with defecation problems, primarily constipation or chronic straining, can suffer from prolapse of the rectal mucosa. The anterior wall of the rectum above the peritoneal reflection is not fixed; it is free to move. This form of prolapse (or intussusception) happens every time the patient attempts to defecate. This prolapse is usually internal and difficult to document. At times even external prolapse (beyond the anal sphincter) occurs and the diagnosis becomes self-evident. Either way, the anterior wall of the rectum becomes a vulnerable structure prone to injury and induration. This, in turn, can lead to mucosal ulceration, which leads to rectal bleeding. This condition, termed *solitary rectal ulcer syndrome,* affects all age groups but particularly younger patients and mostly female patients.

Colitis cystica profunda is a sequela of chronic prolapse and solitary rectal ulcer syndrome. With recurrent prolapse and ulceration, there are stages of ulceration and then healing of the rectal mucosa. Over time, the regenerating mucosa can trap mucus glands underneath the mucosa. These trapped mucus glands continue to secrete mucus but do not drain because of overlying mucosa. Thus, the glands become cystic structures filled with mucin, and hence the name. With time, the cysts produce one of several polypoid structures, typically along the anterior surface of the rectum because this segment is most susceptible to this trauma. This entity is difficult to diagnose in the absence of a history of long-standing defecation dysfunction. Biopsy confirms the diagnosis, and often defecography is helpful in identifying the patient's underlying defecation problems.

Notes

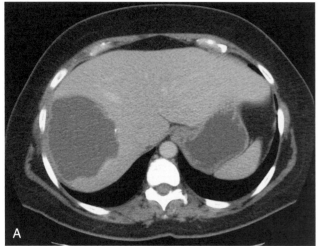

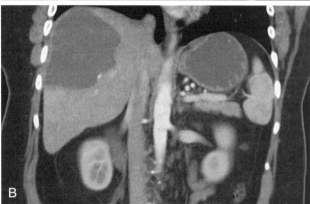

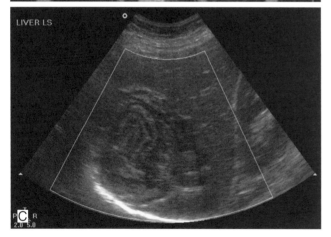

History: A 43-year-old woman presents with dyspepsia.

1. Which of the following should be included in the differential diagnosis of the imaging finding shown in Figure A? (Choose all that apply.)
   A. Candidiasis
   B. Amebic abscess
   C. Echinococcal cyst
   D. Pyogenic abscess
   E. Cystadenocarcinoma

2. The hydatid cyst can rupture spontaneously. Which is the most common direction?
   A. Biliary
   B. Pleural
   C. Peritoneal
   D. Pericardial

3. The liver is the most common site of hydatid disease involvement. What is the next most common site?
   A. Lung
   B. Spleen
   C. Kidneys
   D. Pancreas

4. Which of the following statements regarding infection with *Echinococcus multilocularis* is true?
   A. If left untreated, there is 90% mortality in 10 years.
   B. Primary infection is usually asymptomatic.
   C. The resultant abscess does not calcify.
   D. Imaging shows multiple simple cysts.

Hepatic Hydatid

1. B, C, D, and E

2. A

3. A

4. A

References

Beggs I: The radiology of hydatid disease. *Am J Roentgenol* 1985;145:639-648.

Pedrosa I, Saiz A, Arrazola J, et al: Hydatid disease: radiologic and pathologic features and complications. *Radiographics* 2000;20:795-817.

Cross-Reference

Gastrointestinal Imaging: *THE REQUISITES,* 3rd ed, p 202.

Comment

Echinococcal cysts are produced by two types of tapeworms, *Echinococcus granulosus* and *Echinococcus multilocularis. E. granulosus* is the species most commonly seen in North America. These tapeworms live in the intestinal tract in dogs. Humans, and more commonly, sheep are the intermediate hosts, harboring the parasite in its larval stage. Humans contact the parasite by eating contaminated food, such as unwashed vegetables, or through contact with an infected dog or sheep. When the eggs of the parasite are ingested, they penetrate the mucosa of the intestine and are then carried via the portal vein to the liver. Sometimes the lungs, spleen, and kidneys are involved as well. The embryos then develop in a hydatid stage in which they form cysts in the liver. The life cycle is completed when the intermediate host dies and is consumed by the final host.

Approximately 20% to 30% of the cysts calcify, which is much higher than the percentage of simple hepatic cysts that calcify (see figures). Hydatid cysts consist of three layers. The outer pericyst is a rigid fibrous structure that is vascular and can enhance on CT. There is an intermediate layer, and finally the inner layer or endocyst is the living parasite (see figure). These cysts represent the larval stage, and there are often multiple small cysts seen within the larger cyst. Debris produced by brood capsules may be visible on the dependent potion of the cysts. Most cysts cause no symptoms until they are large enough to create pressure on adjacent structures. Sometimes the cysts spontaneously rupture into the biliary system or the peritoneal, pleural, or pericardial surfaces. Symptoms vary, but this complication can produce cholangitis or inflammation of the structures it comes in contact with. A fatal anaphylactic reaction is also possible. The plain film shown with this case is an example of chronic disease, whereas the CT image indicates a more acute stage.

Hydatid cysts must be drained for treatment. Surgery was once considered necessary treatment for this condition because of the possibility of anaphylactic reaction if the cyst drained into the peritoneum. However, it is now recognized that these cysts can be managed by percutaneous catheter drainage and instillation of scolecidal agents.

Notes

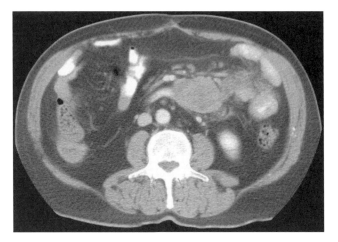

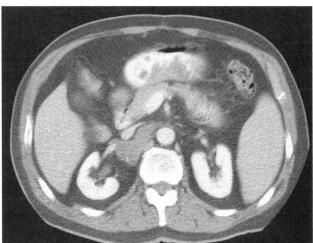

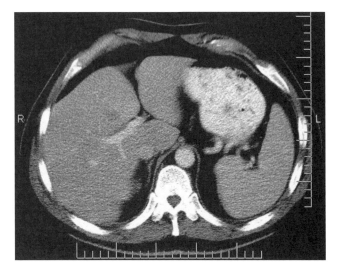

History: A 55-year-old man presents for annual surveillance scan.

1. Which of the following should be included in the differential diagnosis of the imaging finding shown in the figures? (Choose all that apply.)
   A. Leukemia
   B. Lymphoma
   C. Granulomas
   D. Neurofibromatosis
   E. Metastatic melanoma

2. What is the most common radiologic appearance of lymphoma of the small bowel?
   A. Stricture
   B. Infiltrating mass
   C. Multiple nodules
   D. Aneurysmal dilation

3. What is the most common primary site of involvement of the gastrointestinal tract with lymphoma?
   A. Stomach
   B. Small bowel
   C. Colorectal
   D. Multiple GI sites

4. Which of the following predisposing conditions carries the greatest risk of developing lymphoma?
   A. AIDS
   B. Celiac disease
   C. Transplant
   D. Systemic lupus erythematosus

Small Bowel Lymphoma

1. B, C, D, and E

2. B

3. A

4. C

References

Buckley JA, Fishman EK: CT evaluation of small bowel neoplasms: spectrum of disease. *Radiographics* 1998;18:379-392.

Rubesin SE, Gilchrist AM, Bronner M, et al: Non-Hodgkin's lymphoma of the small intestine. *Radiographics* 1990;10:985-998.

Cross-Reference

Gastrointestinal Imaging: *THE REQUISITES,* 3rd ed, p 129.

Comment

Lymphomas occur most commonly in the distal small bowel (compared with adenocarcinoma, which is proximal), but they occur infrequently in other parts of the small bowel. A feature of lymphoma is that it is often multicentric in location (see figures). The majority of small bowel lymphomas are the non-Hodgkin's type, with Hodgkin's disease of the small bowel being considered rare.

Lymphoma is difficult to characterize because of its variable morphologic appearance. Radiologic features include multiple nodules, solitary masses with an excavated cavity that acts as the bowel lumen, infiltrating tumors, and predominant mesenteric masses. The infiltrating or the endoexenteric mass is believed to be the most common type. The excavating form, or aneurysmal dilation, is produced when lymphoma infiltrates, replaces the muscular layer, and destroys the nerves in the area. This results in bulging of the abdominal wall, with resultant dilation. The bowel wall can become completely replaced by tumor with a persistent irregular lumen. Because of this unusual scenario, large masses of the small bowel show no evidence of bowel obstruction. However, perforation is a possibility. The bowel lumen and various layers of the bowel wall can grow back with therapy.

A variety of conditions can lead to the development of lymphoma. Any type of immunosuppression, such as that associated with AIDS, can lead to lymphoma. Perhaps at highest risk are transplant recipients, who are 50 to 100 times more likely to develop lymphoma compared with the general population. Many of these patients have an associated infection with the Epstein-Barr virus. Other conditions that increase the incidence of small bowel lymphoma include celiac disease (sprue) and systemic lupus erythematosus.

Notes

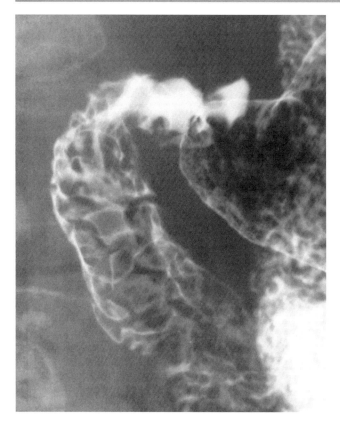

History: A 55-year-old man presents with altered blood in the stool.

1. What should be included in the differential diagnosis of the imaging finding shown in the figure? (Choose all that apply.)
   A. Antral gastritis
   B. Bulbar scarring
   C. Pyloric stenosis
   D. Duodenal ulcer
   E. Post–bulbar deformity

2. The patient has been undertreated for ulcer disease because he has persistent *Helicobacter pylori* infection. Which of the following conditions is associated with the highest prevalence of *H. pylori* infection?
   A. Gastric ulcer
   B. Gastric cancer
   C. Duodenal ulcer
   D. Chronic gastritis

3. What is the most common complication of chronic duodenal ulceration?
   A. Obstruction
   B. Bleeding
   C. Cancer
   D. Pancreatitis

4. Which of the following statements regarding the imaging of complications of duodenal ulceration is true?
   A. On plain radiography, the most common appearance is gastric outlet obstruction.
   B. Patients presenting with GI tract bleeding would benefit from CT to localize the site of bleeding to proceed to optimal endoscopic and angiographic intervention.
   C. Patients with imaging (barium upper GI study or CT) findings of pyloric obstruction should be referred for endoscopy and biopsy.
   D. The absence of pneumoperitoneum excludes perforation.

CASE 111

Duodenal Scarring

1. B, C, D, and E

2. C

3. B

4. C

References

Nadgir RN, Levine MS: Update on *Helicobacter pylori. Appl Radiol* 1999:10-14.
Shaffer HA Jr: Perforation and obstruction of the gastrointestinal tract: assessment by conventional radiology. *Radiol Clin North Am* 1992;30(2):405-426.

Cross-Reference

Gastrointestinal Imaging: *THE REQUISITES,* 3rd ed, p 90.

Comment

There are four major complications of duodenal peptic ulceration: hemorrhage, obstruction, perforation, and penetration. Complications occur in 1% to 2% of patients per year and are more likely to occur in patients with chronic ulceration.

Bleeding from a peptic ulcer is a common medical condition with high patient morbidity and high medical and hospital care costs. Patients present with hematemesis (vomiting of bright or altered blood) or melena (black, tarry stools) or both. Hematochezia may occur if bleeding is massive. Ulcer hemorrhage is usually managed with fluid and blood resuscitation, medical therapy, and endoscopic intervention; a few patients require surgery. Imaging has very little role except in the very few cases in which therapy has been unsuccessful and the patient is unsuitable for surgery. Angiography is used to identify the bleeding vessel and attempt intervention with vasoconstrictors or embolization.

Obstruction is the least frequent complication of duodenal ulceration. In the past, obstruction accounted for at least 10% of patients requiring surgery (see figure). Improvements in medical and endoscopic management have resulted in this decrease. Where the obstruction is pyloric, malignancy rather than peptic disease has become a more prominent cause of obstruction.

Perforation is potentially the most lethal complication. Patients usually present with sudden onset of severe, diffuse abdominal pain. The duodenum is the most common site of perforation, accounting for 60% of perforations secondary to peptic ulcer. Perforation is a more common complication in patients taking nonsteroidal antiinflammatory drugs and in elderly patients. Imaging is usually limited to the detection of free intraperitoneal air on plain radiography. With this finding, the patient proceeds to surgery. The absence of pneumoperitoneum does not exclude a perforated duodenal ulcer because 20% of patients do not have this sign. CT detects small volumes of pneumoperitoneum. Occasionally, a water-soluble contrast (Gastrografin) study is needed to determine the location of perforation and to determine if leakage is ongoing. Although this is a useful confirmatory test, it is unnecessary in most cases and delays surgery.

Penetration occurs when an ulcer erodes into an adjacent viscus or other anatomic structure. Penetration occurs in an estimated 20% of cases, although only a few become clinically evident that require specific imaging and management. The pancreas is the most common site of penetration, which usually results in mild hyperamylasemia; clinical pancreatitis is uncommon. Penetration of a duodenal ulcer into a hollow viscus results in various fistulas (gastric, colic, and biliary). Erosion into a vascular structure may lead to catastrophic hemorrhage. Finally, a localized and clinically silent penetration may progress to an abscess.

Notes

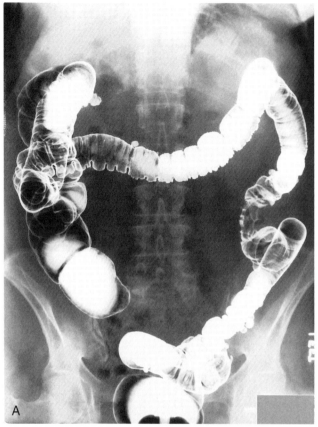

A

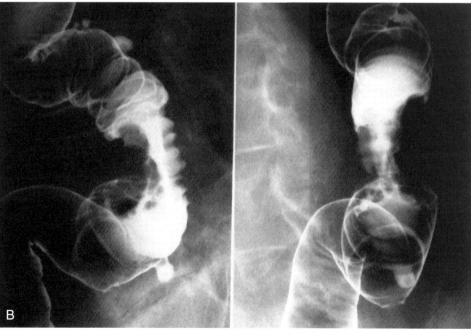

B

History: A 42-year-old woman presents with a positive occult stool test.

1. What should be included in the differential diagnosis of the imaging finding shown in Figure A? (Choose all that apply.)
   A. Focal spasm
   B. Metastatic melanoma
   C. Inflammatory bowel disease
   D. Familial adenomatous polyposis
   E. Primary colonic adenocarcinoma

2. Further family history and genetic testing identify the patient is at high risk for cancer because she has hereditary nonpolyposis colorectal cancer (HNPCC) syndrome. What is another name for this syndrome?
   A. Lynch syndrome
   B. Turcot's syndrome
   C. Cowden's syndrome
   D. Gardner's syndrome

3. Lynch syndrome is associated with an increased risk of developing other cancers. What is the most common extracolonic tumor?
   A. Glioma
   B. Ovarian carcinoma
   C. Endometrial carcinoma
   D. Skin and sebaceous tumors

4. What is the genetic basis of HNPCC syndrome?
   A. Defective DNA mismatch repair sequences
   B. Mutation of the *APC* tumor suppressor gene
   C. Mutation of the *PTEN* tumor suppressor gene
   D. Mutation of the *STK11/LKB1* tumor suppressor gene on chromosome 19

C A S E   1 1 2

Hereditary Nonpolyposis Colorectal Cancer Syndrome

1. A, B, C, and E

2. A

3. C

4. A

References

Lynch HT, Shaw MW, Magnuson CW, et al: Hereditary factors in cancer: study of two large Midwestern kindreds. *Arch Intern Med* 1966;117(2): 206-212.

Lynch HT, Smyrk T: Hereditary nonpolyposis colorectal cancer (Lynch syndrome): an updated review. *Cancer* 1996;78(6):1149-1167.

Cross-Reference

Gastrointestinal Imaging: *THE REQUISITES,* 3rd ed, p 302.

Comment

Approximately 2% of new cases of colorectal cancer fall into the category of HNPCC. Patients with HNPCC syndrome and familial adenomatous polyposis syndrome are considered to be in the high-risk category and should undergo regular screening. Although air contrast barium enema (ACBE) has been shown to be a good screening tool, its impact in cancer screening has decreased, it is not discussed in most literature on the subject, and its use has diminished. ACBE must be performed by competent radiologists with considerable experience and expertise in technique and diagnosis (see figures). The fewer ACBEs done, the less reliable the examination is likely to be, setting up a vicious cycle.

Colonoscopy is becoming the routine examination of choice. However, radiologists have begun to evaluate CT colonography as a far safer option (and, it is hoped, with good accuracy and sensitivity) than colonoscopy. Routine CT is proving to be a good diagnostic tool for detecting bowel lesions. These are usually incidental findings, and except for some polyposis syndromes, high-risk patients or patients with Lynch syndrome cannot be identified radiologically.

Patients with HNPCC are at increased risk for endometrial, ovarian, hepatobiliary, stomach, and small bowel cancers. DNA mismatch repair sequences are normal genetic processes that identify and repair replication errors during cell division. When the mismatch repair sequence is unstable or dysfunctional on certain of several genes, mutation can occur, and the risk of cancer is increased.

Notes

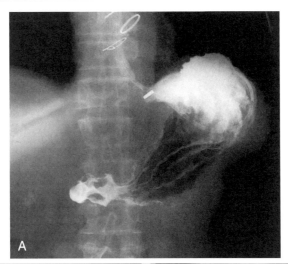

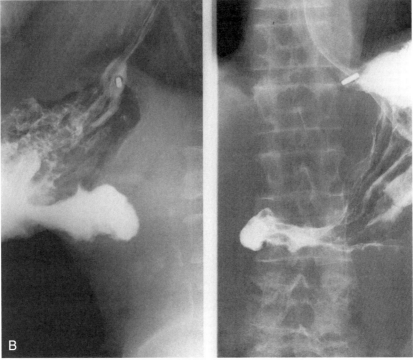

History: A 55-year-old woman presents with vomiting and weight loss.

1. What should be included in the differential diagnosis of the imaging finding shown in Figure A? (Choose all that apply.)
   A. Primary adenocarcinoma
   B. Metastatic carcinoma
   C. Peptic ulcer disease
   D. Gastric volvulus
   E. Gastric atony

2. What is the most common cause of gastric outlet obstruction?
   A. Primary adenocarcinoma
   B. Metastatic carcinoma
   C. Peptic ulcer disease
   D. Pancreatitis

3. Which of the following statements regarding gastric outlet obstruction is *false*?
   A. Caustic ingestion frequently leads to gastric outlet obstruction.
   B. Transpyloric prolapse of gastric mucosa is usually asymptomatic.
   C. Patients with gastroduodenal involvement by Crohn's disease are usually symptomatic.
   D. Gastric outlet obstruction is the most common complication of gastroduodenal tuberculosis.

4. What condition results in gastric obstruction secondary to a gallstone lodged in the pyloric channel?
   A. Rigler's triad
   B. Wilkie's syndrome
   C. Mirizzi's syndrome
   D. Bouveret's syndrome

Gastric Outlet Obstruction Caused by Metastatic Disease

1. A, B, C, and E

2. A

3. C

4. D

References

Dahnert W: *Radiology Review Manual*, 6th ed. Philadelphia: Lippincott Williams & Wilkins, 2007, pp 760-761.

Eisenberg RL, Levine MS: Miscellaneous abnormalities of the stomach and duodenum. In Gore RM, Levine MS (eds): *Textbook of Gastrointestinal Radiology*, 2nd ed. Philadelphia: Saunders, 2000, pp 659-681.

Cross-Reference

Gastrointestinal Imaging: *THE REQUISITES*, 3rd ed, p 49.

Comment

In pediatric patients, especially boys in the first year of life, pyloric hypertrophy with stenosis is a common cause of gastric outlet obstruction and is usually easily diagnosed on ultrasound. However, in older patients, pyloric hypertrophy is very rare. The most common cause of gastric outlet obstruction in adults is probably malignancy, primary and secondary. The usual lesion is pancreatic or peripancreatic. In this case, the lesion was widespread metastatic disease that had invaded the duodenum. Primary carcinoma involving the head of the pancreas is often the obstructing lesion. Pancreatic carcinoma can also invade the stomach itself, but this seldom causes outlet obstruction. Primary duodenal lesions can result in outlet obstruction.

Barium upper GI studies can establish the presence of a mechanical cause of gastric distention and may suggest the cause (see figures). Upper GI endoscopy can do the same with the added benefit of biopsy, if indicated. Multiplanar CT has become an outstanding tool in the work-up of these patients and is being used with increasing frequency. CT evaluation also includes the surrounding structures and the entire peritoneal cavity. Whatever diagnostic pathway is used, multiplanar multidetector CT is usually the eventual imaging choice. MRI is being used with more frequency but is still far behind CT in terms of time, cost, and availability.

Notes

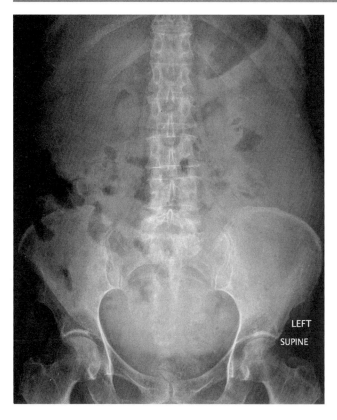

LEFT
SUPINE

History: A 39-year-old woman collapses after complaining of acute abdominal pain and distention.

1. What should be included in the differential diagnosis of the imaging finding shown in the figure? (Choose all that apply.)
   A. Ascites
   B. Adhesions
   C. Uroperitoneum
   D. Hemoperitoneum
   E. Peritoneal metastases

2. This patient with hemoperitoneum had a positive pregnancy test. What is the diagnosis?
   A. Miscarriage
   B. Placenta previa
   C. Molar pregnancy
   D. Ectopic pregnancy

3. What solid organ is most commonly injured by blunt abdominal trauma leading to hemoperitoneum?
   A. Liver
   B. Bowel
   C. Spleen
   D. Pancreas

4. Disease of a retroperitoneal structure does not usually cause free peritoneal fluid. Which of the following diseases of a retroperitoneal viscus frequently produces free peritoneal fluid?
   A. Pancreatitis
   B. Psoas abscess
   C. Renal laceration
   D. Aortic dissection

Hemoperitoneum

1. A, C, D, and E

2. D

3. C

4. A

References

Gore RM, Gore MD: Ascites and peritoneal fluid collections. In Gore RM, Levine MS (eds): *Textbook of Gastrointestinal Radiology*, 2nd ed. Philadelphia: Saunders, 2000, pp 1969-1979.

Lubner M, Menias C, Rucker C, et al: Blood in the belly: CT findings of hemoperitoneum. *Radiographics* 2007;27(1):109-125.

Cross-Reference

Gastrointestinal Imaging: *THE REQUISITES,* 3rd ed, p 132.

Comment

The radiograph shows evidence of free fluid within the abdominal cavity (see figure). Findings include increased density in the pelvis and fluid density in the paracolic gutters between the descending colon and the flank stripe. Fluid within the peritoneal cavity can represent ascites, inflammation, blood, urine, or bile. The appropriate history should be obtained in this situation. Ascites can be the result of various causes and is the most common cause of long-standing fluid accumulation in the abdomen. In the setting of severe symptoms or trauma, all diagnostic possibilities must be considered.

Hemoperitoneum is the most likely cause. In patients who have sustained blunt trauma, the fluid could be the result of laceration of the spleen or the liver. Laceration of bowel or mesentery is less common. Other acute but nontraumatic causes include a ruptured ectopic pregnancy and ruptured blood vessel. A perforated viscus caused by ulceration, inflammation, or trauma usually produces ascitic fluid with little hemorrhage. Urine is another consideration in the setting of trauma, but the only cause is rupture of the bladder. Injury to a retroperitoneal structure almost never causes intraperitoneal bleeding unless it is penetrating. Pancreatitis is the only condition that affects a retroperitoneal structure that produces free intraperitoneal fluid, and this finding occurs only in the setting of acute pancreatitis.

Notes

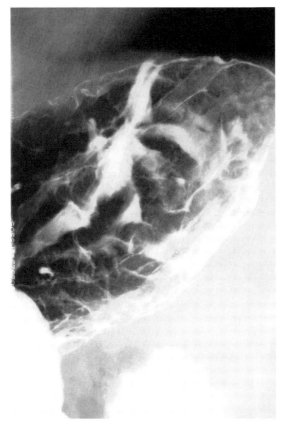

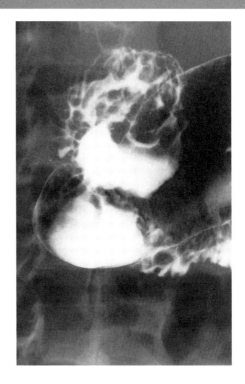

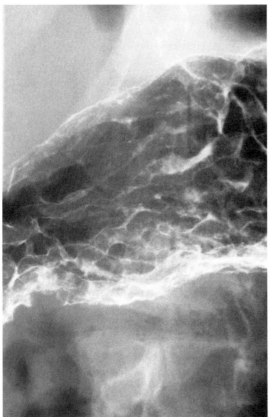

History: A 58-year-old man presents with nausea and dyspepsia.

1. What should be included in the differential diagnosis of the imaging finding shown in the figures? (Choose all that apply.)
   A. Sarcoidosis
   B. Gastric varices
   C. Crohn's gastritis
   D. Ménétrier's disease
   E. Eosinophilic gastritis

2. Which of the following statements regarding Ménétrier's disease is true?
   A. The etiology of Ménétrier's disease is unknown.
   B. Ménétrier's disease progresses to malignancy if uncontrolled.
   C. Ménétrier's disease responds dramatically to steroid treatment.
   D. Fold changes occur only in the proximal stomach.

3. Which of the following statements regarding eosinophilic gastritis is true?
   A. About half of patients have a peripheral eosinophilia.
   B. The small bowel is the most common site of involvement.
   C. There is usually associated colonic disease.
   D. This condition responds well to steroid treatment.

4. Which of the following statements regarding gastric sarcoidosis is true?
   A. There is always associated pulmonary disease.
   B. Gastric involvement is a rare complication of sarcoidosis.
   C. Steroid treatment is valuable for pulmonary disease but not gastric involvement.
   D. The small bowel is the most common site of involvement of the gastrointestinal (GI) tract.

Ménétrier's Disease of the Stomach

1. A, B, D, and E

2. A

3. D

4. A

References

Friedman J, Platnick J, Farruggia S, et al: Ménétrier's disease. *Radiographics* 2009;29(1):297-301.

Tran T, Hung P, Laucirica R, et al: The clinical significance of thickened gastric folds found on upper gastrointestinal series. *J Clin Gastroenterol* 2002;35(2):138-143.

Cross-Reference

Gastrointestinal Imaging: THE REQUISITES, 3rd ed, p 70.

Comment

Thickened gastric folds are a common radiologic finding that can be produced by many unusual disorders. The imaging finding itself is so nonspecific that all of the various disorders cannot be distinguished by their radiologic appearance (see figures).

Ménétrier's disease is a rare condition in which marked glandular hypertrophy of the stomach develops without any underlying cause. There is associated enlargement of the gastric rugae, hypochloremia, and hypoproteinemia. Despite the fact that there is often increased mucus secretion in the stomach, gastric acid output is reduced, which differentiates the disease from other types of hypertrophic gastritis in which acid output is often elevated. Protein-losing enteropathy is another distinguishing characteristic of Ménétrier's disease. Patients often have pain, weight loss, vomiting, and diarrhea. According to the classic description of the disease, the hypertrophic fold changes occur only in the proximal stomach, but it is now known that the thickened folds can be seen throughout the stomach, including the antrum.

Spontaneous remission can occur, but often Ménétrier's disease is a chronic recurrent illness that responds poorly to various therapies (e.g., antibiotics, H2 blockers). In severe cases, gastric resection may be required. There is controversy regarding whether the condition is premalignant. The prevailing thought is that it is not.

In a patient with peripheral eosinophilia and thickened gastric folds, eosinophilic gastritis should be strongly considered. There is often associated small bowel disease in patients with fold thickening. Sarcoidosis of the stomach may be more common than first appreciated; according to some reports, the condition can be identified in 10% of gastric biopsy specimens. With sarcoidosis, there is always associated pulmonary disease, and other portions of the GI tract may be involved. Both of these conditions respond dramatically to steroids, as do a few other gastric conditions.

Notes

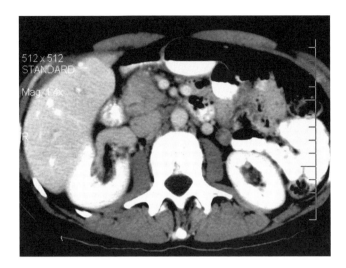
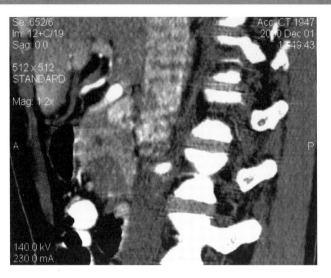

History: A 41-year-old woman presents with abdominal pain.

1. Which of the following should be included in the differential diagnosis of the imaging finding shown in the figures? (Choose all that apply.)
   A. Lymphoma
   B. Pseudoaneurysm
   C. Pancreatic cancer
   D. Lymphadenopathy
   E. Focal acute pancreatitis

2. Which of the following complications of acute pancreatitis usually develops early in the course of the disease?
   A. Abscess
   B. Necrosis
   C. Pseudocyst
   D. Pseudoaneurysm

3. What is the most definitive means to diagnose benign focal pancreatitis in differentiation from pancreatic carcinoma?
   A. Biopsy
   B. MRI scan
   C. PET scan
   D. Follow-up CT

4. Contrast-enhanced CT is the standard imaging modality for evaluating acute pancreatitis and its complications. Which of the following is a contraindication to the performance of a contrast-enhanced CT?
   A. Hepatic insufficiency
   B. The high radiation dose
   C. Allergy to intravenous contrast
   D. When cholelithiasis has not been excluded as the underlying cause

Unusual Presentation of Acute Pancreatitis

1. A, C, D, and E

2. B

3. D

4. C

References

Balthazar EJ, Freeny PC, van Sonnenberg E: Imaging and intervention in acute pancreatitis. *Radiology* 1994;193:297-306.

Neff CC, Simeone JF, Wittenberg J, et al: Inflammatory pancreatic masses. Problems in differentiating focal pancreatitis from carcinoma. *Radiology* 1984;150:35-38.

Cross-Reference

Gastrointestinal Imaging: *THE REQUISITES,* 3rd ed, p 154.

Comment

Acute pancreatitis has a variety of imaging presentations, including disease seemingly limited to the pancreatic head, as seen in this case. In most cases, more of the gland is involved with edema, and hemorrhage and necrosis occur in a few patients. Necrosis and sepsis constitute the leading causes of death in acute pancreatitis.

Most acute pancreatitis involving the pancreatic head can have a very adverse effect on the biliary system, compressing the common bile duct just as a pancreatic malignant mass might. However, that is not always the case, as with this patient. These lesions always present a dilemma and are often biopsied to rule out carcinoma. About 25% to 30% of all cases of pancreatitis manifest with findings limited to the pancreatic head (see figures). Gallstones passing through the shared ampulla of Vater can also give rise to inflammatory changes in the pancreatic head as well as throughout the entire gland. The stone does always have to be present. Some stones lodge, cause havoc with pancreatic drainage, and then pass. More than 80% of patients with gallstone pancreatitis have stones detected in stool. However, most of these have accompanying bile duct obstruction and some degree of distal pancreatic duct obstruction. In this case, the lack of biliary involvement and the normal distal pancreas suggest an inflammatory origin. A calcification in the ampulla of Vater would seal the diagnosis.

In rare instances, pancreatic carcinoma manifests as acute pancreatitis. When there is no etiologic basis for acute pancreatitis in a middle-aged or older adult, cancer is a consideration.

Notes

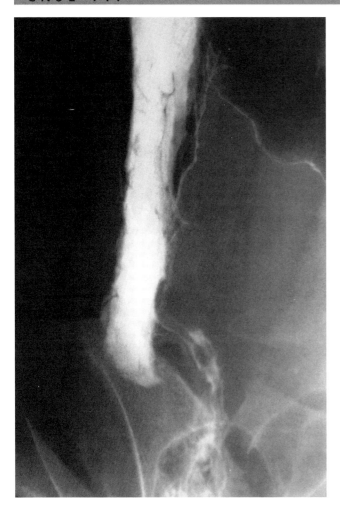

History: A 75-year-old man presents with bloody diarrhea.

1. Which of the following should be included in the differential diagnosis of the imaging finding shown in the figure? (Choose all that apply.)
   A. Cancer
   B. Amebiasis
   C. Tuberculosis
   D. Crohn's disease
   E. Intussusception

2. Which of the following statements regarding colonic amebiasis is true?
   A. Usually involves the left colon
   B. Typically involves the terminal ileum
   C. Usually appears as a diffuse ulcerative colitis
   D. Sometimes occurs as a short masslike narrow segment

3. What is the typical change produced by ulcerative colitis in the terminal ileum?
   A. Dilated gaping terminal ileum
   B. Narrowing, nodular mucosa, fissures, and fistulas
   C. Asymmetrical luminal narrowing with spiculated contour
   D. Mucosal nodularity with fold thickening and superficial ulceration

4. What fungal infection can produce this abnormality?
   A. Actinomycosis
   B. Blastomycosis
   C. Candidiasis
   D. Histoplasmosis

Colonic Amebiasis

1. A, B, C, and D

2. D

3. A

4. B

References

Cardoso JM, Kimura K, Stoopen M, et al: Radiology of invasive amebiasis of the colon. *Am J Roentgenol* 1977;128:935-941.

Kimura K, Stoopen M, Reeder MM, et al: Amebiasis: modern diagnostic imaging with pathological and clinical correlation. *Semin Roentgenol* 1997;32:250-275.

Rogers WF, Ralls PW, Boswell WD, et al: Amebiasis: unusual radiographic manifestations. *Am J Roentgenol* 1980;135:1253-1257.

Cross-Reference

Gastrointestinal Imaging: *THE REQUISITES,* 3rd ed, p 299.

Comment

The coned appearance of the cecum is produced by several diseases, most of which are inflammatory in nature. In determining the exact cause, the radiologist must make a proper evaluation of the region. The most common causative condition encountered in industrialized societies is Crohn's disease. Tuberculosis can manifest with an appearance virtually identical to that of Crohn's disease, with a coned cecum and inflammation of the terminal ileum. Adjacent inflammatory conditions, such as appendicitis and diverticulitis, are considerations.

Amebiasis is an infection of the bowel produced by the protozoan *Entamoeba histolytica.* It is acquired by ingestion of water or soil that contains the cysts. When infection occurs, it can range from very mild or indolent to severe, acute colitis. When cysts spread to the liver or lungs, they can produce abscesses. Changes in the colon include ulceration, which can be either diffuse granularity, collar-button ulcers, or aphthous ulcers. The colon can have skip lesions, with intervening areas of normal bowel, and thus can resemble Crohn's disease. Focal severe inflammation can mimic annular carcinomas. There also may be pronounced granulation tissue, leading to protuberant lesions called amebomas, which can also mimic neoplasia.

The cecum is invariably infected in amebiasis, and the classic appearance is that of the coned cecum (see figure). This abnormality is often seen in the chronic stages of colitis. One strong differential consideration is that amebiasis does not affect the terminal ileum, as do Crohn's disease and tuberculosis. However, amebiasis is seen predominantly in underdeveloped countries and should be considered only if the history is appropriate.

Neoplasms, such as adenocarcinoma and lymphoma, are also in the differential diagnosis. Long-standing ulcerative colitis can produce a coned cecum but often with a dilated terminal ileum, called backwash ileitis. Other rare conditions that can produce this appearance include anisakiasis, blastomycosis, and infection by *Yersinia* species.

Notes

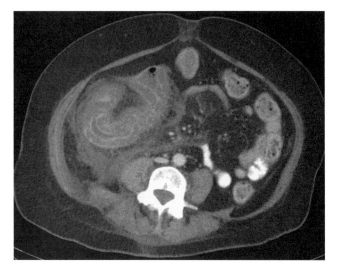

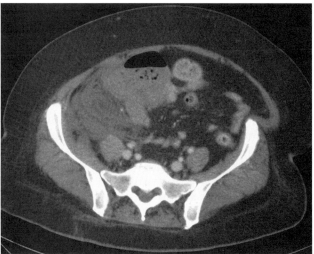

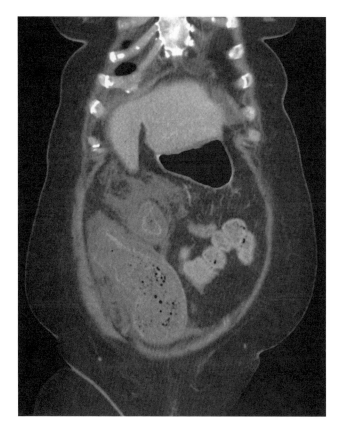

History: A 62-year-old woman presents with abdominal pain that is worse on the right.

1. Which of the following should be included in the differential diagnosis of the imaging finding shown in the figures? (Choose all that apply.)
   A. Typhlitis
   B. Ischemia
   C. Cecal volvulus
   D. Crohn's disease
   E. Pseudomembranous colitis

2. Which of the following statements regarding the epidemiology of typhlitis is true?
   A. Mortality rate of nearly 50%
   B. Predominantly affects female patients
   C. Increased risk with increased age
   D. Most commonly recognized in patients with lymphoma

3. Which of the following statements regarding the investigation of typhlitis is true?
   A. If typhlitis is suspected, colonoscopy is warranted.
   B. CT is the most sensitive modality to detect typhlitis.
   C. Barium enema is useful to assess extent of disease.
   D. The presence of pneumatosis makes typhlitis unlikely.

4. Most inflammatory diseases of the colon demonstrate bowel wall thickening on cross-sectional imaging such as CT. Which is the exception?
   A. Ischemia
   B. Diverticulitis
   C. Epiploic appendagitis
   D. Pseudomembranous colitis

CASE 118

Typhlitis of the Cecum

1. A, B, D, and E

2. A

3. B

4. C

References

Cronin TG, Calandra JD, Del Fava RL: Typhlitis presenting as toxic cecitis. *Radiology* 1981;138:29-30.
Thoeni RF, Cello JP: CT imaging of colitis. *Radiology* 2006;240:623-638.
Vowels M: Typhlitis: neutropaenic colitis. *Australas Radiol* 1988;32:477-479.

Cross-Reference

Gastrointestinal Imaging: *THE REQUISITES,* 3rd ed, p 313.

Comment

Neutropenic colitis, or typhlitis, is an inflammatory condition of the right side of the colon that occurs in patients undergoing treatment for leukemia, lymphoma, and sometimes other malignancies. Typically this condition affects the pediatric population, but in some instances it is encountered in the adult population. The clinical findings include fever, abdominal pain, and sometimes diarrhea. CT is the diagnostic modality of choice, demonstrating thickened bowel wall (sometimes with pneumatosis) and pericolic inflammatory changes in the mesenteric fat (see figures). These changes in the bowel are the result of a combination of edema, hemorrhage, and inflammatory exudate. Neoplastic involvement is not a feature of the disease.

The history of a compromised immune system immediately makes neutropenic colitis the primary diagnostic consideration. Interestingly, the treatment of neutropenic colitis is primarily aggressive antibiotic treatment. Surgery is necessary only for patients with obvious perforation and abscess development. Most patients respond well to antibiotics and supportive treatment and do not require surgery.

Notes

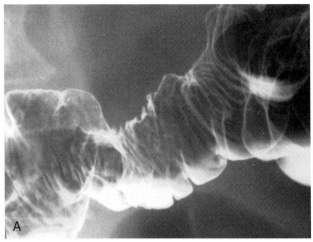
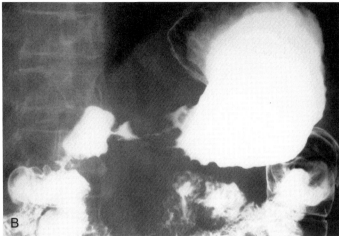

History: A 55-year-old man presents with 2 months of anorexia, nausea, vomiting, and stool test positive for blood.

1. Which of the following should be included in the differential diagnosis of the imaging finding shown in Figure A? (Choose all that apply.)
   A. Metastatic pancreatic malignancy
   B. Metastatic gastric malignancy
   C. Crohn's disease
   D. Villous adenoma
   E. Endometriosis

2. What is the specific component of the omentum that allows spread of cancer from the stomach to the transverse colon?
   A. Lesser omentum
   B. Greater omentum
   C. Gastro-colic ligament
   D. Transverse mesocolon

3. What is the most common tumor of the omentum?
   A. Lymphoma
   B. Mesothelioma
   C. Metastatic melanoma
   D. Metastatic ovarian cancer

4. Which of the following is the most common finding on physical examination indicating metastatic gastric cancer?
   A. Irish node
   B. Virchow's node
   C. Gastrocolic fistula
   D. Sister Mary Joseph's node

Spread of Gastric Carcinoma to the Colon via the Gastrocolic Ligament

1. A, B, C, and E

2. C

3. D

4. B

References

Meyers MA, Oliphant M, Berne AS, Feldberg MAM: The peritoneal ligaments and mesenteries: pathways of intraabdominal spread of disease. *Radiology* 1987;163:593-604.
Sompayrac SW, Mindelzun RE, Silverman PM, Sze R: The greater omentum. *Am J Roentgenol* 1997;168:683.

Cross-Reference

Gastrointestinal Imaging: *THE REQUISITES,* 3rd ed, p 290.

Comment

The "police officer" of the abdomen, the greater omentum (mostly made up of the gastrocolic ligament), encloses the lesser sac anteriorly; the posterior margin is the transverse mesocolon. A small connection between the lesser sac and the peritoneal cavity is located in the region of the duodenum, the epiploic foramen or foramen of Winslow. Processes affecting the lesser curvature of the stomach are therefore able to reach the transverse colon via the gastrocolic ligament, and it would manifest as serosal involvement along the course of the transverse colon, giving the characteristic crenulated margin, as seen in the barium image (see figures).

Peritoneal spread via lymphatics and drop metastases are more common than spread down the gastrocolic ligament. However, there are reports of metastatic disease to the stomach (i.e., melanoma) as well as primary gallbladder carcinoma spreading to the colon via the gastrocolic ligament. However, these are rare, and the first consideration should be the stomach (see figures).

Worldwide, gastric carcinoma is said to be the second most common malignancy after lung cancer, but there has been a significant drop in the incidence in the Western world since the 1980s. In general, the long-accepted "pathway" theory—chronic gastritis, diminished acidity, gastric atrophy, metaplasia, dysplasia, and cancer—is still considered valid. But the pathway may be influenced by several other factors such as *Helicobacter pylori* infection, dietary habits (smoked foods), and of course, long-term cigarette smoking.

Notes

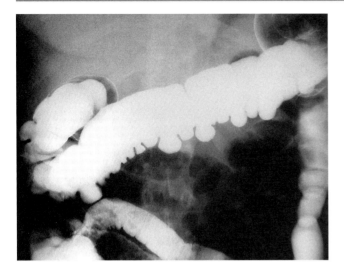

History: A 38-year-old woman presents with diarrhea.

1. Which of the following should be included in the differential diagnosis of the imaging finding shown in the figure? (Choose all that apply.)
   A. Scleroderma
   B. Diverticulosis
   C. Crohn's disease
   D. Previous radiation
   E. Previous ischemia

2. Which of the following lesions of the gastrointestinal tract are "true" diverticula?
   A. Sacculations of scleroderma
   B. Jejunal diverticulosis
   C. Zenker's diverticulum
   D. Colonic diverticula

3. What is the most common gastrointestinal tract site of involvement by scleroderma?
   A. Esophagus
   B. Stomach
   C. Small bowel
   D. Colon

4. Which of the following is the least common complication of colonic scleroderma?
   A. Diarrhea
   B. Constipation
   C. Incontinence
   D. Rectal prolapse

Colonic Scleroderma

1. A, C, D, and E

2. A

3. A

4. A

References

Cohen S, Laufer I, Snape WJ Jr, et al: The gastrointestinal manifestations of scleroderma: pathogenesis and management. *Gastroenterology* 1980;79:155-166.

Rohrmann CA, Ricci MT, Krishnamurthy S, Schuffler MD: Radiologic and histologic differentiation of neuromuscular disorders of the gastrointestinal tract: visceral myopathies, visceral neuropathies, and progressive systemic sclerosis. *Am J Roentgenol* 1981;143:933-941.

Cross-Reference

Gastrointestinal Imaging: THE REQUISITES, 3rd ed, p 312.

Comment

The presence of large wide-mouth sacculations in the colon can be an indication of several diseases (see figure). Many term these wide-mouth diverticula pseudodiverticula because they are not related to the typical diverticula seen in everyday practice. However, they contain all three layers of bowel and thus represent true diverticula. The small diverticula seen in everyday practice are not true diverticula. These large-mouth diverticula or sacculations occur when there is eccentric involvement of the bowel wall by some process, producing fibrosis on one side, with eccentric bulging of the opposite wall.

A variety of processes can result in the loss of the haustral folds, but only some produce the eccentric diverticula. These processes include scleroderma, Crohn's disease, and laxative abuse. Scleroderma does not involve the colon as commonly as it does other portions of the gastrointestinal tract. Just as it does in other portions of the gastrointestinal tract, however, scleroderma of the colon produces patchy smooth muscle atrophy along with fibrotic replacement of the muscle. This effect leads to the formation of wide-mouth sacculations at weakened areas. There are also abnormalities of transit time, and patients often complain of constipation. The haustral fold pattern is often diminished. Fecal impaction is a complication, and patients can develop benign pneumatosis, which could be the result of a combination of steroid therapy and stasis in the colon.

An interesting feature of these wide-mouth sacculations is their ability to retain material. They fail to contract and empty and are found outside the fecal stream in the colon. Thus, develop impacted fecal material or fecaliths sometimes develop within sacculations. These fecaliths can become adherent and resemble polyps or tumors on barium enema studies. Although scleroderma can result in colonic sacculations, the classic hide-bound appearance of scleroderma is limited to small bowel involvement. Fibrosis in the wall and folds of the small bowel give rise to this unusual appearance of atrophic folds, seemingly pulled tightly together by the disease. This should not be confused with the "stack of coins" appearance of small bowel intramural hemorrhage in which the folds show no effacement.

Notes

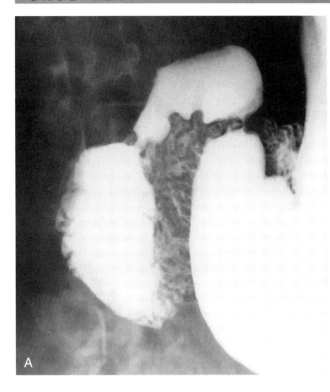

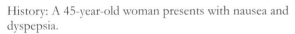

A

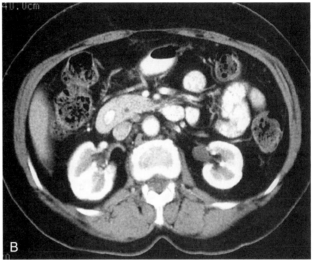

B

History: A 45-year-old woman presents with nausea and dyspepsia.

1. Which of the following should be included in the differential diagnosis of the imaging finding shown in Figure A? (Choose all that apply.)
   A. Peptic scarring
   B. Superior mesenteric artery (SMA) syndrome
   C. Crohn's disease
   D. Annular pancreas
   E. Duodenal diaphragm

2. What is the *most* common presentation of annular pancreas?
   A. Cancer
   B. Jaundice
   C. Pancreatitis
   D. Duodenal obstruction

3. Which of the following statements regarding imaging of annular pancreas is true?
   A. A radiologically incomplete annulus will not result in obstruction.
   B. Pancreas divisum is present in about 3% of patients with annular pancreas.

C. On magnetic resonance cholangiopancreatography (MRCP) or endoscopic retrograde cholangiopancreatography (ERCP), the annulus duct usually drains separately from the main pancreatic duct into the duodenum.
D. The presence of visible pancreatic tissue posterior and lateral to the descending duodenum is diagnostic of annular pancreas.

4. What portion of the embryologic pancreas becomes the uncinate process?
   A. Body
   B. Head
   C. Dorsal
   D. Ventral

Annular Pancreas

1. A, C, D, and E

2. D

3. D

4. D

References

Jayaraman MV, Mayo-Smith WM, Movson JS, et al: CT of the duodenum: an overlooked segment gets its due. *Radiographics* 2001;21:S147-S160.
Sandrasegaran K, Patel A, Fogel EL, et al: Annular pancreas in adults. *Am J Roentgenol* 2009;193:455-460.

Cross-Reference

Gastrointestinal Imaging: *THE REQUISITES,* 3rd ed, p 152.

Comment

The embryologic development of the pancreas is complex and can lead to a variety of anomalies. Some are of no clinical significance, whereas others may present difficulties early or later in life. The pancreas forms as two distinct buds off the biliary or hepatic bud, which comes from the midgut. These buds are the ventral and dorsal pancreatic buds. The dorsal pancreatic bud is to the left of the midline and eventually forms the body and tail of the pancreas. The ventral bud develops to the right of the duodenum. It must rotate, along with the duodenum, to the left. After the ventral and dorsal buds fuse, this ventral bud becomes the head and uncinate process of the pancreas. Failure of fusion results in pancreatic divisum.

Annular pancreas occurs when there is abnormal rotation of the ventral pancreas or the duodenum, both of which must rotate for proper pancreatic positioning. Some believe that the ventral bud adheres to the duodenum, so that as the structures rotate, the ventral pancreas develops and grows around the duodenum rather than in its normal position (see figures). The ventral duct continues to drain into the major papilla and joins with the biliary system, which is its normal embryologic anatomy.

The major pancreatic complication of annular pancreas is the development of acute or chronic pancreatitis. This condition may affect as many as one quarter of patients with annular pancreas. Also, the annular pancreas produces duodenal narrowing or obstruction to varying degrees. About half of the cases of annular pancreas manifest in the neonatal period with duodenal symptoms. There may be other associated anomalies in the neonate as well. If the condition persists until adulthood, the annular pancreas may be discovered incidentally or when symptoms of pancreatitis or duodenal obstruction occur. These patients may become jaundiced as well. Surgery is necessary to correct the condition.

Notes

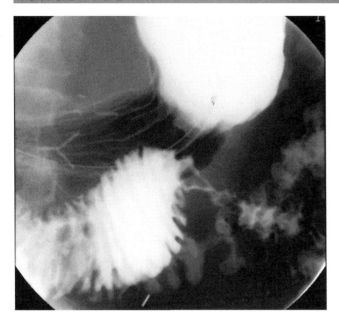

History: A 64-year-old woman presents with nausea and vomiting.

1. What should be included in the differential diagnosis of the imaging finding shown in the figure? (Choose all that apply.)
   A. Lymphoma
   B. Primary cancer
   C. Crohn's disease
   D. Postbulbar ulcer
   E. Metastatic cancer

2. What is the most common primary malignancy of the duodenum?
   A. Carcinoid
   B. Lymphoma
   C. Adenocarcinoma
   D. Malignant stromal tumor

3. What is the most common location of duodenal carcinoma?
   A. Bulbar
   B. Descending
   C. Transverse
   D. Ascending

4. Which of the following diseases places a patient at greatest risk of developing duodenal carcinoma?
   A. Celiac disease
   B. Crohn's disease
   C. Neurofibromatosis
   D. Gardner's syndrome

Duodenal Primary Cancer

1. A, B, C, and E

2. C

3. B

4. D

References

Bradford D, Levine MS, Hoang D, et al: Early duodenal cancer: detection on double-contrast upper gastrointestinal radiography. *Am J Roentgenol* 2000;174(6):1564-1566.

Kim JH, Kim MJ, Chung JJ, et al: Differential diagnosis of periampullary carcinomas at MR imaging. *Radiographics* 2002;22(6):1335-1352.

Cross-Reference

Gastrointestinal Imaging: *THE REQUISITES,* 3rd ed, p 91.

Comment

Primary adenocarcinoma, such as shown in this case (see figure), is uncommon. It is thought to represent 0.3% of all malignancies of the GI tract. Most patients are slow to seek medical attention because the lesion is insidious and the symptoms are nonspecific, and it is often fatal by the time of diagnosis. In one study, the diagnosis was made after death in 25% of cases. At least 50% of patients have metastatic disease at the time of diagnosis. With the increased use of widespread endoscopy and abdominal CT examinations, this percentage should have improved in the last 15 years. However, whether increased use of these imaging examinations has affected long-term survival rates is still unclear. The incidence of primary adenocarcinoma of the duodenum is increased in patients with Gardner's familial polyposis, as is the incidence of adenoma. The more proximal the lesion is located, the earlier a diagnosis is made, and survival is improved. These patients may also present with biliary symptoms.

Notes

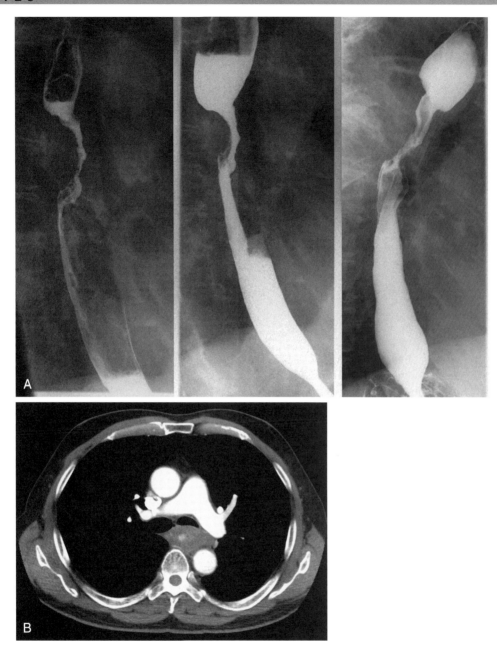

History: A 71-year-old man has a 16-month history of suprasternal dysphagia, which is worse with solids; the dysphagia has been worse in the last 8 months, now requiring food to be chewed to a puree consistency.

1. What should be included in the differential diagnosis of the imaging finding shown in Figure A? (Choose all that apply.)
   A. Radiation
   B. Metastasis
   C. Carcinoma
   D. Stromal tumor
   E. Crohn's disease

2. Endoscopic biopsy confirms a malignant lesion. Which one of the following is most likely?
   A. Adenocarcinoma
   B. Barrett carcinoma

   C. Malignant lymphoma
   D. Squamous cell carcinoma

3. With a diagnosis of esophageal squamous cell carcinoma, what is the best choice of imaging modality to assist in therapeutic planning?
   A. MRI
   B. Bronchoscopy and biopsy
   C. CT
   D. Endoscopic ultrasound

4. Which finding relevant to CT tumor staging is shown in figure 2?
   A. Aortic invasion
   B. Bronchial invasion
   C. Cardiac invasion
   D. Vertebral invasion

Esophageal Squamous Cell Carcinoma

1. A, B, C, and E

2. D

3. C

4. B

References

Iyer R, Dubrow R: Imaging upper gastrointestinal malignancy. *Semin Roentgenol* 2006;41(2):105-112.

Levine MS: Esophageal cancer: radiologic diagnosis. *Radiol Clin North Am* 1997;35(2):265-279.

Cross-Reference

Gastrointestinal Imaging: *THE REQUISITES,* 3rd ed, p 23.

Comment

Most esophageal cancers in Western countries are squamous cell carcinomas. Until the middle of the 20th century, squamous cell carcinomas accounted for more than 90% of esophageal malignancies. The other common tumor is adenocarcinoma, which has increased in frequency in recent decades so that the prevalence of the two primary esophageal tumors is now more equal.

The diagnosis of esophageal cancer is suggested on barium swallow by various appearances. Early esophageal cancer may appear as a superficial plaque or ulceration. Advanced disease is seen as a stricture, a mass, a circumferential infiltration, or an ulceration (see figures).

Prognosis for a patient with esophageal cancer is poor. Accurate staging is required for prognosis and therapeutic planning. Stage I disease is associated with 5-year survival rates of 60% to 70%; stage II disease, 40% to 50%; stage III disease, 15% to 25%; and stage IV disease, less than 10%. The TNM (tumor, node, metastasis) staging system is widely used. Accurate T classification is particularly important to determine tumor resectability. T4 tumors invading local structures are subclassified as T4a or T4b. T4a tumors, which have invaded structures such as pleura, pericardium, or diaphragm, are resectable. T4b tumors are unresectable, having invaded aorta, vertebral body, or trachea or bronchus (see figures).

Notes

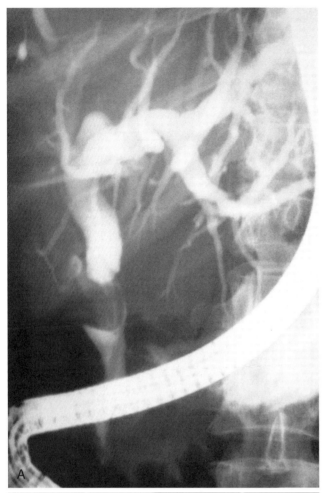

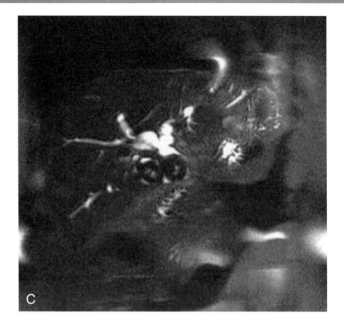

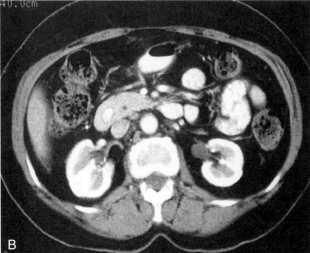

History: A 54-year-old woman presents with right upper quadrant pain, jaundice, and fever.

1. What should be included in the differential diagnosis of the imaging finding shown in Figure A? (Choose all that apply.)
   A. Mirizzi's syndrome
   B. Lymphadenopathy
   C. Bouveret's syndrome
   D. Cholangiocarcinoma
   E. Gallbladder carcinoma

2. What is the mechanism of Mirizzi's syndrome?
   A. A gallstone eroded into the common hepatic duct
   B. A gallstone passed into the common bile duct
   C. A gallstone impacted in the cystic duct
   D. A gallstone eroded into the duodenum

3. What major iatrogenic complication is associated with this condition?
   A. Surgical ligation of the common hepatic duct
   B. Cholecystoduodenal fistula formation
   C. Perforation of the gallbladder
   D. Portal vein thrombosis

4. What is the most common cause of obstructive jaundice?
   A. Viral hepatitis
   B. Choledocholithiasis
   C. Cholangiocarcinoma
   D. Pancreatic carcinoma

Mirizzi's Syndrome

1. A, B, D, and E

2. C

3. A

4. B

References

Becker CD, Hassler H, Terrie F: Preoperative diagnosis of the Mirizzi syndrome: limitations of sonography and computed tomography. *AJR Am J Roentgenol* 1984;143(3):591-596.

Cruz FO, Barriga P, Tocornal J, et al: Radiology of the Mirizzi syndrome: diagnostic importance of the transhepatic cholangiogram. *Gastrointest Radiol* 1983;8(3):249-253.

Cross-Reference

Gastrointestinal Imaging: *THE REQUISITES,* 3rd ed, p 231.

Comment

Mirizzi's syndrome is an uncommon condition that occurs when a stone becomes impacted in the cystic duct or neck of the gallbladder. This type of impaction is very common, but in Mirizzi's syndrome a severe local inflammatory response occurs. The affected area is critical because there are several ducts and crossing vessels in the region. The inflammatory response produces a mass or tumor effect in the area. The inflammatory mass impinges on the common hepatic and bile ducts, producing varying degrees of narrowing or obstruction. The intrahepatic bile ducts may become dilated proximal to the obstruction. Secondary involvement of the major vessels in the area can occur. There is also associated cholecystitis because the gallbladder is now obstructed.

The major concern for physicians encountering this condition is not the inflammation itself but the difficulty in making an appropriate diagnosis and performing corrective surgery. With the inflammatory mass effect and the bile duct dilation, the condition may mimic a neoplasm of either the gallbladder or the bile ducts (see figures). Adenopathy may have a similar appearance. These changes are most confusing on endoscopic retrograde cholangiopancreatography (ERCP).

Prompt surgical intervention is typically warranted. For the surgeon, the difficulty arises in identifying and isolating the correct ducts. Often the common hepatic duct is mistaken for the cystic duct, and ligation of the common hepatic duct ensues, producing disastrous complications. When possible, a stent can be placed in the extrahepatic ducts at ERCP to help identify them for the surgeon. The syndrome is named for Mirizzi, an Argentinian physician who described it in 1948.

Notes

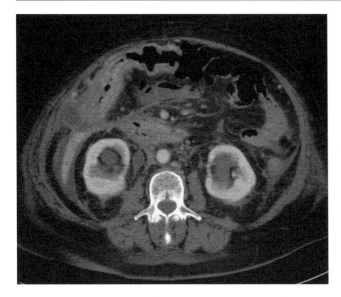

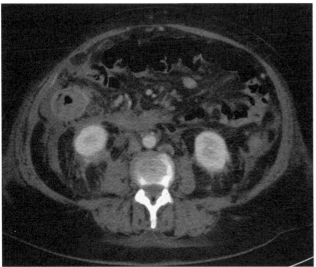

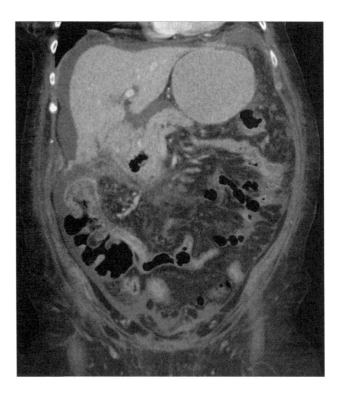

History: A 68-year-old woman presents with right upper quadrant abdominal pain of 4 weeks' duration associated with nausea and vomiting.

1. What should be included in the differential diagnosis of the imaging finding shown in the figures? (Choose all that apply.)
   A. Metastatic carcinoma
   B. Crohn's disease
   C. Colon carcinoma
   D. Pneumatosis coli
   E. Ischemic colitis

2. What is the most common origin of hematogenous metastases to the colon?
   A. Melanoma
   B. Lung carcinoma
   C. Breast carcinoma
   D. Gastric carcinoma

3. What is the most common site of metastatic disease to the gastrointestinal (GI) tract from a breast cancer primary?
   A. Colon
   B. Stomach
   C. Esophagus
   D. Small bowel

4. Lobular carcinoma is the most common type of breast carcinoma to metastasize to the GI tract. What is the most common morphology of these lesions?
   A. Perforation
   B. Linitis plastica
   C. Aneurysmal dilation
   D. Submucosal nodules

Metastatic Disease to the Colon

1. A, B, C, and E

2. C

3. B

4. B

References

Cifuentes N, Pickren JW: Metastases from carcinoma of mammary gland: an autopsy study. *J Surg Oncol* 1979;11(3):193-205.

Kim SY, Kim KW, Kim AY, et al: Bloodborne metastatic tumors to the gastrointestinal tract: CT findings with clinicopathologic correlation. *AJR Am J Roentgenol* 2006;186(6):1618-1626.

Rubesin SE, Furth EE: Other tumors of the colon. In Gore RM, Levine MS (eds): *Textbook of Gastrointestinal Radiology*, 2nd ed. Philadelphia: Saunders, 2000, pp 1049-1074.

Cross-Reference

Gastrointestinal Imaging: THE REQUISITES, 3rd ed, p 290.

Comment

Breast cancer is the most common malignant lesion in women. Metastatic disease is common; most secondary spread involves the bone, liver, lungs, brain, adrenals, and pleural or peritoneal cavities. Metastatic disease can result in serosal invasion of the colon, which is well known. However, a very few spread to the gut directly. The most common site for the direct spread of breast carcinoma is the stomach. It can appear as metastatic masses, sometimes with ulceration giving the "bull's eye" lesion of the stomach. In other cases, spread can be infiltrative in the stomach, and this is one of the causes of linitis plastica.

Direct spread to the colon is rare. When it does occur, it has the same manifestation as seen in the stomach. There can be one mass or several masses, or the metastasis can manifest as an infiltrative mural process such as in this case. The wall of the cecum is thickened. The infiltrative involvement of the ileocecal valve has resulted in an unusual presentation in this case. The CT images also clearly show the small bowel obstruction that gave rise to this patient's abdominal complaints.

Most malignant lesions of the breast are of the ductal infiltrative type. A smaller number, 10% to 12%, are lobular carcinomas. Some investigators believe that the lobular types are more likely to metastasize, and the lobular type almost always results in the uncommon direct metastatic spread to sites in the GI tract such as the stomach and colon. Colonic spread is said to occur in more than 5% of breast carcinomas (see figures). However, this number may include serosal spread as well as direct spread. There are several cases in the literature of direct spread to the colon masquerading as primary colon carcinoma.

Notes

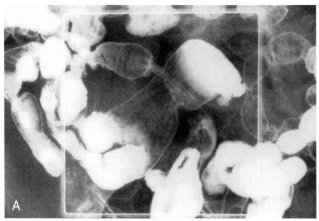

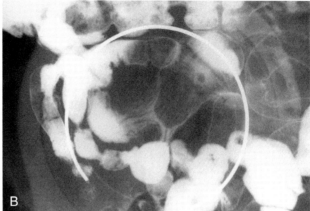

History: A 26-year-old woman presents with a 1-year history of dyspepsia, nausea, vomiting, dark stools, and diarrhea.

1. What should be included in the differential diagnosis of the imaging finding shown in Figure A? (Choose all that apply.)
   A. Scleroderma
   B. Ileal dysgenesis
   C. Urachal diverticulum
   D. Meckel's diverticulum
   E. Postsurgical deformity

2. Which of the following statements about Meckel's diverticula is true?
   A. If a Meckel's diverticulum is symptomatic, the most common manifestation is obstruction.
   B. Meckel's diverticula can contain ectopic pancreatic tissue.
   C. Meckel's diverticula are more common in women.
   D. Of Meckel's diverticula, 80% are asymptomatic.

3. Which of the following statements about the imaging findings of Meckel's diverticula is *false*?
   A. A Meckel's diverticulum may appear on CT scan as an elongated ileal polyp.
   B. Plain radiographs visualize about 50% of Meckel's enteroliths.
   C. A persistent vitelline artery on angiography is diagnostic.
   D. An inverted diverticulum has a "picket fence" appearance on enteroclysis.

4. Which of the following statements about the scintigraphic diagnosis of Meckel's diverticula is true?
   A. The administered agent (^{99m}Tc pertechnetate) is specifically taken up by gastric mucosa only.
   B. Of Meckel's diverticula, 90% contain gastric mucosa allowing scintigraphic detection.
   C. Pentagastrin and glucagon are useful.
   D. Cimetidine increases tracer secretion.

Meckel's Diverticulum

1. A, B, D, and E

2. B

3. D

4. C

References

Elsayes KM, Menias CO, Harvin HJ, et al: Imaging manifestations of Meckel's diverticulum. *AJR Am J Roentgenol* 2007;189(1):81-88.

Herlinger H, Maglinte DDT, Birnbaum B: *Clinical Imaging of the Small Intestine,* 2nd ed. New York: Springer-Verlag, 1999, pp 235-239.

Cross-Reference

Gastrointestinal Imaging: *THE REQUISITES,* 3rd ed, p 142.

Comment

Meckel's diverticulum is the most common congenital anomaly of the intestines; it occurs in 3% of the population. Meckel's diverticulum represents incomplete obliteration of the omphalomesenteric duct (also called vitelline duct), which is an embryologic structure. Most Meckel's diverticula do not cause symptoms. However, almost half of these diverticula contain gastric mucosa that may be functional and may produce pain, ulceration, and bleeding (see figures). Meckel's diverticulum scan, in which ^{99m}Tc pertechnetate is used and is taken up by the gastric mucosa, can detect areas of ectopic gastric mucosa. However, this test is not always reliable. Other complications of Meckel's diverticula include obstruction caused by either invagination and intussusceptions or formation of a large enterolith. Malignancy is rarely encountered.

Enteroliths are rare, forming in less than 10% of cases of symptomatic Meckel's diverticula, and do not always calcify. When they do calcify, enteroliths may produce bleeding or obstruction. Major differential considerations include a gallstone that has eroded into the gastrointestinal tract, the so-called gallstone ileus syndrome, or a calcified appendicolith.

Notes

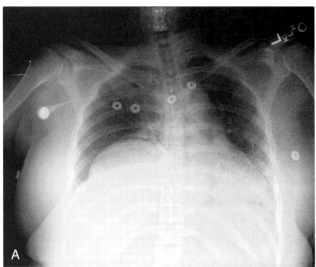

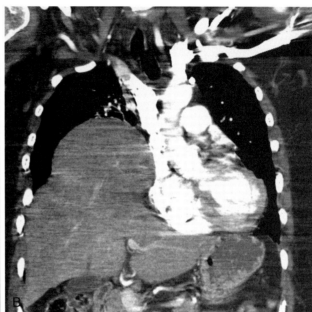

History: A woman was involved in a high-speed motor vehicle accident.

1. What should be included in the differential diagnosis of the imaging finding shown in Figure A? (Choose all that apply.)
   A. Pleural mass
   B. Phrenic nerve injury
   C. Diaphragmatic rupture
   D. Right lower lobe collapse
   E. Loculated pleural effusion

2. What is the common perception error in right-sided rupture?
   A. Mistaken for right basal contusion
   B. Mistaken for right pleural effusion
   C. Mistaken for right lower lobe collapse
   D. Mistaken for elevation or eventration of the intact hemidiaphragm

3. Which of the following statements regarding blunt traumatic diaphragmatic injury is true?
   A. Injury is usually a small linear tear.
   B. Most are posterolateral and radial.
   C. Injury usually involves the peripheral diaphragm.
   D. Right diaphragm rupture is more common than left.

4. What other visceral injury occurs most commonly with left diaphragmatic injury?
   A. Aorta
   B. Liver
   C. Spleen
   D. Stomach

Diaphragmatic Rupture with the Liver in the Chest

1. A, B, C, and E

2. D

3. B

4. C

References

Eren S, Kantarci M, Okur A: Imaging of diaphragmatic rupture after trauma. *Clin Radiol* 2006;61(6):467-477.

Van Hise M, Primack S: CT in blunt chest trauma: indications and limitations. *Radiographics* 1998;18(5):1071-1084.

Cross-Reference

Gastrointestinal Imaging: THE REQUISITES, 3rd ed, p 326.

Comment

Most diaphragmatic ruptures are not as dramatic as the one shown in this case. This patient was involved in a high-speed motor collision. The supine portable image of the chest ought to arouse suspicion immediately because of what appears to be a high, rounded right-sided diaphragm (see figures). CT is the examination of choice (see figures), but it can miss small diaphragmatic tears. The likelihood of a diaphragmatic tear is eight times greater on the left side compared with the right side. It is believed that the liver absorbs some of the traumatic shock that would have been otherwise transmitted in its entirety to the diaphragm.

Although autopsy results put the incidence of diaphragmatic rupture at 5% to 6%, it is much lower clinically and radiologically. The reasons are that many of the patients die before reaching the hospital and the diagnosis is often difficult, even with CT. When discovered, a diaphragmatic tear should be surgically repaired. Most tears result in bowel in the lower chest, and the risk of future bowel obstruction, ischemia, or gastric volvulus is increased; this is generally applicable to right-sided tears as well. Almost every practicing radiologist has examined patients with bowel and in some cases liver in their chest who have no complaints relative to that finding. It is more than an "incidental" finding and should be handled as a significant finding. Other CT findings include discontinuation of the diaphragmatic stripe; this should be evaluated in cases of blunt severe abdominal trauma, especially so if a liver laceration is identified.

Notes

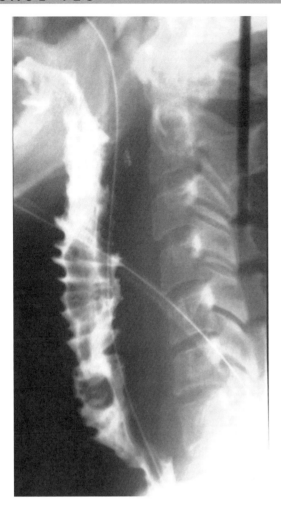

History: A 47-year-old woman presents with dysphagia.

1. What should be included in the differential diagnosis of the imaging finding shown in the figure? (Choose all that apply.)
   A. Esophagectomy
   B. Crohn's disease
   C. Feline esophagus
   D. Severe esophagitis
   E. Corrugated esophagus

2. What is the most common surgical technique used for the management of esophageal carcinoma?
   A. Bypass with colonic conduit
   B. McKeown procedure
   C. Ivor Lewis procedure
   D. Jejunal interposition

3. What is the most common intraoperative complication of esophagectomy?
   A. Anastomotic leak
   B. Acid reflux disease
   C. Tracheobronchial tree injury
   D. Recurrent laryngeal nerve injury

4. The most common nonmalignant reason for performing an esophagectomy in a pediatric patient is esophageal atresia. Which is the most common of the types of esophageal atresia (EA), often associated with a tracheoesophageal fistula (TEF)?
   A. EA without TEF
   B. EA with proximal TEF
   C. EA with distal TEF
   D. EA with proximal and distal TEF

Esophagectomy with Small Bowel Transposition

1. A, B, D, and E

2. C

3. D

4. C

References

Kim TF, Lee KH, Kim YH, et al: Postoperative imaging of esophageal cancer: what chest radiologists need to know. *Radiographics* 2007;27(2):409-429.

Rubesin SE, Williams NW: Postoperative esophagus. In Gore RM, Levine MS (eds): *Textbook of Gastrointestinal Radiology*, 2nd ed. Philadelphia: Saunders; 2000, pp 495-508.

Cross-Reference

Gastrointestinal Imaging: *THE REQUISITES,* 3rd ed, p 39.

Comment

The surgical repair of esophageal resection can present the unsuspecting radiologist with some perplexing esophageal findings later in life when the patient undergoes an upper GI examination. Radiologists practice the specialty of radiologic imaging in the profession of medicine. It is crucial when possible to talk to the patient before any examination, to answer all questions or concerns, and to take a concise past and current medical history. Such an approach would greatly reduce the likelihood of the resident being startled by the findings.

In this case, the patient had a pharyngoesophageal carcinoma that was treated with resection and jejunal interposition between the pharynx and the distal esophagus (see figure). In an attempt to maintain the continuity of the bowel, most of these surgeries today are done using colonic interposition. Such procedures may also be seen in patients who have fibrosis and marked generalized strictures of the esophagus. The haustral fold pattern of the interposed colon is retained to some extent and is usually easily recognizable. In the case of jejunal interposition, the normal jejunal pattern alters and is more difficult to recognize. The major long-term problem is gastric acid reflux, which is severe in almost 25% of these patients. A few cases (< 5%) develop a tracheoesophageal fistula. There is an increased risk of malignancy in patients whose interpositions were performed for malignancy. There has been some discussion in the literature about the risk of malignancy in interposition done for nonmalignant diseases; it seems to be minimal.

Notes

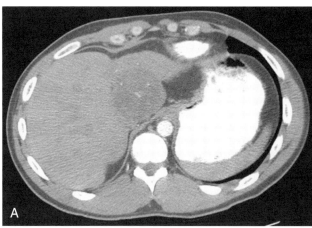

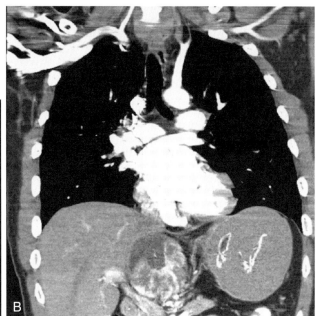

History: A 26-year-old man presents with dyspepsia. A liver abnormality is noted on ultrasound.

1. What should be included in the differential diagnosis of the imaging finding shown in Figure A? (Choose all that apply.)
   A. Cyst
   B. Hepatoma
   C. Metastasis
   D. Hemangioma
   E. Focal nodular hyperplasia

2. What type of hepatoma occurs in young adults?
   A. Hepatoblastoma
   B. Hepatic adenoma
   C. Fibrolamellar hepatoma
   D. Focal nodular hyperplasia

3. What conditions predispose an individual to develop fibrolamellar hepatoma?
   A. Alcoholism
   B. Viral hepatitis
   C. Male predominance
   D. None known

4. Which of the following statements regarding imaging of fibrolamellar hepatoma is true?
   A. Calcification is rare.
   B. On CT, the central scar is best seen during the arterial phase scan.
   C. On MRI, the central scar is usually hypointense on all sequences.
   D. Scanning with ^{99m}Tc–labeled sulfur colloid, the tumor often exhibits uptake.

Fibrolamellar Hepatoma

1. B, C, D, and E

2. C

3. D

4. C

References

McLarney JK, Rucker PT, Bender GN, et al: Fibrolamellar carcinoma of the liver: radiologic-pathologic correlation. *Radiographics* 1999;19(2):453-471.

Wong LK, Link DP, Frey CF, et al: Fibrolamellar hepatocarcinoma: radiology, management and pathology. *AJR Am J Roentgenol* 1982;139(1):172-175.

Cross-Reference

Gastrointestinal Imaging: *THE REQUISITES,* 3rd ed, p 196.

Comment

Neoplasms of the liver in young patients can be caused by several different cell types. The most commonly encountered are FNH and hepatic adenoma. Hemangiomas and metastases also must be considered. The appearance of this tumor in conjunction with a central scar or low-density areas is suggestive of FNH, but this appearance also can occur in other conditions.

Fibrolamellar carcinoma is an unusual variant of conventional hepatocellular carcinoma seen almost exclusively in younger patients. Also, the usual predisposing factors associated with hepatocellular carcinoma, such as cirrhosis or long-standing hepatitis, are not associated with fibrolamellar carcinoma. The development of fibrolamellar hepatoma is not believed to be associated with any etiologic risk factors, but this possibility must be a strong consideration when liver masses are encountered in a young adult.

The radiologic diagnosis can be difficult to make because the lesion may resemble other liver tumors. It typically has a central "scar" or area of fibrous or necrotic tissue that can resemble FNH in its appearance. Fibrolamellar hepatoma does calcify, as in this case, and has been described in 50% of patients (see figures). On CT scans, the tumor is often hypodense, particularly its central scar. However, delayed images show increasing homogeneity or enhancement of the lesion with the surrounding liver, simulating a hemangioma. A poorly performed CT scan may underestimate the size of the lesion. Nuclear scanning may help differentiate the mass from FNH because fibrolamellar hepatoma does not have Kupffer cells.

The prognosis for patients with fibrolamellar hepatoma is much better than the prognosis for patients with hepatocellular carcinoma, and the lesion is potentially curable with surgery. Vascular invasion and other abnormalities of hepatocellular carcinoma are much less common in fibrolamellar hepatoma. This lesion also responds well to chemotherapy.

Notes

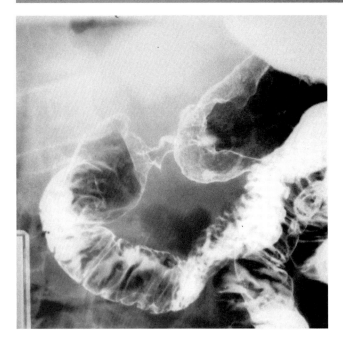

History: A 68-year-old man presents with anorexia, weight loss, and vomiting.

1. What should be included in the differential diagnosis of the imaging finding shown in the figure? (Choose all that apply.)
   A. Crohn's disease
   B. Pancreatic carcinoma
   C. Gastric mucosal prolapse
   D. Transpyloric spread of lymphoma
   E. Transpyloric spread of gastric cancer

2. What is the most common gastric malignancy?
   A. Adenocarcinoma
   B. Stromal tumor
   C. Lymphoma
   D. Metastasis

3. This was a case of a malignancy crossing the pylorus. What is the most likely malignancy to cross the pylorus?
   A. Adenocarcinoma
   B. Stromal tumor
   C. Lymphoma
   D. Metastasis

4. What is the most common gross morphology of gastric adenocarcinoma?
   A. Ulcer
   B. Mass lesion
   C. Linitis plastica
   D. Thickened folds

Gastric Carcinoma Crossing the Pylorus

1. A, B, D, and E

2. A

3. A

4. B

References

Iyer R, Dubrow R: Imaging upper gastrointestinal malignancy. *Semin Roentgenol* 2006;41(2):105-112.

Low VH, Levine MS, Rubesin SE, et al: Diagnosis of gastric carcinoma: sensitivity of double-contrast barium studies. *AJR Am J Roentgenol* 1994;162(2):329-334.

Cross-Reference

Gastrointestinal Imaging: *THE REQUISITES,* 3rd ed, p 68.

Comment

About 90% to 95% of gastric malignancies are adenocarcinomas; about 4% are lymphomas; and the rest are a rare assortment of other lesions, mostly malignant gastrointestinal stromal tumors. It has long been taught that adenocarcinomas crossing the pylorus are very rare. Residents are taught that lymphomas have a greater disposition to cross the pylorus and affect the duodenum, with adenocarcinomas doing this much less often. Although this teaching is true, when the question which lesions are found to have crossed the pylorus in more cases is posed, the answer is found by simple logic. Although lymphomas have a greater tendency to cross the pylorus, they constitute only a tiny fraction of gastric malignancies compared with adenocarcinomas. The specific answer to a question phrased in such a manner is adenocarcinoma.

The idea that adenocarcinomas only rarely cross into the duodenum comes from early radiologic literature. Residents were taught that the pylorus was a "barrier" to the extension of the gastric lesion in that direction. However, more recent observations with microscopic support have suggested that transpyloric extension of gastric carcinomas may be more common than we believed. Studies have found that transpyloric extension may be 20%. This case demonstrates the point (see figure). Lesions in the prepyloric gastric antrum can result in two significant complications. Gastric outlet obstruction (often in a patient with no past history of peptic ulcer disease) is more common, but we must consider the possibility of transpyloric extension, even when not macroscopically visible.

Notes

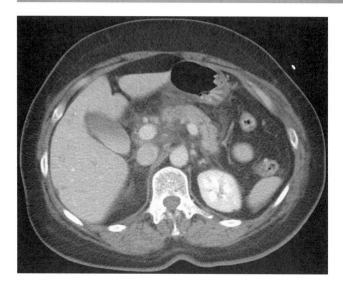

History: A 17-year-old girl presents to the emergency department inebriated and complaining of abdominal pain.

1. What should be included in the differential diagnosis of the imaging finding shown in the figure? (Choose all that apply.)
   A. Pancreatic contusion
   B. Acute pancreatitis
   C. Duodenal ulcer
   D. Edema
   E. Normal

2. Which of the following statements regarding the clinical aspects of pancreatic trauma is true?
   A. Pancreatic injury is more common with blunt trauma than with penetrating injuries.
   B. Adults are more likely to sustain pancreatic injury in the same clinical scenario.
   C. Pancreatic injury occurs in about 10% of blunt abdominal trauma cases.
   D. Elevated serum amylase is a reliable indicator of pancreatic injury.

3. What is the most important issue in suspected pancreatic injury?
   A. Injury of the main pancreatic duct.
   B. There is often associated skeletal injury.
   C. Delayed mortality is usually pancreatic endocrine and exocrine failure.
   D. Acute mortality related to pancreatic injury is usually due to duodenal perforation.

4. Which of the following statements regarding imaging of pancreatic injury is true?
   A. The pancreatic head is the most common site of injury.
   B. There are almost always associated injuries of other upper abdominal viscera.
   C. Early CT scanning is important; if CT is normal, pancreatic injury is reliably excluded.
   D. The presence of peripancreatic fluid is a highly sensitive and specific finding on CT scan, indicating pancreatic injury.

Subtle Pancreatic Trauma

1. A, B, C, and D

2. C

3. A

4. B

References

Fischer J, Carpenter K, O'Keefe G: CT diagnosis of an isolated blunt pancreatic injury. *AJR Am J Roentgenol* 1996;167(5):1152.

Gupta A, Stuhlfaut J, Fleming K, et al: Blunt trauma of the pancreas and biliary tract: a multimodality imaging approach to diagnosis. *Radiographics* 2004;24(5):1381-1395.

Cross-Reference

Gastrointestinal Imaging: *THE REQUISITES,* 3rd ed, p 174.

Comment

Pancreatic blunt trauma is uncommon; the pancreas is ninth or tenth on the list of organs most commonly injured in blunt trauma. It seems to be more common in penetrating trauma. Multidetector CT (and in some cases clinical suspicions of subtle injury may require thin sections through the pancreas) is the examination of choice at the present time. The pancreas lying across the bony spine would seem to be the most obvious candidate for contusion or fracture in blunt trauma. The fact that it is not injured more often is puzzling. It may be that subtle cases are missed or that subtle cases are not seen with current CT technique.

Most subtle injuries are located in the body of the pancreas. The intimate relationship of vascular structures to the pancreatic head makes diagnosis and the morbidity and mortality rates of pancreatic injury greater than at other sites in the pancreas. The aorta, subhepatic inferior vena cava, superior mesenteric artery and superior mesenteric vein, and confluence of the portal vein all are found around and contiguous with the substance of the pancreatic head. In this case, the evidence for pancreatic injury is the fluid seen close to the pancreas (see figure). In cases such as this, specific treatment is not required, and the outcome, as in this patient, is excellent. However, follow-up is recommended to ensure complete healing without complication.

Notes

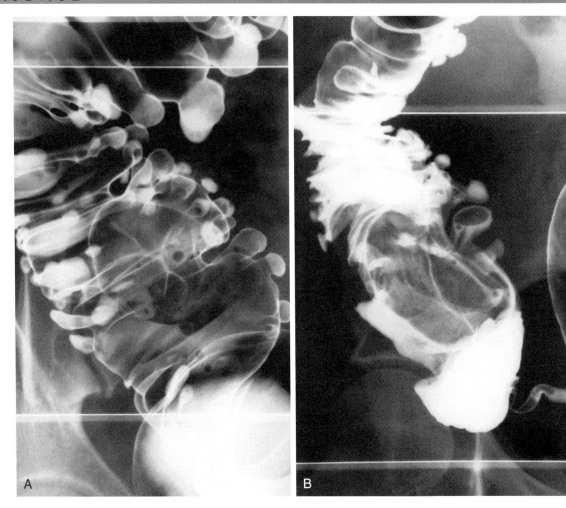

History: A 43-year-old woman underwent a CT scan for renal colic, and findings suspicious for a mass in the cecum were incidentally noted.

1. What should be included in the differential diagnosis of the imaging finding shown in Figure A? (Choose all that apply.)
   A. Fatty infiltration of the ileocecal valve
   B. Lipoma of the ileocecal valve
   C. Primary colonic carcinoma
   D. Ileocolic intussusception
   E. Mucocele of the appendix

2. Which of the following statements regarding the ileocecal valve at barium enema is true?
   A. The ileocecal valve is usually directly visible.
   B. A lobulated mucosal surface is suspicious for malignancy.
   C. Asymmetry of the valve lips indicates infiltration by disease.
   D. Filling of the terminal ileum is required to identify the ileocecal valve.

3. Which of the following statements regarding disease at the ileocecal valve is true?
   A. In chronic ulcerative colitis, the resultant scarring prevents demonstration of the terminal ileum by reflux of barium.
   B. With diseases of the appendix, there is usually deformity of the wall of the cecum opposite from the ileocecal valve.
   C. The ileocecal valve is the most common site of development of cancer of the right colon.
   D. A lipoma results in an asymmetric deformity of the ileocecal valve.

4. Which infective disease of the small bowel typically involves the terminal ileum?
   A. Cryptosporidiosis
   B. Candidiasis
   C. Giardiasis
   D. Yersiniosis

Fatty Infiltration of the Ileocecal Valve

1. A, C, and D

2. A

3. D

4. D

References

Dahnert W: *Radiology Review Manual*, 6th ed. Philadelphia: Lippincott Williams & Wilkins, 2007, p 780.

El-Amin LC, Levine MS, Rubesin SE, et al: Ileocecal valve: spectrum of normal findings at double-contrast barium enema examination. *Radiology* 2003;227(1):52-58.

Cross-Reference

Gastrointestinal Imaging: *THE REQUISITES,* 3rd ed, p 279.

Comment

With the development of CT, the opportunity to detect ileocecal disease has increased. Although a true ileocecal valve mass or cecal mass is the principal concern, other possibilities might warrant consideration. In this case, the "mass" proved to be fatty infiltration of the ileocecal valve, which is a benign condition.

A functional phenomenon of prolapse is sometimes the cause, which is visible with static imaging. It has long been suspected by fluoroscopists that prolapse through the ileocecal valve occurs when the right colon, and in particular, the ileocecal valve, is empty. Conversely, when the cecum becomes distended, the prolapsed ileum returns to its normal position, and there may be reflux of colonic material into the terminal ileum in some patients with incompetent ileocecal valves.

This condition must be distinguished from an ileocolonic intussusception, which is truly pathologic and almost always has an underlying cause and is invariably symptomatic. There are things to look for on CT studies of the abdomen: Evaluate the surrounding pericolic fat looking for stranding or small nodes. Evaluate the serosal wall of the bowel to ensure it is crisp. Make sure there is no suggestion of obstruction. If there is any concern, ask for a barium enema or dedicated colonography for confirmation (see figures).

Notes

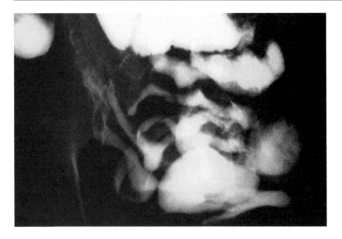

History: A 24-year-old woman presents with nausea and diarrhea 52 days after bone marrow transplant for leukemia.

1. What should be included in the differential diagnosis of the imaging finding shown in the figure? (Choose all that apply.)
   A. Graft-versus-host disease (GVHD)
   B. Radiation enteritis
   C. Crohn's disease
   D. Tropical sprue
   E. Ischemia

2. What is the most common site of involvement with acute GVHD?
   A. Skin
   B. Liver
   C. Esophagus
   D. Small bowel

3. When does subacute GVHD occur?
   A. Within 100 days after bone marrow transplant
   B. In 1 to 4 months after bone marrow transplant
   C. In 3 to 6 months after bone marrow transplant
   D. In 3 to 12 months after bone marrow transplant

4. What is the most common site of GI tract chronic GVHD?
   A. Colon
   B. Oral cavity
   C. Esophagus
   D. Small bowel

Small Bowel Graft-Versus-Host Disease

1. A, B, C, and E

2. A

3. B

4. B

References

Coy DL, Ormazabal A, Godwin FD, et al: Imaging evaluation of pulmonary and abdominal complications following hematopoietic stem cell transplantation. *Radiographics* 2005;25(2):305-318.

Kalantari BN, Mortele KJ, Cantisani V, et al: CT features with pathologic correlation of gastrointestinal graft-versus-host disease after bone marrow transplantation in adults. *AJR Am J Roentgenol* 2003;181(6):1621-1625.

Cross-Reference

Gastrointestinal Imaging: *THE REQUISITES,* 3rd ed, p 125.

Comment

Transplant recipients face a variety of GI complications, which are typically related to the immunosuppressive drugs taken to prevent rejection. Peptic ulcer disease, bowel perforation, and opportunistic infections are common. Pancreatitis and hepatitis also occur more frequently in these patients. In patients who undergo bone marrow transplants for various diseases, other complications can occur in addition to those already mentioned. In the initial induction phase of therapy, during which the native bone marrow is destroyed, the patient receives high-dose radiation or chemotherapy. During this phase, acute enteritis with diarrhea, pain, and bleeding may develop because of the loss of mucosal cells lining the bowel. In the latter stages, the transplanted marrow (graft) may mount an immune response against the body (host), producing GVHD. This rejection typically occurs within the first few months of bone marrow transplant, although later development is possible.

The major organs involved in GVHD include the skin, GI tract, lungs, and liver. Patients develop a diffuse rash, protein-losing diarrhea, and jaundice. Abnormalities encountered in the small bowel include fold thickening, which may progress to complete effacement of the folds; luminal narrowing; and separation of the bowel loops (see figure). Similar changes also may occur in the colon, resembling chronic ulcerative colitis. Pneumatosis of the bowel also has been reported. Gastric abnormalities include dilation and delayed gastric emptying. An unusual radiologic abnormality is prolonged barium coating of the mucosa. CT findings include bowel wall thickening, the "halo" sign caused by bowel wall edema, pericolic inflammation, and mesenteric thickening.

Notes

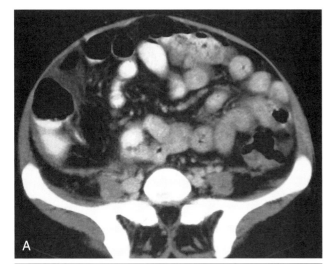

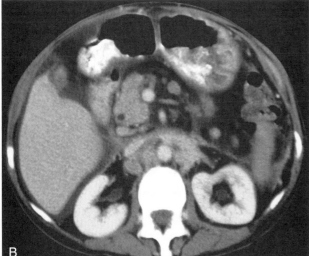

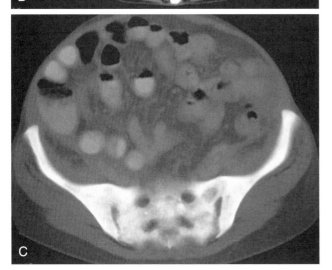

History: A 58-year-old woman presents with pruritus, rash, dyspepsia, and diarrhea.

1. What should be included in the differential diagnosis of the imaging finding shown in Figure A? (Choose all that apply.)
   A. Nontropical sprue
   B. Lymphangiectasia
   C. Cryptosporidiosis
   D. Mastocytosis
   E. Giardiasis

2. What is the most common site of involvement with mastocytosis?
   A. Skin
   B. Liver
   C. Esophagus
   D. Small bowel

3. Which of the following conditions produces the greatest elevation of serum gastrin levels?
   A. Zollinger-Ellison syndrome
   B. Pernicious anemia
   C. G-cell hyperplasia
   D. Mastocytosis

4. What is the most common abnormal finding in barium studies of the GI tract affected by mastocytosis?
   A. Distal duodenal ulceration
   B. Jejunal mucosal nodules
   C. Ileal mucosal fold thickening
   D. Colorectal strictures

C A S E 1 3 4

Mastocytosis of the Small Bowel

1. B, C, D, and E

2. A

3. A

4. B

References

Avila NA, Ling A, Worobec AS, et al: Systemic mastocytosis: CT and US features of abdominal manifestations. *Radiology* 1997;202(2):367-372.

Herlinger H: Malabsorption. In Gore RM, Levine MS (eds): *Textbook of Gastrointestinal Radiology*, 2nd ed. Philadelphia: Saunders, 2000, pp 759-784.

Cross-Reference

Gastrointestinal Imaging: *THE REQUISITES,* 3rd ed, p 127.

Comment

Numerous clinical conditions produce elevated serum gastrin levels. The best-known cause is Zollinger-Ellison syndrome, which results from a gastrin-producing tumor. Another condition associated with elevated gastrin is mastocytosis. Mastocytosis is an accumulation of mast cells in the skin and various other organs. Mast cells are responsible for storage and release of histamine. Histamine increases gastrin levels, although not to the extent seen in patients with Zollinger-Ellison syndrome (often >1000 pg/mL).

Mastocytosis typically involves the skin. When the mast cells are disturbed and release histamine, they produce yellow, red, or brown macules or papules, accounting for the disease description *urticaria pigmentosa.* It is less commonly known that other organs may be involved with a mast cell infiltrate; this occurrence is termed *systemic mastocytosis.* The GI tract (small bowel) is the second most commonly involved organ after the skin; the bone, liver, and spleen also can be involved. There can be both local and systemic release of histamine. Clinically, patients complain of bouts of diarrhea caused by malabsorption, flushing, and tachycardia. Alcohol consumption may precipitate the symptoms, and the condition is treated with histamine receptor antagonists.

Radiologically, small bowel examination shows thickened folds and sometimes bowel wall thickening (see figures). Because of increased gastrin levels, there is a higher incidence of peptic ulcer disease and increased secretions in the small bowel. All these abnormalities may be present in a patient with Zollinger-Ellison syndrome. Other findings in patients with systemic mastocytosis include hepatosplenomegaly and lymphadenopathy (see figures). Mastocytosis can involve the bone marrow, producing diffuse sclerotic changes (see figures). In this case, all the visualized bones are quite dense.

Notes

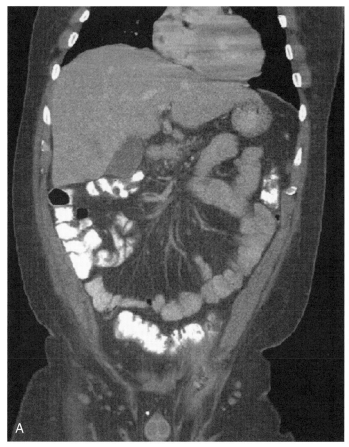

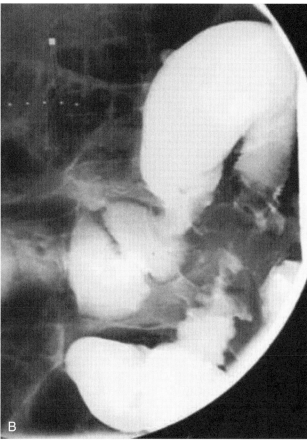

History: A 45-year-old woman presents with fever, weight loss, lower abdominal pain, and an area of redness and swelling at the left iliac fossa.

1. What should be included in the differential diagnosis of the imaging finding shown in Figure A? (Choose all that apply.)
   A. Actinomycosis
   B. Colon carcinoma
   C. Crohn's disease
   D. Diverticular abscess
   E. Pseudomembranous colitis

2. Which of the following statements regarding actinomycosis is true?
   A. Penicillin is the treatment of choice.
   B. The most common site of infection is in the chest.
   C. The diagnosis is usually made by aspirate and culture.
   D. Lymphatic and hematogenous spread readily occurs.

3. What is the most common site of actinomycosis of the gastrointestinal tract?
   A. Ileocecal region
   B. Sigmoid colon
   C. Small bowel
   D. Esophagus

4. With what iatrogenic intervention is this infection in the pelvis associated?
   A. Intrauterine contraceptive devices
   B. Tubal ligation
   C. Abortion
   D. Tampon

CASE 135

Actinomycosis of the Sigmoid Colon

1. A, B, C, and D

2. A

3. A

4. A

References

Ha HK, Lee HJ, Kim H, et al: Abdominal actinomycosis: CT findings in 10 patients. *AJR Am J Roentgenol* 1993;161(4):791-794.

Kim SH, Kim SH, Yang DM, et al: Unusual causes of tubo-ovarian abscess: CT and MR imaging findings. *Radiographics* 2004;24(6):1575-1589.

Cross-Reference

Gastrointestinal Imaging: *THE REQUISITES,* 3rd ed, p 317.

Comment

Actinomycosis is an uncommon inflammatory entity caused by the commonly found anaerobic bacterium, *Actinomyces israelii,* a gram-positive bacillus, which is a component of the normal human flora and can be found in the mouths of most people. When the cellular environment is conducive for anaerobic proliferation, it is possible for *Actinomyces* to proliferate, migrate, and infect tissue. It can occur almost anywhere in the body. Bowel involvement is uncommon, although it has increased in frequency over the last few decades. The most common site of the disease is the ileocolic junction. Involvement of the sigmoid colon has been described in patients with use of intrauterine contraceptive devices. Actinomycosis, similar to syphilis, can mimic other diseases, such as colonic diverticulitis, abscesses, appendagitis, and malignant tumors, presenting a diagnostic challenge and often being identified postoperatively in many cases.

The diagnosis can be determined with endoscopy and imaging techniques such as CT and MRI, where the striking characteristic of actinomycosis is best displayed: the tendency of the disease routinely to breach normal barriers to disease such as muscle and fascial planes (see figures). Other common findings in CT scan and barium study include mural invasion with stricture formation, mass effect with tapered narrowing of the lumen, and thickened mucosal folds (see figures). In many cases, the radiologic findings are similar to findings of intestinal tuberculosis and destructive malignant tumors.

Notes

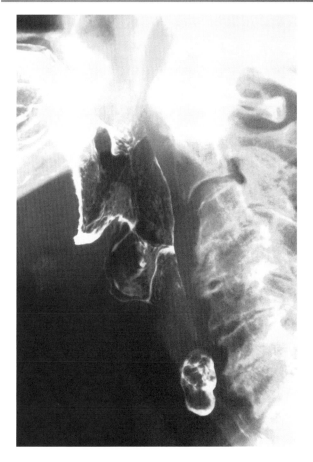

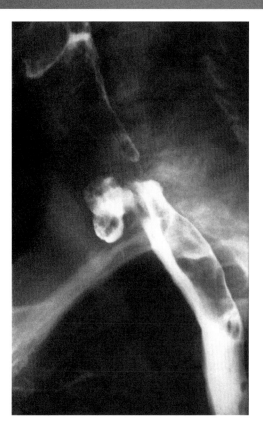

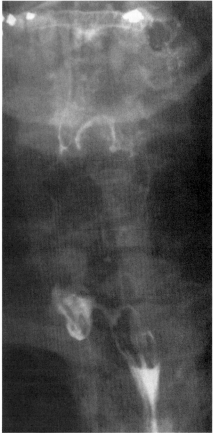

History: An 83-year-old woman presents with suprasternal dysphagia.

1. What should be included in the differential diagnosis of the imaging finding shown in the figures? (Choose all that apply.)
   A. Laryngocele
   B. Traction diverticulum
   C. Zenker's diverticulum
   D. Killian-Jamieson diverticulum
   E. Lateral hypopharyngeal pouch

2. What is the anatomy of the site of weakness where a Killian-Jamieson diverticulum occurs?
   A. Killian's dehiscence
   B. Between the oblique and transverse fibers of the cricopharyngeus muscle
   C. Between the inferior pharyngeal constrictor muscle and the thyrohyoid muscle
   D. Lateral to the insertion of the longitudinal muscles of the esophagus to the upper esophageal sphincter

3. What specific complication is a patient at risk of with treatment of this lesion?
   A. Stricture formation
   B. Mediastinal infection
   C. Esophagopharyngeal reflux
   D. Injury of the recurrent laryngeal nerve

4. Which of the following is a *true* diverticulum?
   A. Traction diverticulum
   B. Zenker's diverticulum
   C. Killian-Jamieson diverticulum
   D. Intramural pseudodiverticulum

Killian-Jamieson Diverticulum

1. B, C, D, and E

2. D

3. D

4. A

References

Ekberg O, Nylander G: Lateral diverticula from the pharyngo-esophageal junction area. *Radiology* 1983;146(1):117-122.

Rodgers PJ, Armstrong WB, Dana E: Killian-Jamieson diverticulum: a case report and a review of the literature. *Ann Otol Rhinol Laryngol* 2000;109(11):1087-1091.

Rubesin SE, Levine MS: Killian-Jamieson diverticula: radiographic findings in 16 patients. *AJR Am J Roentgenol* 2001;177(1):85-89.

Cross-Reference

Gastrointestinal Imaging: THE REQUISITES, 3rd ed, p 28.

Comment

Also known as a proximal lateral cervical esophageal diverticulum, a Killian-Jamieson diverticulum is a pulsion diverticulum. It arises from an anatomic weak spot below the level of the cricopharyngeus muscle and lateral to the longitudinal muscles of the esophagus, just below its insertion into the cricoid cartilage.

Compared with the more common Zenker's diverticulum, a Killian-Jamieson diverticulum is usually smaller in size and less likely to be symptomatic. Clinical distinction between the two types of diverticula is difficult because their symptoms are very similar. Radiologically, Zenker's diverticulum can be confused with a Killian-Jamieson diverticulum (see figures). However, it is important to distinguish between the two because surgical management differs. A Killian-Jamieson diverticulum is in close proximity to the recurrent laryngeal nerve, and there is a tendency for surgical rather than endoscopic management of this diverticulum because of concerns regarding potential nerve injury.

Identification of the cricopharyngeus muscle is key to the diagnosis. The opening of a Zenker's diverticulum lies *above* the protruding cricopharyngeus bar. The sac of a Zenker's diverticulum is *posterior* to the cervical esophagus on lateral images and in the *midline* on frontal images. In contrast, the opening of a Killian-Jamieson diverticulum is *below* the cricopharyngeus bar. The sac of diverticulum overlaps the *anterior* wall of the cervical esophagus on lateral images and projects *laterally* on frontal images.

Notes

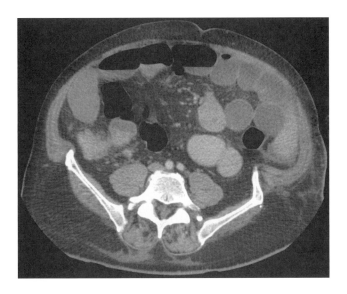

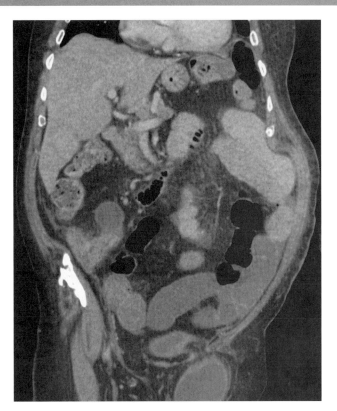

History: A 54-year-old man undergoes assessment for swelling of the left groin.

1. What should be included in the differential diagnosis of the imaging finding in the right lower quadrant shown in the figures? (Choose all that apply.)
   A. Appendiceal tumor
   B. Crohn's disease
   C. Appendicolith
   D. Appendicitis
   E. Mucocele

2. What is the most common cause of an appendiceal mucocele?
   A. Obstruction
   B. Mucosal hyperplasia
   C. Mucinous cystadenoma
   D. Mucinous cystadenocarcinoma

3. What is the most common neoplasm of the appendix?
   A. Adenocarcinoma
   B. Metastases
   C. Lymphoma
   D. Carcinoid

4. What is the most common abnormality seen on CT in appendicitis?
   A. Abscess
   B. Appendicolith
   C. Abnormal appendix
   D. Pericecal inflammation

Appendix Carcinoma

1. A, B, D, and E

2. C

3. D

4. D

References

Duran JC, Beidle TR, Perret R, et al: CT imaging of acute right lower quadrant disease. *AJR Amer J Roentgenol* 1997;168(2):411-416.

Pickhardt PJ, Levy AD, Rohrmann CA, et al: Primary neoplasms of the appendix: radiologic spectrum of disease with pathologic correlation. *Radiographics* 2003;23(3):645-662.

Cross-Reference

Gastrointestinal Imaging: *THE REQUISITES,* 3rd ed, p 318.

Comment

Primary neoplasms of the appendix are uncommon, accounting for less than 1% of all gastrointestinal tumors. The most common are benign carcinoids. The most common primary malignant lesion of the appendix is adenocarcinoma, most frequently mucinous adenocarcinoma. Because of this and other mucoid lesions of the appendix, the presence of pseudomyxoma peritonei is always a possibility. Lesions are often found on routine appendectomy. Most carcinoids are found incidentally during postmortem examination.

The primary lesions are often small. At surgery, the appendix is found to be thickened and hard, and the leaves of the mesentery are studded with innumerable tiny yellow metastatic deposits. CT is the examination of choice (see figures). Although the disease is rare, if the thickened wall of the appendix does not look like edema, or there are adjacent nodes, hazy density of the mesentery, or evidence of distal disease, the diagnosis of neoplasia should be considered instead of the much more common diagnosis of appendicitis. Ascitic fluid is often present. An inflamed appendix may weep small amounts of fluid into the peritoneal cavity, which collects in the pelvic recesses; unless the ascites is significant, this is a less significant sign.

Notes

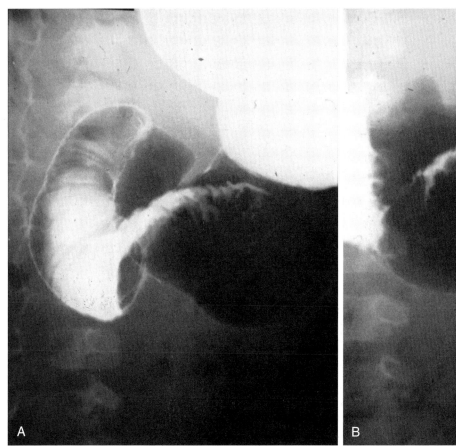

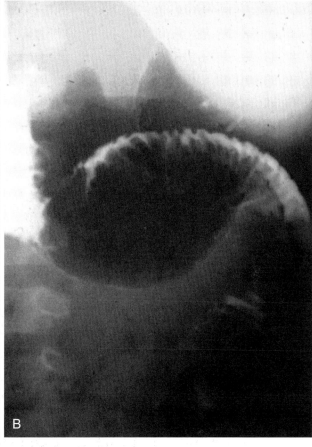

History: A 3-year-old boy presents with vomiting.

1. What should be included in the differential diagnosis of the imaging finding shown in Figure A? (Choose all that apply.)
   A. Annular pancreas
   B. Duodenal hematoma
   C. Retroperitoneal mass
   D. Pancreatic pseudocyst
   E. Duodenal intraluminal diverticulum

2. Which of the following patterns is diagnostic of a duodenal hematoma on CT scan?
   A. Grossly thickened folds
   B. Retroperitoneal stranding
   C. "Coiled spring" appearance
   D. Asymmetric ovoid intramural mass

3. What is the most common cause of a duodenal hematoma?
   A. Trauma
   B. Coagulation disorder
   C. Tumoral hemorrhage
   D. Vascular malformation

4. Which of the following statements regarding blunt abdominal trauma in children is true?
   A. Abdominal wall bruising indicates significant intraabdominal injury in children involved in motor vehicle crashes.
   B. The most common intestinal injury is hematoma formation and obstruction.
   C. There is a higher mortality with pancreatic than with intestinal tract injury.
   D. The most common site of injury is the duodenum.

Duodenal Hematoma

1. B, C, and D

2. D

3. A

4. A

References

Iuchtman M, Steiner T, Faierman T, et al: Post-traumatic intramural duodenal hematoma in children. *Isr Med Assoc J* 2006;8(2):95-97.

Linsenmaier U, Wirth S, Reiser M, et al: Diagnosis and classification of pancreatic and duodenal injuries in emergency radiology. *Radiographics* 2008;28(6):1591-1602.

Cross-Reference

Gastrointestinal Imaging: *THE REQUISITES,* 3rd ed, p 97.

Comment

Numerous references in the literature discuss large duodenal hematomas being mistakenly diagnosed as upper abdominal masses (see figures). These hematomas may be present without a history of trauma. Huge lymphomatous masses (root of mesentery and retroperitoneal adenopathy) through which the duodenum passes unobstructed—the so-called sandwich sign—are a good example. The patient in this case experienced both gastric outlet obstruction and a degree of obstruction of the biliary duct, had decompression of the obstruction performed with a nasogastric tube, and was treated conservatively and continuously improved. No bile duct intervention was required, and a repeat study obtained 6 weeks later showed almost complete resolution of the hematoma. Not all large upper abdominal hematomas manifest with a history of trauma. Sometimes the history is suppressed. Sometimes the patient has a coagulability problem. Sometimes the hematoma is entirely idiopathic. Some of these patients are diagnosed at surgery.

Notes

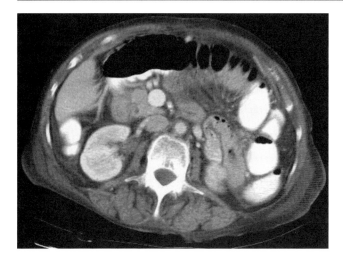

History: A 42-year-old woman presents with a 2-week history of vomiting and diarrhea.

1. What should be included in the differential diagnosis of the imaging finding shown in the figure? (Choose all that apply.)
   A. Scleroderma
   B. Paralytic ileus
   C. Celiac disease
   D. Ileal dysgenesis
   E. Small bowel obstruction

2. What is the most common cause of small bowel obstruction in young adults?
   A. Adhesions
   B. Intussusception
   C. Small bowel tumor
   D. Inflammatory disease

3. What finding is most consistently recognized in cross-sectional imaging of active Crohn's disease?
   A. Enhancement
   B. Lymphadenopathy
   C. Perienteric stranding
   D. Bowel wall thickening

4. Which of the following statements regarding Crohn's disease is true?
   A. The populations with the highest incidence of Crohn's disease are in Spain, South America, and Asia.
   B. The incidence among blacks and Native Americans is higher than in whites in North America.
   C. A person with Crohn's disease is more likely to have a relative with IBD.
   D. The highest prevalence is among individuals 50 to 80 years old.

Crohn's Disease Small Bowel Obstruction

1. A, B, C, and E

2. A

3. D

4. C

References

Horsthuis K, Bipat S, Bennink RJ, et al: Inflammatory bowel disease diagnosed with US, MR, scintigraphy, and CT: meta-analysis of prospective studies. *Radiology* 2008;247(1):64-79.

Wills JS, Lobis IF, Denstman FJ: Crohn disease: state of the art. *Radiology* 1997;202(3):597-610.

Cross-Reference

Gastrointestinal Imaging: *THE REQUISITES,* 3rd ed, p 114

Comment

It is unusual for Crohn's disease to manifest as a small bowel obstruction. However, a small percentage of patients present with small bowel obstruction, which often creates some diagnostic confusion. Why this obstruction occurs is unclear. It is probably a true inflammatory stricture further complicated by additional inflammation and edema, possibly around the site of a developing sinus or fistulous tract. CT, especially multidetector CT multiplanar imaging, has greatly increased the diagnostic capability of the physician (see figure). Although uncommon, a young patient presenting with small bowel obstruction and no history of prior abdominal surgery should raise the possibility of Crohn's disease or acute appendicitis. Patients with Crohn's disease presenting with acute small bowel obstruction represent about 2% of all newly seen disease. Acute small bowel obstruction is one of the few reasons that the treatment of these patients may be surgical. In some patients, nasogastric suction and high-dose steroids may relieve obstructive symptoms.

Notes

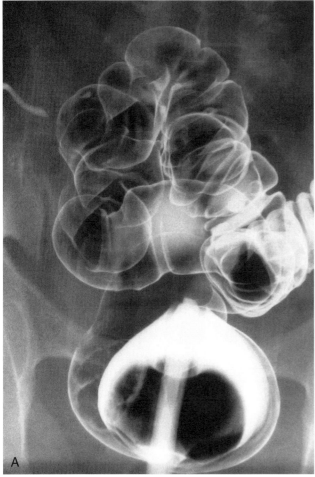

A

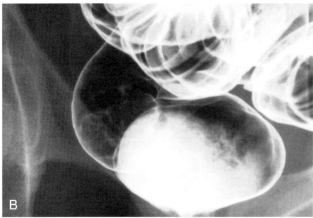

B

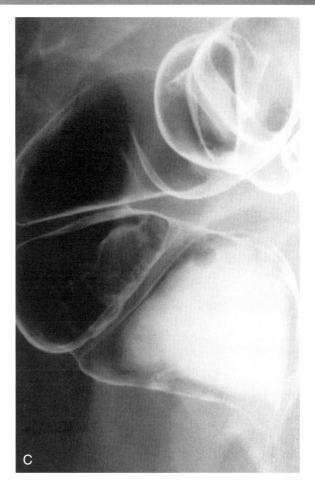

C

History: A 54-year-old man presents with rectal bleeding.

1. What should be included in the differential diagnosis of the imaging finding shown in Figure A? (Choose all that apply.)
   A. Proctitis
   B. Rectocele
   C. Rectal varices
   D. Colonic urticaria
   E. Villous adenoma

2. What is the most common site of colonic villous adenomas?
   A. Ascending colon
   B. Sigmoid colon
   C. Rectum
   D. Cecum

3. Which of the following statements regarding colonic polyps is true?
   A. Of colonic polyps, 10% are adenomas.
   B. Of colonic polyps, 10% are of flat morphology.
   C. Of colonic polyps, 10% are found in the rectum.
   D. Of colonic adenomas 1 to 2 cm in diameter, 10% contain carcinoma.

4. Which of these signs on barium enema describes a pedunculated polyp?
   A. Apple core sign
   B. Bowler hat sign
   C. Mexican hat sign
   D. Spiculation sign

Rectal Villous Adenoma

1. A, C, and E

2. C

3. D

4. C

References

O'Brien MJ, Winawer SJ, Zauber AG, et al: The National Polyp Study. Patient and polyp characteristics associated with high-grade dysplasia in colorectal adenomas. *Gastroenterology* 1990;98(2):371-379.

Rubesin SE, Saul SH, Laufer I, et al: Carpet lesions of the colon. *Radiographics* 1985;5:537-552.

Cross-Reference

Gastrointestinal Imaging: *THE REQUISITES,* 3rd ed, p 268.

Comment

Neoplastic lesions of the colon usually manifest as polypoid protuberances into the lumen of the bowel. They occasionally grow superficially or even infiltrate through the wall of the bowel. The "carpet" lesion of the colon results when a neoplastic growth develops superficially along the mucosa rather than growing in a polypoid fashion. This growth produces a subtle irregularity of the mucosal surface, and the barium that becomes entrapped within the interstices of the lesion has the appearance of shag carpet—hence the terminology.

This subtle lesion is on the lateral rectal wall, is flat (instead of having the usual concavity), and is slightly irregular (see figures). Tumors that develop in this fashion typically occur in areas of the colon where the diameter is quite large. Most are found in the rectum and cecum and to a lesser extent in the ascending colon. These areas are where peristaltic activity is least likely to push an intraluminal lesion distally, which may promote intraluminal growth as seen in other areas.

Pathologically, these tumors tend to be predominantly villous adenomas and are potentially dangerous because many contain foci of malignancy. Some investigators consider villous adenoma as a premalignant lesion. It would be unusual for these lesions to be simple adenomas. The lesions typically are larger than 3 cm because they are often difficult to diagnose when they are small. Lacking the intraluminal component, the subtle mucosal irregularity can be appreciated only with good double-contrast technique. The incidence of carcinoma in colonic adenomas increases with increasing size and with villous histologic findings. Some large carpet lesions may have villous histologic features but turn out not to be malignant.

These lesions are usually too large to be removed endoscopically. Because of their lack of intraluminal components, they are not amendable to endoscopic removal.

Notes

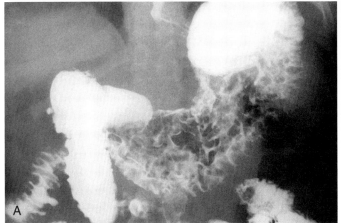
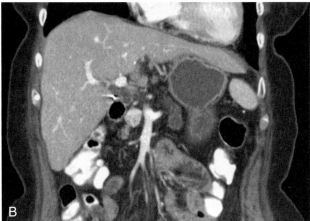

History: A 41-year-old man presents with dyspepsia and diarrhea.

1. What should be included in the differential diagnosis of the imaging finding shown in Figure A? (Choose all that apply.)
   A. Lymphoma
   B. Stromal tumor
   C. Infective gastritis
   D. Hypertrophic gastritis
   E. Zollinger-Ellison syndrome (ZES)

2. What is the most common location of extrapancreatic gastrinomas?
   A. Para-aortic retroperitoneum
   B. Urinary bladder
   C. Duodenum
   D. Ovaries

3. Besides multiple ulcers, what is another common presentation of gastrinomas?
   A. Weight loss
   B. Heartburn
   C. Vomiting
   D. Diarrhea

4. Which of the following statements regarding gastrinomas is true?
   A. The most sensitive test for the diagnosis of a gastrinoma is elevation of the fasting serum gastrin above the normal value of 150 pg/mL.
   B. Somatostatin receptor scintigraphy is the most sensitive noninvasive method for localizing primary tumors and metastases.
   C. The best screening test for follow-up of patients after curative resection of a malignant gastrinoma is CT.
   D. Endoscopy with ultrasound is an optimal means to assess the duodenal site after resection.

Zollinger-Ellison Syndrome

1. A, C, D, and E

2. C

3. D

4. B

References

Thompson WM, Norton G, Kelvin FM, et al: Unusual manifestations of peptic ulcer disease. *Radiographics* 1981;1:1-16.

Yu J, Fulcher AS, Turner MA, et al: Normal anatomy and disease processes of the pancreatoduodenal groove: imaging features. *AJR Am J Roentgenol* 2004;183(3):839-846.

Cross-Reference

Gastrointestinal Imaging: *THE REQUISITES*, 3rd ed, p 98.

Comment

ZES is caused by gastrin secretion from non–islet cell tumors of the pancreas, so-called gastrinomas (see figures). Most (>75%) occur in the pancreas, but this tumor is also known to occur in ectopic locations. Approximately 15% of gastrinomas are found in the duodenum, and the remainder are in the para-aortic region, bladder, ovaries, and liver. About one fourth are associated with multiple endocrine neoplasia type I (MEN-I) syndrome, which also causes tumors of the parathyroid, pituitary, and adrenal glands. Most (approximately 60%) gastrinomas are malignant and have a propensity for early metastasis. The tumors associated with tumors of the parathyroid, pituitary, and adrenal gland in MEN-I syndrome have a smaller incidence of malignancy, however.

On CT, gastrinomas are usually hypervascular and are best seen on the arterial phase of scanning. The small enhancing mass is seen in the pancreatic head just to the right of the origin of the superior mesenteric artery on the coronal CT image in this case (see figures).

Clinically, patients develop peptic ulcer disease because of the acid hypersecretion related to the elevated gastrin levels. Most ulcers in patients with ZES occur in the gastric antrum and duodenal bulb. Occasionally, ulcers occur in the distal duodenum. Although they are uncommon even in patients with ZES, distal duodenal ulcers are so rare in healthy patients that they are considered a feature of the disease. Serum gastrin levels can be variable in patients with ZES, although any level greater than 1000 pg/mL is indicative of the condition. Often a provocative test using secretin is necessary to determine the presence of a gastrinoma. (This test produces a dramatic increase in serum gastrin levels in affected patients.)

Gastric acid hypersecretion may manifest as increased fluid in the stomach, along with thickened rugal folds (see figures). Many patients with gastrinoma also complain of diarrhea. The increased acidity in the small bowel interferes with the function of the small bowel enzymes, resulting in diminished intestinal absorption. In severe cases, a spruelike condition may ensue, with villous atrophy, malabsorption, and steatorrhea.

Notes

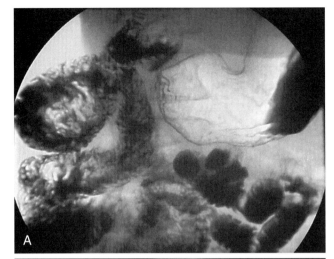

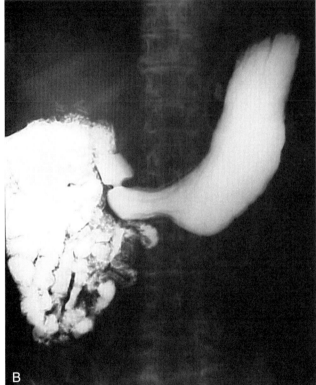

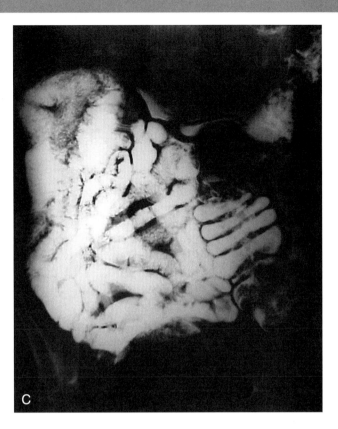

History: A 38-year-old woman presents with dyspepsia.

1. What should be included in the differential diagnosis of the imaging finding shown in Figure A? (Choose all that apply.)
   A. Malrotation
   B. Mislabeling
   C. Duodenal volvulus
   D. Surgical mobilization
   E. Right paraduodenal hernia

2. What is the key vascular finding on CT that suggests midgut malrotation?
   A. Relationship between the superior mesenteric artery and vein
   B. Left-sided inferior vena cava
   C. Congenital heart disease
   D. Persistent vitelline artery

3. What is the most common presentation of symptomatic midgut malrotation?
   A. Newborn less than 1 month old with acute vomiting
   B. Child less than 1 year old with abdominal pain
   C. Child more than 1 year old with intermittent vomiting
   D. Adult with malabsorption

4. Malrotation is associated with heterotaxy and various other congenital abnormalities. What is the leading cause of death in these patients?
   A. Polysplenia
   B. Midgut volvulus
   C. Congenital heart disease
   D. Absence of the pancreatic uncinate process

Midgut Malrotation

1. A and D

2. A

3. A

4. C

References

Applegate KE, Anderson JM, Klatte EC: Intestinal malrotation in children: a problem-solving approach to the upper gastrointestinal series. *Radiographics* 2006;26(5):1485-1500.

Long FR, Kramer SS, Markowitz RI, et al: Radiographic patterns of intestinal malrotation in children. *Radiographics* 1996;16(3):547-556.

Pickhardt PJ, Bhalla S: Intestinal malrotation in adolescents and adults: spectrum of clinical and imaging features. *AJR Am J Roentgenol* 2002;179(6):1429-1435.

Cross-Reference

Gastrointestinal Imaging: *THE REQUISITES,* 3rd ed, p 146.

Comment

The human gut herniates into the umbilicus at about 6 weeks of intrauterine life. This herniation results in 270 degrees of counterclockwise rotation around the superior mesenteric artery before reentering the coelomic cavity at 12 weeks. The process can be faulty in about 1 in 500 live births with failure of achieving the full 270 degrees, resulting in degrees of malrotation abnormality.

In adults, midgut malrotation often is an incidental finding. The colon is usually found on the left. The small bowel is on the right, and the positions of the superior mesenteric artery and superior mesenteric vein are reversed. In addition, the position of the ligament of Treitz can be located in the midline or the right upper abdomen. About 60% of all symptomatic midgut malrotations are diagnosed by 1 year of age. A barium upper GI study is still the fastest and most inexpensive method of diagnosis (see figures). In some adults, vague symptoms, such as low-grade chronic recurrent abdominal pain and symptoms suggestive of malabsorption, may be present that bring the patient to a diagnostic work-up.

Notes

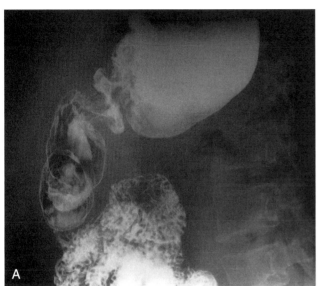

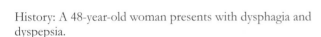

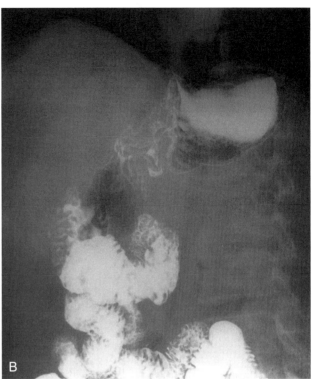

History: A 48-year-old woman presents with dysphagia and dyspepsia.

1. What should be included in the differential diagnosis of the imaging finding shown in Figure A? (Choose all that apply.)
   A. Postoperative deformity
   B. Benign stromal tumor
   C. Peptic ulceration
   D. Malignant tumor
   E. Gastric volvulus

2. What is the most serious complication of partial gastrectomy?
   A. Cancer
   B. Bile reflux
   C. Perforation
   D. Gastroesophageal reflux

3. What operation causes a gastric fundal pseudotumor?
   A. Fundoplication
   B. Gastric banding
   C. Sleeve gastrectomy
   D. Bilroth (1 or 2) operations

4. What is a pseudolymphoma of the stomach?
   A. Thickened rugal folds secondary to varices
   B. Gastric adenocarcinoma that resembles lymphoma
   C. Lymphoid tissue proliferation that simulates lymphoma
   D. Lymphoma developing from chronic *Helicobacter* gastritis

Pseudotumor of the Stomach

1. A, C, and D

2. A

3. A

4. C

References

Kim KW, Choi BI, Han JK, et al: Postoperative anatomic and pathologic findings at CT following gastrectomy. *Radiographics* 2002;22(2):323-336.

Ott DJ, Munitz HA, Gelfand DW, et al: The sensitivity of radiography of the postoperative stomach. *Radiology* 1982;144(4):741-743.

Smith C, Deziel DJ, Kubicka RA: Evaluation of the postoperative stomach and duodenum. *Radiographics* 1994;14(1):67-86.

Cross-Reference

Gastrointestinal Imaging: THE REQUISITES, 3rd ed, p 86.

Comment

This case emphasizes the importance of having a correct and relevant patient history before doing a procedure. In this case, the history was not given with the imaging request, and the radiologist failed to obtain the history of prior gastric surgery from the patient. The stricture of the distal stomach was misdiagnosed as a possible malignancy (see figures). The stricture is actually a pseudotumor of the stomach caused by the large deformity that results from anastomosing a large lumen. This case is a reminder to residents in training that they are physicians and that no procedure should ever be undertaken without first talking to the patient (if possible) and obtaining a short, concise, and relevant history.

Pseudotumor of the stomach should not be confused with pseudolymphoma of the stomach, the appearance of which mimics an aggressive lymphoma or adenocarcinoma. Pseudolymphomas of the stomach are rare but should be included (near the bottom of the list) in the differential diagnosis of any large, seemingly aggressive lesion of the stomach.

Notes

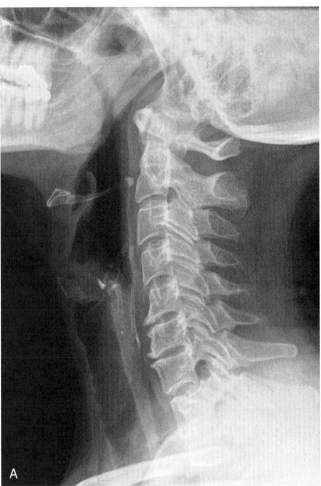

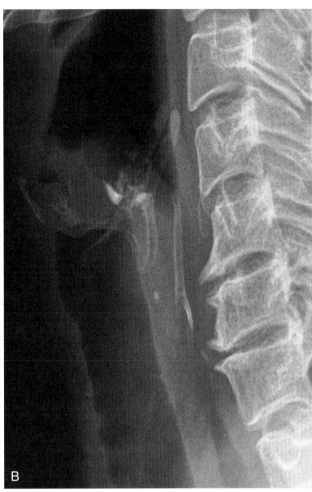

History: A 61-year-old woman experiences acute pharyngeal pain during a meal of chicken.

1. What should be included in the differential diagnosis of the imaging finding shown in Figure A? (Choose all that apply.)
   A. Impacted chicken bone
   B. Calcified carotid plaque
   C. Lymph node calcification
   D. Calcified cervical osteophyte
   E. Laryngeal cartilage calcification

2. In cases of suspected impacted pharyngeal chicken bone or other foreign body with inconclusive physical examination findings, what is the appropriate next step?
   A. Barium swallow
   B. Lateral radiograph
   C. Upper GI endoscopy
   D. Multidetector CT scan

3. What is the most common site of impaction of an ingested foreign body?
   A. Pharynx
   B. Esophagus
   C. Pylorus
   D. Ileocecal valve

4. After an impacted foreign body passes into the stomach, it usually continues through the intestinal tract without further hold-up. However, there are situations where endoscopic retrieval from the stomach is indicated. Which of the following is *not* such an indication?
   A. Batteries
   B. Long objects
   C. Large food bolus
   D. Narcotic packages

Chicken Bone Stuck at the Pharyngoesophageal Junction

1. A, B, C, and E

2. B

3. A

4. C

References

Low VHS, Killius JS: Animal, vegetable, or mineral: a collection of abdominal and alimentary foreign bodies. *Appl Radiol* 2000;29:23-30.

Macpherson RI, Hill JG, Othersen HB: Esophageal foreign bodies in children: diagnosis, treatment, and complications. *AJR Am J Roentgenol* 1996;166(4):919-924.

Cross-Reference

Gastrointestinal Imaging: *THE REQUISITES,* 3rd ed, p 37.

Comment

Fish or chicken bones caught in the cervical esophagus are a problem (1) because they are the most common foreign body seen in the upper esophagus, and (2) because they are among the hardest to see on routine imaging. The bones may not be radiopaque enough to see. There may be laryngeal calcifications that obscure them (see figures). Plain images of the neck have a low yield (approximately 20%). The contrast agent–soaked cotton pledgets employed before the advent of high-quality CT were virtually useless and a waste of time and radiation. I have been asked many times to do this examination for the suspicion of a fish or chicken bone lodged in the upper esophagus, and I have never seen a positive result. The idea was that the contrast agent–soaked pledget would hang up on the bone.

Plain images are still used as a screening tool, but ultimately the examination of choice is CT scan of the neck and upper esophagus. CT not only identifies the foreign body in almost every case but also assesses the area around the bone for penetration and complication. When a fish or chicken bone passes and is in the distal gastrointestinal tract, the problem is usually solved. However, the lodging and then passing of sharp objects may cause an abrasion of the upper esophageal mucosa. In these cases, the patient's symptoms do not abate with the passing of the bone but may continue until the healing of the abrasion.

Notes

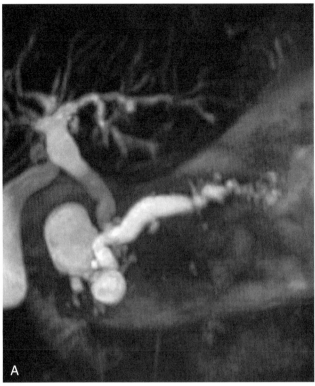

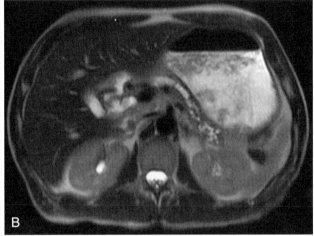

History: A 49-year-old man with chronic alcoholic pancreatitis presents with increasing right upper quadrant pain. Liver function tests show increased bilirubin.

1. What should be included in the differential diagnosis of the imaging finding shown in Figure A? (Choose all that apply.)
   A. Acute pancreatitis
   B. Pancreas divisum
   C. Chronic pancreatitis
   D. Senile pancreatic atrophy
   E. Patulous sphincter of Oddi

2. What is the tumor most commonly diagnosed in association with dilation of the pancreatic duct?
   A. Glucagonoma of the pancreaticoduodenal groove
   B. Ductal adenocarcinoma of the pancreatic head
   C. Ampullary duodenal adenocarcinoma
   D. Intraductal papillary mucinous tumor

3. What is the significance of signal poor filling defects within a dilated pancreatic duct on magnetic resonance cholangiopancreatography (MRCP)?
   A. Clots
   B. Mucin
   C. Calculi
   D. Papilloma

4. Which statement regarding imaging of chronic pancreatitis is true?
   A. Pancreatic calcification visible on plain film radiographs occurs most commonly with idiopathic pancreatitis.
   B. Although MRCP has many advantages over CT and endoscopic retrograde cholangiopancreatography (ERCP), its main disadvantage is the lower spatial resolution.
   C. The feature on endoscopic ultrasound most predictive of chronic pancreatitis is the degree of pancreatic atrophy.
   D. ERCP is the traditional gold standard for the diagnosis of chronic pancreatitis because a normal study excludes the disease.

MRCP of Chronic Pancreatitis

1. C and D

2. B

3. C

4. B

References

Matos C, Winant C, Deviere J: Magnetic resonance pancreatography. *Abdom Imaging* 2001;26(3):243-253.

Vitellas KM, Keogan MT, Spritzer CE, et al: MR cholangiopancreatography of bile and pancreatic duct abnormalities with emphasis on the single-shot fast spin-echo technique. *Radiographics* 2000;20(4):939-957.

Cross-Reference

Gastrointestinal Imaging: *THE REQUISITES,* 3rd ed, p 158.

Comment

The considerable controversy regarding the role of MRCP in the work-up of biliary and pancreatic lesions can be summed up with this straightforward question: Will MRCP replace ERCP? The question begs an answer, in that any noninvasive diagnostic procedure that has the potential to replace an invasive procedure and achieve the same results is a straightforward patient care issue. ERCP is currently considered the gold standard for diagnosis of biliary obstruction and some pancreatic processes. However, ERCP carries with it the same risks of bowel perforation as routine endoscopy.

MRCP is often used after failed ERCP or in patients who might not tolerate ERCP. However, this situation may change. No patient preparation is required for MRCP, usually no sedation is necessary, and contraindications of MRCP are fewer than ERCP. Because of all this, studies to compare the sensitivity and specificity of the two techniques are ongoing. The initial results suggest that MRCP is a comparable examination for diagnostic purposes to ERCP without many of the associated risks (see figures). However, ERCP can also be an interventional procedure (e.g., used to place a stent or remove a stone) and will remain an important part of biliary-pancreatic medicine.

Notes

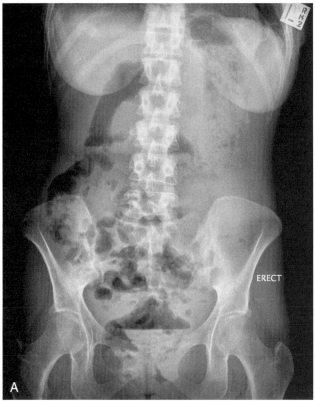

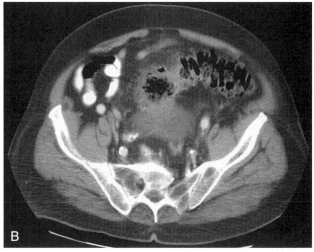

History: A 73-year-old woman presents with lower abdominal pain.

1. What should be included in the differential diagnosis of the imaging finding shown in Figure A? (Choose all that apply.)
   A. Fluid level in an ovarian dermoid
   B. Gas in the urinary bladder
   C. Gas in a pelvic abscess
   D. Fluid level in the rectum
   E. Fournier's gangrene

2. What is the most common etiology for a colovesical fistula?
   A. Bladder diverticulum
   B. Ulcerative colitis
   C. Colon cancer
   D. Diverticulitis

3. What is the most common of the various fistulas of the lower urinary tract?
   A. Fistula to skin
   B. Fistula to colon
   C. Fistula to vagina
   D. Fistula to small bowel

4. What is the most common cause of lower urinary tract fistulas?
   A. Pelvic malignancy
   B. Nonsurgical trauma
   C. Gynecologic surgery
   D. Inflammatory bowel disease

Colovesical Fistula

1. B, C, and D

2. D

3. C

4. C

References

Avritscher R, Madoff DC, Ramirez PT, et al: Fistulas of the lower urinary tract: percutaneous approaches for management of a difficult clinical entity. *Radiographics* 2004;24(Suppl 1):S217-S236.

Pickhardt PJ, Bhalla S, Balfe DM: Acquired gastrointestinal fistulas: classification, etiologies, and imaging evaluation. *Radiology* 2002;224(1):9-23.

Cross-Reference

Gastrointestinal Imaging: *THE REQUISITES,* 3rd ed, p 316.

Comment

Of the many things to consider in radiologic evaluation of a plain image of the abdomen is the question, "Is there air in unexpected places?" In this case, allowing for exclusion of other innocuous causes such as bladder catheterization, air is seen in the urinary bladder (see figures) and must be considered abnormal, and a pathologic fistulous connection to an air-containing adjacent hollow organ viscus is a prime diagnostic consideration.

When considering the diagnosis, patient age and medical history become important. In a young patient, one might consider Crohn's disease and possibly tuberculosis. If the patient has had a pelvic neoplasm treated with pelvic radiation, there is the possibility of a radiation-induced fistulous connection to bowel. Older patients would be more likely to have colonic diverticulitis as the underlying process. From the plain film, it is not difficult to ascertain that this is an older patient (73-year-old woman). The transaxial image confirms pericolonic inflammation with sigmoid diverticulitis as the underlying cause. The paracolic abscess pointed to and connected with the bladder (see figures). With the naturally occurring abscess drainage, the patient reported feeling better, but she experienced pneumaturia.

Notes

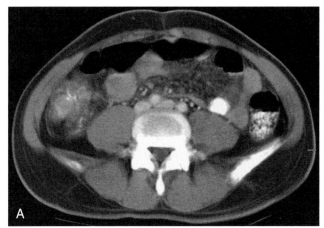

A

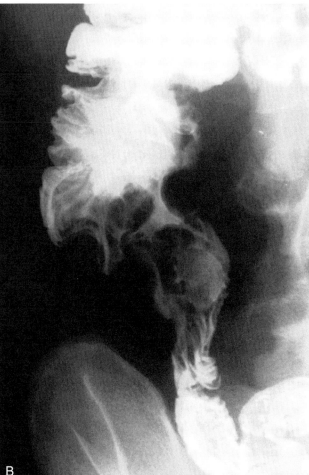

B

History: A 41-year-old Malaysian man presents with fever.

1. What should be included in the differential diagnosis of the imaging finding showing an abnormal cecum in Figure A? (Choose all that apply.)
   A. Carcinoma
   B. Tuberculosis
   C. Crohn's disease
   D. Epiploic appendagitis
   E. Undistended normal bowel

2. What is the most common site of involvement of abdominal tuberculosis?
   A. Ileocecal region
   B. Lymph nodes
   C. Peritoneum
   D. Stomach

3. Which statement regarding tuberculosis of the gastrointestinal tract is true?
   A. Esophageal involvement usually occurs secondary to traction from the pulmonary apical sites of fibrosis.
   B. Tuberculosis of the small bowel apart from the terminal ileum most frequently involves the duodenum.
   C. Chest radiographs are almost always abnormal in patients with tuberculosis of the gastrointestinal tract.
   D. Thickening of the lips of the ileocecal valve with gaping of the valve and narrowing of the terminal ileum is characteristic of tuberculosis.

4. Several other infections favor the ileocecal region; which of the following infections does *not*?
   A. Giardiasis
   B. Amebiasis
   C. Yersiniasis
   D. Actinomycosis

Tuberculosis of the Cecum

1. A, B, and C

2. B

3. D

4. A

References

Burrill J, Williams CJ, Bain G, et al: Tuberculosis: a radiologic review. *Radiographics* 2007;27(5):1255-1273.
Leder RA, Low VH: Tuberculosis of the abdomen. *Radiol Clin North Am* 1995;33(4):691-705.

Cross-Reference

Gastrointestinal Imaging: *THE REQUISITES,* 3rd ed, p 300.

Comment

The CT image shows thickening and deformity of the cecum with a narrowed lumen (see figures). The image from the barium small bowel follow-through in this case shows some deformity of the cecum (see figures). One of the most common inflammatory processes of the ileocecal region is Crohn's disease. It also can affect any portion of the gastrointestinal tract, and the colon is a likely area for further involvement. Possible infectious processes include amebiasis and tuberculosis. Both of these conditions can affect the ileocecal area and the rest of the colon. Of the possible neoplastic processes, the most likely is serosal metastasis, which has an affinity for the cecal region. Lymphoma must always be considered in the differential diagnosis of gastrointestinal lesions.

The final correct diagnosis for this patient was tuberculosis. When a chest radiograph was obtained, it was normal. A normal chest x-ray film should not preclude this diagnosis because intestinal tuberculosis can occur without an abnormal chest film, especially in patients with human immunodeficiency virus. Most intestinal tuberculosis occurs as a result of a patient with pulmonary tuberculosis swallowing infected sputum; intestinal tuberculosis is usually secondary. Although adenopathy may occur in patients with intestinal tuberculosis, it also occurs in patients with Crohn's disease or lymphoma and does not help differentiate the conditions. Patients with these findings in the right lower quadrant are often misdiagnosed as having Crohn's disease.

Notes

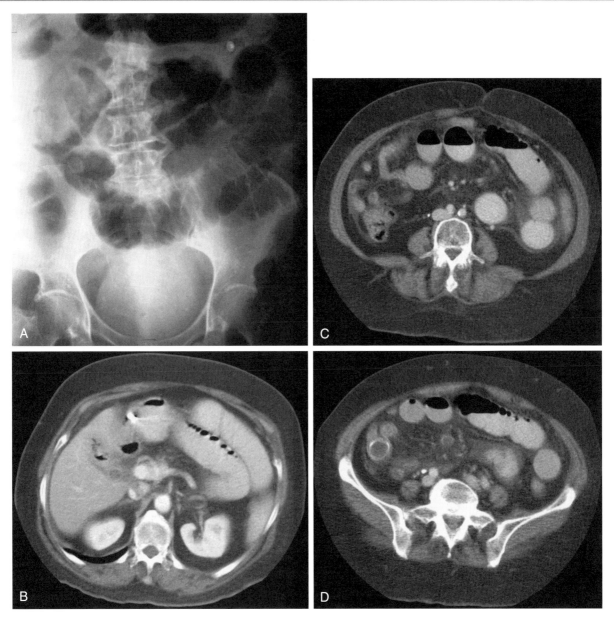

History: A 72-year-old woman presents with abdominal distention and pain and tenderness in the right upper quadrant.

1. What should be included in the differential diagnosis of the imaging finding of the right lower quadrant calcification relevant to the abnormal appearance of the bowel shown in Figure A? (Choose all that apply.)
   A. Gallstone
   B. Appendicolith
   C. Renal calculus
   D. Ovarian teratoma
   E. Mesenteric lymph node calcification

2. There are three radiographic features associated with gallstone ileus: an ectopic gallstone in the bowel, small bowel obstruction, and gas in the biliary system. What is the eponym for these signs?
   A. Rigler's triad
   B. Courvoisier's sign

   C. Mirizzi's syndrome
   D. Bouveret's syndrome

3. In gallstone ileus, where does the stone most often impact itself?
   A. Pylorus
   B. Terminal ileum
   C. Ligament of Treitz
   D. Transverse duodenum

4. Which statement regarding gallstone ileus is true?
   A. Gallstone ileus causes 10% of cases of small bowel obstruction.
   B. Gallstone ileus most commonly occurs in women older than 40 years.
   C. Rigler's triad, comprising signs of gallstone ileus, is seen on plain radiography in 10% of cases.
   D. Gallstone ileus occurs as a complication in 10% of patients with cholelithiasis.

Gallstone Ileus

1. A and B

2. A

3. B

4. C

References

Lassandro F, Romano S, Ragozzino A, et al: Role of helical CT in diagnosis of gallstone ileus and related conditions. *AJR Am J Roentgenol* 2005;185(5): 1159-1165.

Lobo DN, Jobling JC, Balfour TW: Gallstone ileus: diagnostic pitfalls and therapeutic successes. *J Clin Gastroenterol* 2000;30(1):72-76.

Cross-Reference

Gastrointestinal Imaging: *THE REQUISITES,* 3rd ed, p 136.

Comment

The term *gallstone ileus* refers to an unusual set of circumstances that develop in conjunction with chronic gallbladder disease and stone formation. In this condition, a large gallstone or gallstones develop. There must also be associated chronic cholecystitis. During this inflammation, a portion of the bowel becomes adherent to the gallbladder, which is a common occurrence in patients with chronic gallbladder inflammation. With time, the gallstone erodes through the gallbladder wall and into the lumen of the bowel, resulting in a cholecystenteric fistula. The fistula most commonly extends into the duodenum, but extension into the colon and the stomach also has been reported. As the large gallstone travels through the bowel lumen, it becomes impacted at a site where the lumen narrows, resulting in bowel dilation or obstruction.

The classic triad in this condition consists of gas in the biliary system, bowel obstruction, and a radiopaque stone evident in the abdomen (see figures). The biliary gas is seen in about 50% of cases and is secondary to the fistula that is open between the gallbladder and bowel. The amount of gas is often quite small. The stone is the most difficult finding to establish because of the bowel dilation. If it is not obscured by the contrast material, the stone often can be shown on CT (see figures). Finally, the bowel obstruction usually occurs in the terminal ileum at the ileocecal valve. Rarely, the stone obstructs the third portion of the duodenum, or the sigmoid colon. Infrequently (probably less than a third of the time), the entire triad of radiologic findings is present. Any time two of the entities are visible, the diagnosis of gallstone ileus should be considered.

Notes

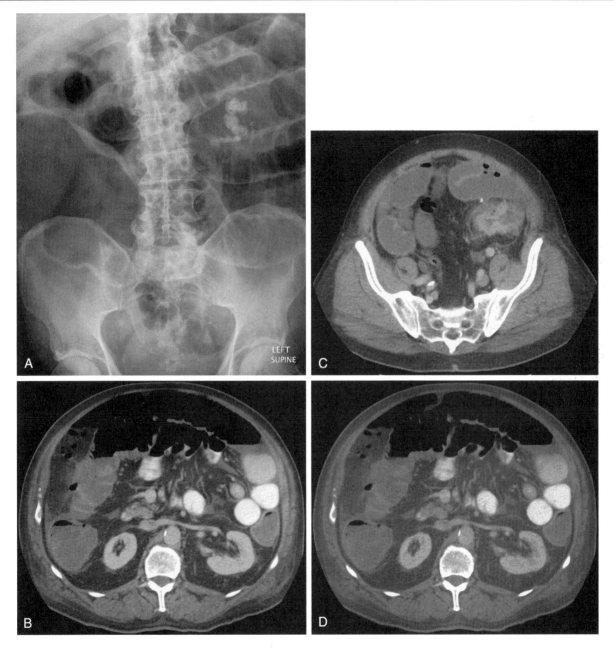

History: A 68-year-old man with 5 months of constipation now presents with 3 days of acute lower abdominal pain and distention.

1. What should be included in the differential diagnosis of the imaging finding shown in Figure A? (Choose all that apply.)
   A. Small bowel obstruction
   B. Large bowel obstruction
   C. Diffuse adynamic ileus
   D. Jejunal dysgenesis
   E. Celiac disease

2. Which of the following complications of colon cancer is most frequently observed?
   A. Perforation
   B. Intussusception
   C. Bowel obstruction
   D. Abscess formation

3. Sigmoid diverticulitis and carcinoma can appear similar on CT scan. Which feature favors a diagnosis of carcinoma?
   A. Engorgement of pericolonic vessels
   B. Fluid in the mesenteric root
   C. Pericolic lymph nodes
   D. Perforation

4. To differentiate colonic perforation that is caused by cancer from perforation caused by various benign conditions, which of the following features is *most* suggestive of malignancy?
   A. Irregular thickening of the colonic wall
   B. Focal defect in the colon wall
   C. Pericolic fat stranding
   D. Pneumoperitoneum

Left-Sided Colonic Cancer Obstruction with Perforation

1. B and C

2. C

3. C

4. A

References

Horton KM, Abrams RA, Fishman EK: Spiral CT of colon cancer: imaging features and role in management. *Radiographics* 2000;20(2):419-430.

Kim SW, Shin HC, Kim IY, et al: CT findings of colonic complications associated with colon cancer. *Korean J Radiol* 2010;11(2):211-221.

Cross-Reference

Gastrointestinal Imaging: *THE REQUISITES,* 3rd ed, p 302.

Comment

The general thinking regarding the clinical differences in right versus left colonic carcinomas relates to the following factors:

- The wider right-sided lumen and relatively thinner wall of the left colon
- The fact that the bowel content being delivered to the right colon from the terminal ileum is mostly fluid in nature
- The fact that one of the main physiologic functions of the colon is water reabsorption

Most right-sided lesions can grow quite large and still not be obstructive. Most left-sided lesions manifest with rectal bleeding. The lumen of the left side is smaller and water absorption has resulted in stool formation, and as a result a left-sided lesion often manifests as an obstructive process such as seen on the CT images in this case (see figures).

However, a slowly growing indolent lesion of the left colon may manifest as an exception to the rule. Because of slow growth, the luminal contours of the lesions are affected by the fecal stream and develop a "flap valve" configuration. As a result, such patients may be shown to have complete retrograde obstruction to the flow of barium, with no evidence of antegrade obstruction (i.e., dilated fluid-filled loops of bowel, air-fluid levels). This situation addresses the age-old issue of "should I stop the barium flow when I encounter an incomplete colonic obstruction?" The answer is clear. If there is evidence of antegrade obstruction, one should cease the barium flow immediately. Putting barium on the proximal side of an obstructing lesion can complicate the situation. However, if there is no evidence of antegrade obstruction on plain images of the abdomen, one can continue to examine the proximal colon without fear of causing harm.

Notes

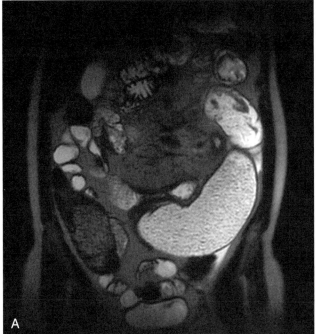
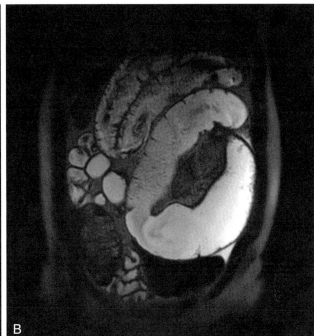

History: A 32-year-old woman presents with abdominal pain.

1. What should be included in the differential diagnosis of the imaging finding shown in Figure A? (Choose all that apply.)
   A. Mucocele of the appendix
   B. Large bowel feces
   C. Small bowel feces
   D. Cecal volvulus
   E. Abscess

2. What finding on MRI most reflects active pathologic inflammation of the bowel in Crohn's disease?
   A. Mesenteric lymphadenopathy
   B. Bowel wall stratification
   C. Contrast enhancement
   D. Perienteric stranding

3. What is the main advantage of MRI over CT for the evaluation of Crohn's disease?
   A. Multiplanar capability
   B. Contrast enhancement
   C. Lack of ionizing radiation
   D. Improved spatial resolution

4. In this case, small bowel feces has occurred secondary to Crohn's disease. With which of the following conditions would you *not* expect small bowel feces to occur?
   A. Ischemia
   B. Adhesions
   C. Cystic fibrosis
   D. Mesenteric volvulus

Small Bowel Feces Sign in Crohn's Disease

1. B, C, and E

2. C

3. C

4. D

References

Sempere GA, Martinez Sanjuan V, Medina Chulia E, et al: MRI evaluation of inflammatory activity in Crohn's disease. *AJR Am J Roentgenol* 2005;184(6):1829-1835.

Wills JS, Lobis IF, Denstman FJ: Crohn disease: state of the art. *Radiology* 1997;202(3):597-610.

Cross-Reference

Gastrointestinal Imaging: THE REQUISITES, 3rd ed, p 137.

Comment

Despite its appearance, what looks like stool in the loop of bowel is actually fecal-like material backed up behind a stricture in the ileum of a young woman with Crohn's disease. Note the thickened inflamed bowel and a stricture with proximal dilation and feces-like material distending the loop of obstructed small bowel (see figures). This finding, the small bowel feces sign (SBFS), although not rare, is relatively uncommon. It is most likely to occur in patients with long-standing moderate to severe narrowing of the small bowel. SBFS is often seen in patients with Crohn's disease. However, it has also been described in patients with small bowel obstruction secondary to adhesions, ischemia, hernias, and cystic fibrosis.

Any chronic, slow-developing obstruction may result in this finding. The SBFS is helpful in that it occurs at the level of the obstruction, with the distal tip of the feces-like material tapering down to the exact obstructive site. Generally, CT is a fast and effective way to evaluate for potential small bowel or even colonic obstruction. It can be done quickly without luminal contrast because dilated bowel proximal to the obstructing site is usually distended with air or, more likely, fluid. The identification of normal-caliber bowel and its relationship to fluid-filled distended bowel can often detect the obstructing site and, in some cases, the offending agent. Adhesions are difficult to see with CT; the absence of any other cause of a sudden transition is suggestive of adhesions. Because adhesions are the most common cause of small bowel obstruction, and approximately 20% of hospital admissions are the result of some form of small bowel obstruction, CT evaluation is becoming an increasingly important diagnostic tool in these cases.

Notes

Challenge

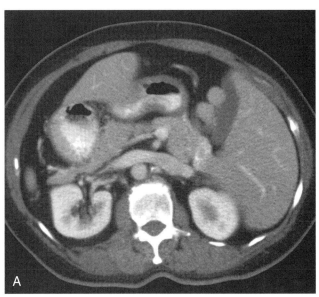

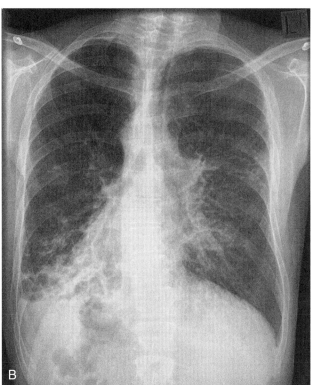

History: A 47-year-old man presents with abdominal pain.

1. What should be included in the differential diagnosis of the imaging finding shown in Figure A? (Choose all that apply.)
   A. Malrotation
   B. Postoperative
   C. Situs inversus
   D. Splenomegaly
   E. Mislabeled image

2. Chest x-ray shows dextrocardia and right lower lobe bronchiectasis. What chronic disease does this patient have?
   A. Cystic fibrosis
   B. Recurrent aspiration
   C. Kartagener's syndrome
   D. Tracheoesophageal fistula

3. What is the most serious disease associated with situs ambiguus (heterotaxy syndrome)?
   A. Recurrent chest infections
   B. Congenital heart disease
   C. Pancreatic insufficiency
   D. Thrombocytopenia

4. Which of the following statements regarding situs inversus is true?
   A. Kartagener's syndrome is characterized by situs inversus, bronchiectasis, and chronic mastoiditis.
   B. The incidence of congenital heart disease in patients with situs inversus is about 5%.
   C. The underlying condition causing situs inversus is primary ciliary dyskinesia.
   D. Prevalence of Kartagener's syndrome is about 1 in 10,000.

Situs Inversus

1. C and E

2. C

3. B

4. B

References

Applegate KE, Goske MJ, Pierce G, et al: Situs revisited: imaging of the heterotaxy syndrome. *Radiographics* 1999;19(4):837-852.

Fulcher AS, Turner MA: Abdominal manifestations of situs anomalies in adults. *Radiographics* 2002;22(6):1439-1456.

Cross-Reference

Gastrointestinal Imaging: THE REQUISITES, 3rd ed, p 146.

Comment

The reverse of the normal arrangement of organs in the chest and abdomen (situs solitus) is called situs inversus and sometimes situs ambiguus, although situs ambiguus (heterotaxy) is usually reserved for conditions that fall outside the mere orderly mirror arrangement of situs inversus, such as seen in this patient (see figures). Situs ambiguus would include an array of anomalies that may or may not be present in any predictable frequency, such as discontinuous inferior vena cava, azygos continuation, and common or shared trunk for the celiac and superior mesenteric arteries. Situs ambiguus can also occur with asplenia, and these patients have an extremely high incidence of congenital heart disease (85% to 95%); situs ambiguus is more commonly seen in pediatric patients. The other main division of situs ambiguus is situs ambiguus with polysplenia. The incidence of heart disease is much lower. Most of these patients have levocardia. This patient has dextrocardia (see figures).

Situs ambiguus with asplenia is almost universally associated with some form of congenital heart disease and is uncommon in adults. This probably relates to the high mortality of situs ambiguus and asplenia in infancy. Situs ambiguus with polysplenia may be an asymptomatic condition if not associated with a congenital cardiac defect. The organ arrangement may be an incidental discovery. Occasionally these patients are referred for vague abdominal pain.

Notes

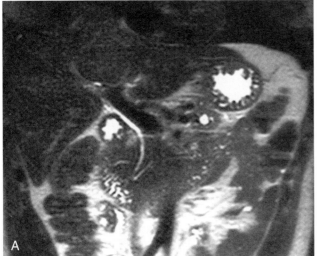

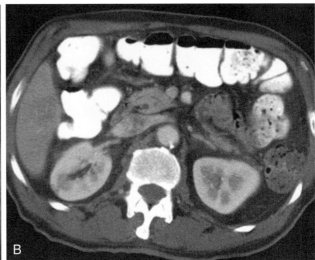

History: A 42-year-old man presents with epigastric pain.

1. What is the diagnosis of the imaging finding shown in Figure A?
   A. Annular pancreas
   B. Pancreas divisum
   C. Chronic pancreatitis
   D. "Double-duct" sign
   E. Normal anatomy

2. What is the most common congenital abnormality of the pancreatic gland and ducts?
   A. Pancreatic ectopia
   B. Pancreas divisum
   C. Annular pancreas
   D. Pancreatic cysts

3. What is the most common clinical scenario associated with pancreas divisum?
   A. Asymptomatic
   B. Pancreatitis
   C. Carcinoma
   D. Diabetes

4. Pancreas divisum is characterized at endoscopic retrograde cholangiopancreatography (ERCP) by a duct in the head and uncinate of the pancreas with a foreshortened, arborizing appearance. What is the embryologic origin of this duct?
   A. Vaterian duct
   B. Duct of Wirsung
   C. Duct of Santorini
   D. Dorsal pancreatic duct

CASE 152

Pancreas Divisum

1. B

2. B

3. A

4. B

References

Chalazonitis NA, Lachanis BS, Laspas F, et al: Pancreas divisum: magnetic resonance cholangiopancreatography findings. *Singapore Med J* 2008;49(11):951-954.

Soto JA, Lucey BC, Stuhlfaut JW: Pancreas divisum: depiction with multidetector row CT. *Radiology* 2005;235(2):503-508.

Cross-Reference

Gastrointestinal Imaging: *THE REQUISITES,* 3rd ed, p 152.

Comment

The pancreas develops as two separate buds from the midgut that appear at about 5 weeks of gestation and fuse together shortly thereafter to form a single pancreas. Not only do the two buds fuse their tissue, but also the associated ductal structures must join. Because of the complex nature of the ductal structures, anomalies affecting the drainage of the pancreatic ducts occur in a large percentage of individuals. Embryologically, the major, or ventral, pancreatic bud develops into the ventral pancreas. In situations in which the ventral and dorsal buds do not fuse, as the ventral pancreas rotates, its duct becomes the major duct in the head of the pancreas with a foreshortened, arborizing appearance. It also is joined to the biliary system, and these ducts drain through the major papilla. The minor ventral bud of the pancreas develops separately and drains via the minor papilla. Under normal circumstances, the duct of Santorini fuses to the duct of Wirsung, and the Santorini duct goes on to drain through the Wirsung duct and into the major papilla. The portion of the Santorini duct that did drain into the duodenum usually involutes, and there is no separate papilla.

Pancreas divisum (seen in 4% to 7% of autopsy cases) may have several variations, the most common of which is when the less prominent ventral duct maintains its separate drainage, along with the bile duct, into the duodenum via the major papilla. The minor papilla is usually proximal to the major papilla and drains the greater dorsal duct. The dorsal duct drains the body and tail, and the ventral duct drains the head and uncinate. In some instances, as in this case, there may be a tiny communicating branch between the two systems.

Most cases of pancreas divisum are discovered incidentally during ERCP or, as in this case (see figures), magnetic resonance cholangiopancreatography (MRCP). However, there is a higher than normal incidence of pancreatitis in these patients. The exact etiology of pancreatitis in pancreatic divisum, excluding all other factors (e.g., stones, alcohol), is unclear. Some researchers think it relates to the major duct attempting to empty its exocrine content into the duodenum via a tiny minor papilla. Acute pancreatitis in a young person should arouse some suspicion for this condition. Although ERCP or MRCP would be the examination of choice, a CT scan showing what appears to be three ducts in the pancreatic head is suggestive, as in the CT image of this case (see figures).

Notes

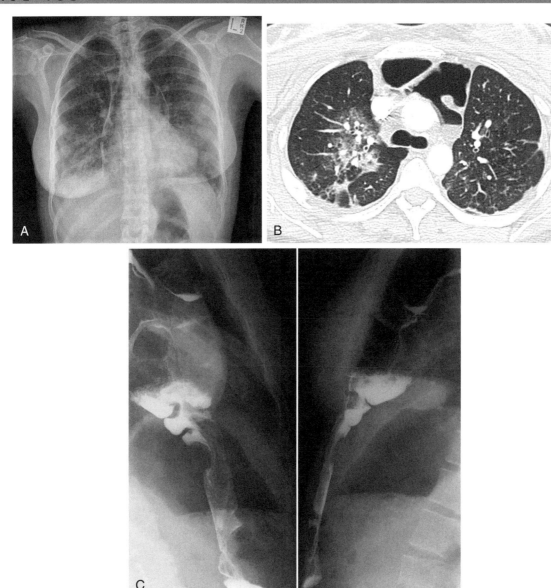

History: A 35-year-old woman presents with heartburn and dyspnea.

1. What should be included in the differential diagnosis of the imaging finding shown in Figure A? (Choose all that apply.)
   A. Hiatal hernia
   B. Morgagni hernia
   C. Bochdalek hernia
   D. Colonic interposition
   E. Pneumomediastinum

2. What is the most common viscus used for esophageal interposition surgery?
   A. Stomach
   B. Duodenum
   C. Jejunum
   D. Colon

3. What is the most common serious postoperative complication of esophageal interposition surgery?
   A. Leak
   B. Stricture
   C. Mucocele
   D. Aspiration

4. Esophagectomy with interposition is also performed for management of esophageal carcinoma; however, tumors recur in 60% to 75% of cases. Where do tumors most commonly recur?
   A. Anastomosis
   B. Distant metastases
   C. Interposed segment
   D. Regional metastases

Colonic Interposition

1. A, B, D, and E

2. A

3. A

4. B

References

Kim SH, Lee KS, Shim YM, et al: Esophageal resection: indications, techniques, and radiologic assessment. *Radiographics* 2001;21(5):1119-1137.

Meloni GB, Feo CF, Profili S, et al: Postoperative radiologic evaluation of the esophagus. *Eur J Radiol* 2005;53(3):331-340.

Cross-Reference

Gastrointestinal Imaging: *THE REQUISITES,* 3rd ed, p 39.

Comment

A patient with severe esophageal disease may require surgical bypass when the native esophagus is obstructed or no longer functional. Some surgeons use a length of colon and anastomose it from the upper thoracic or cervical esophagus to the stomach (see figures). Alternatively, jejunum may be used, bypassing the diseased esophagus. The remaining esophagus may be surgically isolated but usually is not removed because of potential damage to nerves, lymphatics, and collateral blood flow. Colonic interposition is commonly performed in patients with benign diseases, such as caustic or peptic strictures, or severe motor disorders. Occasionally, this procedure is performed in patients with malignant disease, in particular, if there is a good chance of survival or if a complication, such as perforation, has occurred.

Complications are common because of the complexity of the surgery. Early complications include anastomotic leakage and possible fistula formation. Stenoses also may develop at the anastomotic sites, typically the proximal site. Aspiration of ingested contents is another problem. Later problems include stasis of swallowed material within the interposed segment and reflux of gastric contents into the colonic interposition. Malignancy has been described in these colonic interpositions, but it is rare.

In the course of the surgery, if the surgeon isolates the esophagus by surgically closing its ends, a mucocele of the esophagus may develop. This mucocele consists of mucous or proteinaceous secretions that fill the lumen of the isolated esophagus and have nowhere to drain. The phenomenon is usually self-limited because increasing pressure within the lumen causes cessation of the mucous secretion. Rarely, the mass continues to increase in size, leading to symptoms. However, in the absence of an adequate history, the presence of a transposed colon or jejunum in the chest may surprise the resident or radiologist. Talking to the patient before the examination is very good; being surprised during the performance of the examination is not.

Notes

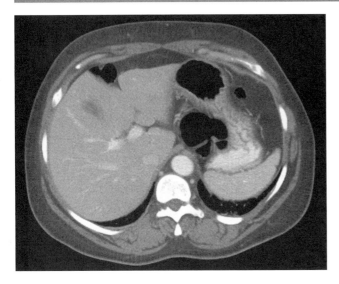

History: A 54-year-old woman presents with abdominal pain.

1. What should be included in the differential diagnosis of the imaging finding shown in the figure? (Choose all that apply.)
   A. Paraduodenal hernia
   B. Pancreatic pseudocyst
   C. Transmesenteric hernia
   D. Perivaterian diverticulum
   E. Foramen of Winslow hernia

2. What is the peritoneal space posterior to the stomach and anterior to the pancreas called?
   A. Lesser sac
   B. Greater sac
   C. Morison's pouch
   D. Pouch of Douglas

3. Which of the following is the viscus most commonly herniated through the foramen of Winslow?
   A. Right colon
   B. Small bowel
   C. Gallbladder
   D. Transverse colon

4. Which of the following is the most common of the various internal hernias?
   A. Pericecal
   B. Paraduodenal
   C. Transmesenteric
   D. Foramen of Winslow

Foramen of Winslow Internal Bowel Hernia

1. A, C, and E

2. A

3. B

4. B

References

Martin LC, Merkle EM, Thompson WM: Review of internal hernias: radiographic and clinical findings. *AJR Am J Roentgenol* 2006;186(3):703-717.
Takeyama N, Gokan T, Ohgiya Y, et al: CT of internal hernias. *Radiographics* 2005;25(4):997-1015.

Cross-Reference

Gastrointestinal Imaging: *THE REQUISITES,* 3rd ed, p 331.

Comment

The foramen of Winslow (also known as the epiploic foramen) lies at the right free edge of the hepatogastric and hepatoduodenal ligaments in the region of the underside of the liver. It is posterior to the edge of the lesser omentum, just to the right of the spine. It is normally a little larger than the width of a finger but can be much larger in some people. It is unusual to see bowel herniation via the foramen into the lesser sac. The clinician must take time to evaluate carefully because a right paraduodenal hernia can have a similar appearance. If the herniated bowel crosses the midline to the right, it is evidence of a hernia of the foramen of Winslow. In some cases, such as this case, it is redundant transverse colon or right colon with little or no retroperitonization that herniates through the foramen. If the bowel becomes strangulated, it becomes a surgical emergency.

A barium enema would be very helpful, but as seen in this case, CT suggests the diagnosis (see figure). On plain film, the gastric air bubble is seen along with a collection of air overlying but not in the stomach. On this CT image, air is seen behind the stomach in the region of the gastrohepatic ligament and the foramen itself.

Internal bowel hernias are uncommon, and hernias of the foramen of Winslow are even less common. Most internal hernias are paraduodenal or transmesenteric. Many hernias are asymptomatic and are discovered incidentally. The hernia can also be transient and be the cause of endless work-ups for a patient with vague abdominal complaints and transient obstructive symptoms. It is also possible for the herniated bowel to compress the common bile duct, and a few cases of jaundice relating to hernias of the foramen of Winslow have been reported.

Notes

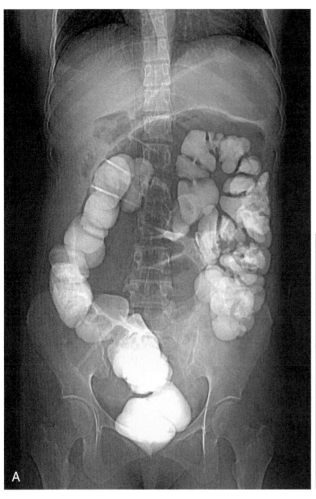

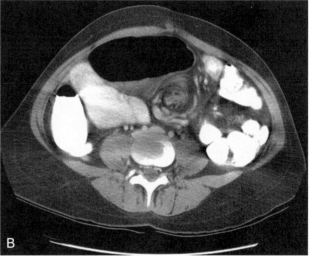

History: A 25-year-old woman presents with sudden onset of severe abdominal pain after several episodes of intermittent abdominal pain and swelling.

1. What should be included in the differential diagnosis of the imaging finding shown in Figure A? (Choose all that apply.)
   A. Cecal volvulus
   B. Umbilical hernia
   C. Small bowel volvulus
   D. Appendiceal mucocele
   E. Paraesophageal hernia

2. What name best describes the type of obstruction that results in the marked dilation seen in this case?
   A. High grade
   B. Mechanical
   C. Closed loop
   D. Incarcerated

3. In what age group is this condition of mesenteric volvulus most commonly seen?
   A. Prenatal
   B. Infancy
   C. Adolescence
   D. Adulthood

4. What imaging examination would you consider next?
   A. None
   B. B-mode ultrasound
   C. Doppler ultrasound
   D. Mesenteric angiography

Mesenteric Volvulus

1. A, B, and C

2. C

3. B

4. A

References

Peterson CM, Anderson JS, Hara AK, et al: Volvulus of the gastrointestinal tract: appearances at multi-modality imaging. *Radiographics* 2009;29(5): 1281-1293.

Pickhardt PJ, Bhalla S: Intestinal malrotation in adolescents and adults: spectrum of clinical and imaging features. *AJR Am J Roentgenol* 2002;179(6): 1429-1435.

Cross-Reference

Gastrointestinal Imaging: *THE REQUISITES,* 3rd ed, p 110.

Comment

Small bowel, or mesenteric, volvulus is a life-threatening condition that occurs when a loop or loops of small bowel twist around its mesenteric root. When complete occlusion occurs, it is, in effect, a "closed-loop obstruction" and requires immediate treatment to avoid compromise of the vascular pedicle, bowel necrosis, perforation, peritonitis, and death. The condition may be transitory in some cases. However, even when the bowel is unobstructed, CT may suggest the possibility of the diagnosis by the swirling appearance of the root of the mesentery, even if the patient is unobstructed. In this case, the swirling configuration of the mesenteric root is quite pronounced, and the patient is experiencing a closed-loop obstruction with gross dilation of loops of small bowel in the midabdomen (see figures).

The condition is most frequently seen in infants with midgut malrotation, Ladd's bands, and the attendant increase risk of midgut volvulus. This condition is sometimes referred to as secondary mesenteric volvulus because there are underlying congenital causes for the volvulus. However, mesenteric volvulus is occasionally seen in older individuals as a primary volvulus in which no congenital abnormalities are present. Conditions such as an extra long mesentery, high-fiber diet, or anorexia may contribute to the development of the condition; however, this is speculation and it is unknown why some patients develop this condition.

Mesenteric volvulus is uncommon and represents about 1% to 2% of small bowel obstructions. However, a full-blown twist of the mesenteric root and the resulting closed-loop obstruction can lead to mesenteric infarction in almost half of patients. There is probably a direct correlation of morbidity to the length of the interval between diagnosis and treatment.

Not all swirling seen at the mesenteric root is a small bowel volvulus. As indicated, it may be a transient process that results in complicated work-ups without significant results. Similar to cases of transient intussusception, seeing the patient between episodes can be problematic.

Notes

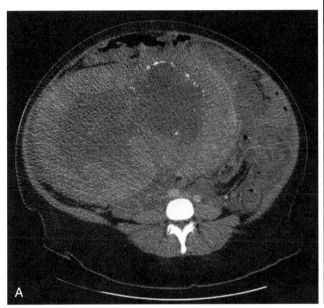

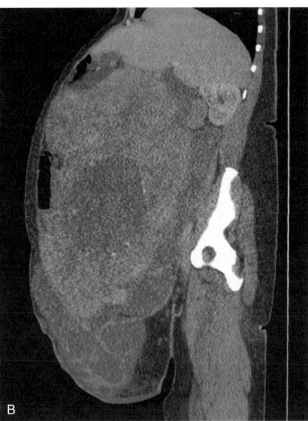

History: A 56-year-old woman presents with abdominal distention.

1. What should be included in the differential diagnosis of the site of origin of the imaging finding shown in Figure A? (Choose all that apply.)
   A. Renal
   B. Hepatic
   C. Body wall
   D. Mesenteric
   E. Gynecologic

2. What is the most common gynecologic tumor in women older than 30 years?
   A. Endometrial carcinoma
   B. Ovarian dermoid
   C. Uterine fibroid
   D. Hydrosalpinx

3. What is the most common mode of presentation of uterine fibroids?
   A. Asymptomatic
   B. Uterine bleeding
   C. Bulk-related symptoms
   D. Reproductive dysfunction

4. What imaging modality would you recommend to visualize uterine fibroids best when planning for surgery or intervention?
   A. Hysterosalpingography
   B. Transvaginal ultrasound
   C. Saline infusion sonography
   D. MRI

Huge Myometrial Leiomyomas

1. A, B, D, and E

2. C

3. A

4. D

References

Fielding JR: MR imaging of the female pelvis. *Radiol Clin North Am* 2003;41(1):179-192.

Murase E, Siegelman EV, Outwater EK, et al: Uterine leiomyomas: histopathologic features, MR imaging findings, differential diagnosis, and treatment. *Radiographics* 1999;19(5):1179-1197.

Ueda H, Togashi K, Konishi I, et al: Unusual appearances of uterine leiomyomas: MR imaging findings and their histopathologic backgrounds. *Radiographics* 1999;19(Spec No):S131-S145.

Cross-Reference

Gastrointestinal Imaging: *THE REQUISITES,* 3rd ed, p 308.

Comment

Uterine fibroids do not usually present a problem for either patients or radiologists. They are commonly a secondary finding noted at the time of examination (especially in CT). This patient's huge myometrial leiomyoma is unusual, and malignancy was suspected (see figures). A 30-lb fibroid and adhesions and fluid were found at surgery, and pathologic examination showed no evidence of malignancy. There is a small malignant risk in uterine fibroids usually reported as about 1%. Most are asymptomatic. Some are implicated in infertility states.

Common treatments include selective resection or total hysterectomy, if deemed necessary. An estimated 600,000 hysterectomies are performed annually in the United States, and approximately one-third are for uterine leiomyomas (fibroid). In recent years, treatment by uterine artery embolization has proved helpful in the treatment of symptomatic lesions.

CT and ultrasound are often used in the evaluation of this condition. However, MRI may also be very helpful. Fibroids tend to enhance on the margins when gadolinium enhancement is used. The rim may be seen in unenhanced cases with T2 imaging. The tissue signal is usually lower than the surrounding tissue on both T1 and T2 imaging. Small linear arrangements of calcification can be seen in this lesion, which might suggest benignity but cannot rule out malignancy. Alternative diagnostic considerations in this patient would be ovarian mass, tumor originating from ovary or uterus, uterine leiomyosarcoma, and adenomyosis of the uterus.

Notes

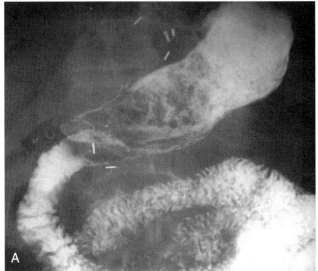

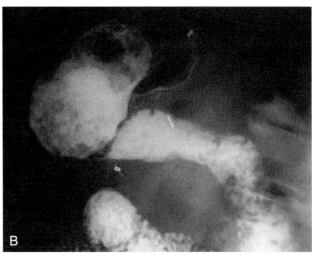

History: A 67-year-old man presents for evaluation of choking episodes.

1. What should be included in the differential diagnosis of the imaging finding shown in Figure A? (Choose all that apply.)
   A. Bezoar
   B. Large polyp
   C. Diverticulum
   D. Linitis plastica
   E. Poor preparation

2. The stomach has an abnormal configuration as a result of previous surgery. What operation has been performed?
   A. Billroth I operation
   B. Billroth II operation
   C. Whipple operation
   D. Sleeve gastrectomy

3. Which of the following is the most common material found in bezoars?
   A. Persimmon fruit
   B. Vegetable fiber
   C. Psyllium fiber
   D. Hair

4. Which of the following postgastrectomy complications is more common after the Billroth II operation compared with the Billroth I operation?
   A. Gastric stump carcinoma
   B. Afferent loop syndrome
   C. Stomal ulceration
   D. Gastroparesis

Gastric Bezoar in Post–Billroth I Stomach

1. A, B, and E

2. A

3. B

4. B

References

Ripolles T, Garcia-Aguayo J, Martinez M, et al: Gastrointestinal bezoars: sono-graphic and CT characteristics. *AJR Am J Roentgenol* 2001;177(1):65-69.

Woodfield CA, Levine MS: The postoperative stomach. *Eur J Radiol* 2005;53(3):341-352.

Cross-Reference

Gastrointestinal Imaging: *THE REQUISITES*, 3rd ed, p 78.

Comment

Gastric bezoars represent a complication of gastric surgery relating to disordered motility. However, bezoars can be seen in stomachs with normal anatomy as well. A bezoar is a ball of foreign or nondigestible material that does not pass the pylorus or the stoma in a postoperative stomach (see figures). Most bezoars are seen as a complication of gastric surgery or as the result of the ingestion of nonfood items, such as hair (trichobezoars) or indigestible fiber (phytobezoars). The fruit of the persimmon tree is almost always used as an example and is probably the most common cause of bezoars in non-surgical stomachs in the United States. Bezoars have been reported with other accumulations of fiber in the stomach as well, including psyllium fiber powder laxatives ingested with insufficient water.

After gastric surgery, the occurrence of bezoars is thought to range from 5% to 12%; this can seem high given day-to-day experience with these patients. Such indigestible items as orange peels, potato peels, and laxative fiber probably account for most bezoars in this setting. Bilateral vagotomy, which usually accompanies gastric resection, leading to the resultant alteration in gastric empty-ing, is largely the source of the problem.

After gastric surgery, patients with a gastric bezoar often complain of abdominal discomfort, pain, fullness, and vomit-ing. Rarely, bezoars can occur in other parts of the gastrointes-tinal tract. Also found in the literature are reports of unusual types of bezoars such as varnish bezoars in detail painters for fine furniture.

Notes

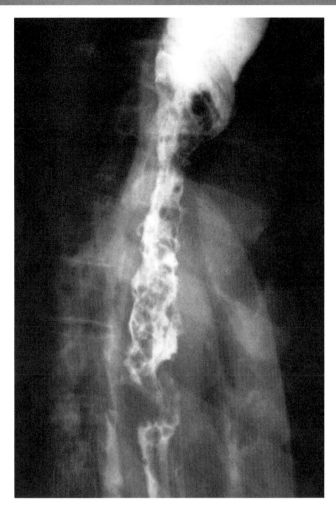

History: A 57-year-old male alcoholic presents with a 6-month history of retrosternal dysphagia and 10-kg weight loss.

1. What should be included in the differential diagnosis of the imaging finding shown in the figure? (Choose all that apply.)
   A. Esophagitis
   B. Esophageal carcinoma
   C. Downhill esophageal varices
   D. Uphill esophageal varices
   E. Lymphoma

2. What part of the bowel wall present in other segments of the GI tract is not found in the esophagus?
   A. Longitudinal muscularis
   B. Transverse muscularis
   C. Lymphatics
   D. Serosa

3. Why do "jump" metastases occur in esophageal carcinoma?
   A. Portosystemic venous collaterals
   B. Network of lymphatic channels
   C. Absence of esophageal serosa
   D. Metachronous tumor deposits

4. What disease is the world's most common cause of portal hypertension and varices?
   A. Bronchogenic carcinoma
   B. Alcoholic cirrhosis
   C. Schistosomiasis
   D. Tuberculosis

CASE 158

Esophageal Varicoid Cancer

1. A, B, C, and E

2. D

3. B

4. C

References

Iyer R, Dubrow R: Imaging upper gastrointestinal malignancy. *Semin Roentgenol* 2006;41(2):105-112.

Levine MS: Esophageal cancer: radiologic diagnosis. *Radiol Clin North Am* 1997;35(2):265-279.

Sabedotti G, Dreweck MO, Sabedotti V, et al: Best cases from the AFIP: Carcinoma of the esophagus: varicoid pattern. *Radiographics* 2006;26(1):271-274.

Cross-Reference

Gastrointestinal Imaging: THE REQUISITES, 3rd ed, p 32.

Comment

Esophageal carcinoma can appear in many different forms. The most common form is a stricture, usually irregular in nature. It also may be an eccentric mass or a polypoid mass within the lumen. It may ulcerate, with resultant bleeding. The anatomy of the esophagus is different from the anatomy of the remainder of the GI tract, which results in the rapid spread of the neoplasm and the resultant poor prognosis.

In contrast to the rest of the GI tract, there is no serosal layer in the esophagus, and neoplasms invade the adjacent structures directly, resulting in a high rate of morbidity. Also, the lymphatic drainage of the esophagus is complex. There is an extensive network of lymphatic channels in all layers of the esophagus. This characteristic results in metastases spreading circumferentially and to adjacent lymph node groups in the mediastinum. The tumor may "jump" or disseminate throughout the length of the esophagus via these channels. There may be intervening normal mucosa between these areas of tumor. This pattern of spread is believed to result in the varicoid appearance of esophageal carcinoma seen in this patient (see the figure). Despite the history of alcoholism in this patient, varicoid carcinoma of the esophagus can be distinguished by the fact that the pattern does not change whether the patient is upright or recumbent, does not change with Valsalva respiration, is not pliable, and carries no peristaltic waves.

Varicoid carcinoma is an unusual variant of esophageal carcinoma. The tumor spreads submucosally down the length of the esophagus, producing thickened folds. The appearance closely mimics esophageal varices—hence the name. Because of this pattern of spread, dysphagia is usually a late symptom, and the disease has usually spread extensively before being diagnosed. A patient with this form of esophageal neoplasm has a poor prognosis.

Notes

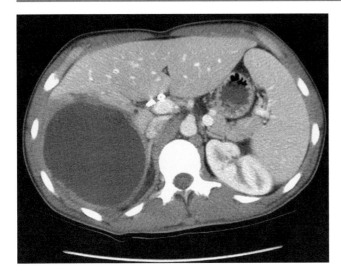

History: A 49-year-old man presents with right upper quadrant pain and a relevant past history of laparoscopic cholecystectomy 5 years ago.

1. What should be included in the differential diagnosis of the imaging finding shown in the figure? (Choose all that apply.)
   A. Hemangioma
   B. Choledochocele
   C. Echinococcal cyst
   D. Intrahepatic biloma
   E. Biliary cystadenoma

2. What imaging modality would you recommend to evaluate further for bile duct injury related to this lesion in planning for intervention?
   A. Endoscopic retrograde cholangiopancreatography (ERCP)
   B. Ultrasound
   C. MRI with magnetic resonance cholangiopancreatography (MRCP)
   D. Percutaneous cholangiography

3. What is the most common complication of laparoscopic cholecystectomy?
   A. Bleeding
   B. Bowel injury
   C. Bile duct injury
   D. Retained stone

4. What is the most common benign neoplasm of the liver?
   A. Simple cyst
   B. Hemangioma
   C. Intrahepatic biloma
   D. Biliary cystadenoma

Intrahepatic Biloma

1. C, D, and E

2. C

3. D

4. B

References

Thurley PD, Dhingsa R: Laparoscopic cholecystectomy: postoperative imaging. *AJR Am J Roentgenol* 2008;191(3):794-801.

Wright TB, Bertino RB, Bishop AF, et al: Complications of laparoscopic cholecystectomy and their interventional radiologic management. *Radiographics* 1993;13(1):119-128.

Cross-Reference

Gastrointestinal Imaging: *THE REQUISITES,* 3rd ed, p 241.

Comment

The CT image shows a large cystic, well-defined lesion taking up considerable space in the liver (see the figure). Major diagnostic considerations include some type of cystic structure communicating with the biliary system. Simple hepatic cysts, although lined by biliary tract epithelium, rarely communicate with the biliary system, despite their common occurrence. Echinococcal cysts may communicate with the biliary system, and a major complication is spontaneous rupture into the bile ducts or peritoneal cavity. Necrotic tumors or metastases rarely communicate with the biliary tract.

The most common cause for this intrahepatic cystic lesion, which was later drained, is the accumulation of bile as a result of a ruptured bile duct sustained in the initial injury. This injury may be seen following the course of cholecystectomy. During cholecystectomy, the surgeon often inserts probes or catheters into the bile ducts to identify possible retained calculi or debris. Sometimes a small endoscope is inserted into the ducts. Because intrahepatic ducts often taper rapidly, some of these small intrahepatic ducts may rupture during passage of some of these instruments. If a cholangiogram is obtained in the immediate postoperative period, a small area of extravasation may be identified.

Usually these small intrahepatic duct perforations close spontaneously after 2 to 3 weeks. Problems arise if pressure in the biliary system is increased because of obstruction, as in this patient. In this scenario, the bile collection may increase in size and form a biloma. If the biliary tract also is infected, the bile may become infected and form an abscess. The radiologist must recognize this complication and identify its true nature accurately. This study usually can be followed by drainage of the biloma and injection into the evacuated cavity to see if the leaking bile duct can be identified. If so, repeat injections of the drained biloma over the course of the next few weeks may be undertaken to show healing and integrity of the biliary system. Similar but more expensive mechanisms for following the healing biliary system would be serial CT and MRI studies. The most worrisome complications of a biloma are infection and leakage into the peritoneal cavity.

Notes

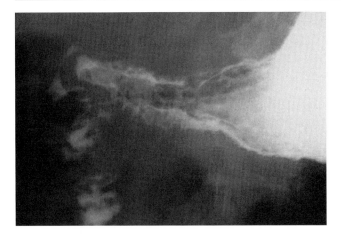

History: A 54-year-old woman presents with intermittent nausea, vomiting, and diarrhea.

1. What should be included in the differential diagnosis of the imaging finding shown in the figure? (Choose all that apply.)
   A. Tuberculosis
   B. Gastric varices
   C. Crohn's disease
   D. Metastatic carcinoma
   E. Primary gastric carcinoma

2. In patients with Crohn's disease, what area of the stomach is most commonly involved?
   A. Body
   B. Antrum
   C. Fundus
   D. Whole stomach

3. When Crohn's disease is long-standing, the antrum and duodenum become a featureless rigid tube. What is the name given to this sign?
   A. "Cobblestone" sign
   B. "Ram's horn" sign
   C. "Rose thorn" sign
   D. "String" sign

4. Crohn's disease is one of many granulomatous diseases that may involve the stomach. Which is the most common in a Western hemisphere population?
   A. Sarcoidosis
   B. Tuberculosis
   C. Crohn's disease
   D. Wegener's granulomatosis

Crohn's Disease of the Stomach

1. A, C, D, and E

2. B

3. B

4. C

References

Horsthuis K, Bipat S, Bennink RJ, et al: Inflammatory bowel disease diagnosed with US, MR, scintigraphy, and CT: meta-analysis of prospective studies. *Radiology* 2008;247(1):64-79.

Wills JS, Lobis IF, Denstman FJ: Crohn disease: state of the art. *Radiology* 1997;202(3):597-610.

Cross-Reference

Gastrointestinal Imaging: THE REQUISITES, 3rd ed, p 69.

Comment

Crohn's disease of the stomach is usually found in the distal aspect of the stomach but rarely may involve the entire organ. The antrum is first to become involved, and the disease may spread more proximally. Fundal involvement is unusual. Many patients also have associated involvement of the duodenum (see the figure). The stomach is rarely the only part of the gut that is involved by Crohn's disease; most often, there is ileal or colonic Crohn's disease as well, and it should be assumed that there is disease in other portions of the GI tract, too. The incidence of Crohn's disease involving the stomach ranges from 5% to 40% of cases. A much higher incidence is reported in Japan than in North America.

The most common manifestation of Crohn's disease in the stomach is gastric erosions. These erosions are identical to other types of erosions in the stomach, and there is no way to distinguish them radiologically. As the disease progresses, the severity of the inflammation may increase, and ulcers may become confluent and linear or stellate in configuration. As with other portions of the GI tract, the inflammation is transmural, resulting in fibrosis and scarring. Typically (according to some reports, in more than half of the cases of gastric Crohn's disease), there may be involvement of the adjacent duodenum.

When Crohn's disease is long-standing, the antrum and duodenum become a featureless rigid tube; this presentation is called the "ram's horn" sign because of the conical antrum and widening funnel of the body and fundus. This configuration may be so severe that it resembles a scirrhous carcinoma or any condition that might give a linitis plastica appearance to the stomach. Fistulas are a rare complication of gastric Crohn's disease but can develop into the transverse colon. Postinflammatory polyps may develop as a sequela of Crohn's disease of the stomach as they do elsewhere in the gut, especially in the colon.

Notes

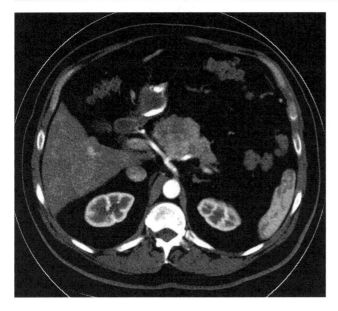
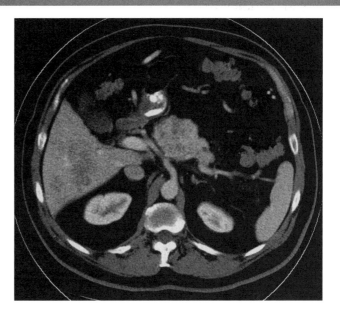

History: A 61-year-old woman presents for evaluation of fainting episodes.

1. What should be included in the differential diagnosis of the imaging finding shown in the figures? (Choose all that apply.)
   A. Metastases from a neuroendocrine tumor
   B. Metastases from a mucinous carcinoma
   C. Multifocal hepatocellular carcinoma
   D. Multifocal hemangiomas
   E. Lymphoma

2. Which of the following is the most common pancreatic islet cell tumor?
   A. VIPoma
   B. Insulinoma
   C. Gastrinoma
   D. Nonfunctioning islet cell tumor

3. What is the most common malignancy that results in hypervascular liver metastases?
   A. Carcinoid
   B. Melanoma
   C. Renal cell carcinoma
   D. Pancreatic islet cell tumor

4. If this patient exhibits palpitations, sweating, and headache, what clinical diagnosis should be suspected?
   A. VIPoma
   B. Insulinoma
   C. Gastrinoma
   D. Glucagonoma

Islet Cell Tumor of the Pancreas

1. A, B, C, and D

2. D

3. A

4. B

References

Horton KM, Hruban RH, Yeo C, et al: Multi-detector row CT of pancreatic islet cell tumors. *Radiographics* 2006;26(2):453-464.

Ichikawa T, Peterson MS, Federle MP, et al: Islet cell tumor of the pancreas: biphasic CT versus MR imaging in tumor detection. *Radiology* 2000;216(1):163-171.

Lee DS, Brooke Jeffrey R, Kamaya A: Islet-cell tumors of the pancreas: spectrum of MDCT findings. *Appl Radiol* 2009;38:10-28.

Cross-Reference

Gastrointestinal Imaging: *THE REQUISITES,* 3rd ed, p 164.

Comment

About 50% of all islet cell tumors of the pancreas are non-functioning islet cell tumors. Because they are relatively asymptomatic (they do not produce and secrete endocrine products), they can grow to large size, such as in this case (see figures). The biliary system is not invaded, and there is no biliary dilation within the liver. Because these tumors grow slowly and quietly over a long period, they are quite large when discovered and may be malignant. Studies have shown that almost 50% of islet cell tumors of the pancreas are malignant at the time of discovery, mostly by contiguous spread or from metastatic disease to the liver.

Most tumors are large enough to have necrotic centers at the time of discovery. In addition, nonfunctioning islet cell tumors may have a cystic component, which can confuse and delay diagnosis. Nonfunctioning islet cell tumors can occur anywhere in the pancreas, with the most popular sites being the head and tail. They can reach sizes of 8 to 20 cm.

Even with the high potential of malignancy, the prognosis remains good, which is not the case for ductal adenocarcinomas of the pancreas. Of all islet cell tumors, functioning or nonfunctioning, 20% to 25% have some calcifications within them, whereas only 1% to 2% of ductal carcinomas show any sign of calcification. The treatment is surgical.

Notes

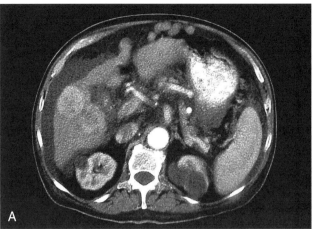

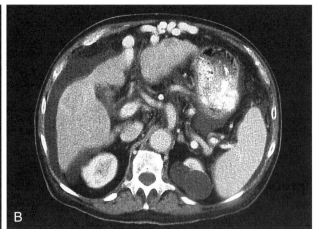

History: An 83-year-old man presents with lower limb pitting edema.

1. What should be included in the differential diagnosis of the imaging finding shown in Figure A? (Choose all that apply.)
   A. Amebic abscesses
   B. Hepatocellular carcinoma (HCC)
   C. Focal nodular hyperplasia
   D. Hypervascular metastases
   E. Mesenchymal hamartomas

2. What is the predisposing condition most commonly associated with this diagnosis in whites in the United States?
   A. α₁-Antitrypsin deficiency
   B. Hemochromatosis
   C. Alcoholic cirrhosis
   D. Diabetes mellitus

3. What is the predisposing condition most commonly associated with this diagnosis in Asians?
   A. Viral hepatitis
   B. Alcoholic cirrhosis
   C. Parasitic liver infections
   D. Environmental contamination

4. What elevated serum factor is commonly seen with this disease?
   A. Alpha-fetoprotein (AFP)
   B. Carcinoembryonic antigen (CEA)
   C. Gamma-glutamyl transferase
   D. Beta-human chorionic gonadotropin

Hepatocellular Carcinoma

1. B, C, and D

2. C

3. A

4. A

References

Clark HP, Forrest Carson WF, Kavanagh PV, et al: Staging and current treatment of hepatocellular carcinoma. *Radiographics* 2005;25(Suppl 1):S3-S24.

Szklaruk J, Silverman PM, Charnsangavej C: Imaging in the diagnosis, staging, treatment, and surveillance of hepatocellular carcinoma. *AJR Am J Roentgenol* 2003;180(2):441-454.

Cross-Reference

Gastrointestinal Imaging: *THE REQUISITES,* 3rd ed, p 195.

Comment

HCC is a primary malignancy of the hepatocyte. In the West, the disease is uncommon compared with Asia. However, it is usually associated with alcoholism and cirrhosis in the West. Hepatic infections, especially hepatitis B, and parasitic infections of the liver are thought to be the major etiologic factors in Asia. The disease has a dismal prognosis with survival usually not exceeding 6 to 18 months after diagnosis. At the time of diagnosis, at least 50% of patients have tumor spread to the portal veins. There seems to be an increasing incidence of HCC in the West, possibly relating to an increasing incidence of hepatitis B and C. The disease is more commonly seen in men, especially in Asia.

The advent of high-quality multidetector CT and MRI has not changed the mortality rate. The CT image in this case shows typical HCC mass lesions of the right lobe of the liver (see figures). Generally, distortion of the liver architecture by cirrhosis further complicates the process of detecting subtle or early lesions (see figures). An elevated AFP level is helpful for its positive predictive value, but if serum AFP is normal, it does not exclude the disease. In practice, the higher the AFP levels, the greater the likelihood of HCC. CT-guided liver biopsy, if not contraindicated by the possibility of abnormal bleeding and clotting issues, is the most efficient method of diagnosis.

Notes

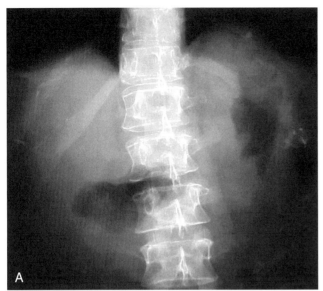

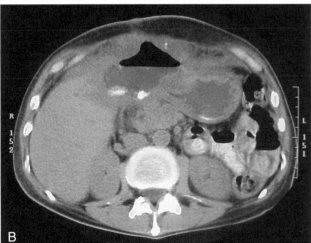

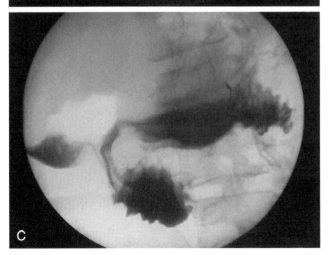

History: A 55-year-old man presents with abdominal pain.

1. What should be included in the differential diagnosis of the imaging finding shown in Figures A and B? (Choose all that apply.)
   A. Abscess
   B. Duodenal hematoma
   C. Localized perforation
   D. Giant duodenal ulcer
   E. Duodenal diverticulum

2. Which of the following is a mucosal defect replacing two thirds of the duodenal bulb?
   A. Giant duodenal ulcer
   B. Duodenal perforation
   C. Duodenal penetration
   D. Duodenal diverticulum

3. Where do perforating ulcers most commonly occur?
   A. Gastric body
   B. Gastric antrum
   C. Duodenal bulb
   D. Postbulbar duodenum

4. Which of the following duodenal neoplasms can be specifically diagnosed with CT?
   A. Lipoma
   B. Hematoma
   C. Lymphoma
   D. Villous adenoma

Giant Duodenal Ulcer

1. A, C, D, and E

2. A

3. C

4. A

References

Kirsh IE, Brendel T: The importance of giant duodenal ulcer. *Radiology* 1968;91(1):14-19.

Zissin R, Osadchy A, Gayer G, et al: Pictorial review. CT of duodenal pathology. *Br J Radiol* 2002;75(889):78-84.

Cross-Reference

Gastrointestinal Imaging: *THE REQUISITES,* 3rd ed, p 99.

Comment

This patient has a giant duodenal ulcer (see figures). The luminal (Gastrografin) study shows retained contrast material within what appears to be a duodenal configuration (see figures). However, no fold pattern is detected. Postbulbar narrowing can also be seen frequently in giant duodenal ulcer disease. The most important complications are bleeding and perforation. The CT image shows large amounts of gas and oral contrast agent in a dependent position within the cavity of the giant ulcer (see figures). CT is very useful to diagnose perforation complicating the ulcer. CT may show 1 to 2 mL of free intraperitoneal air. Studies have indicated that upright or decubitus radiographs also may show similarly tiny amounts of free intraperitoneal air (see figures).

In practice, CT has proved more sensitive than other modalities in showing small amounts of free intraperitoneal air. Also, patients are often too sick to obtain adequate positional views for abdominal studies, and the demonstration of free intraperitoneal air on CT is not dependent on upright positioning. Although the indirect signs of pneumoperitoneum may be seen on conventional images in patients who are too ill to stand, CT is very sensitive for the detection of free air regardless of the patient position. A diagnosis of free intraperitoneal air may be easy to make, but the exact site of perforation may not be so easy to determine. Sometimes the site of perforation is identified at the time of surgery.

Plain radiographs of the abdomen reveal only the presence of free intraperitoneal air, which is a nonspecific finding. However, with the increased use of CT in the emergency setting, the detection of contrast material leaking into the peritoneal cavity and the presence of free intraperitoneal air has become possible. In the right clinical setting, it is unnecessary to perform further studies, and surgery should be performed promptly.

Notes

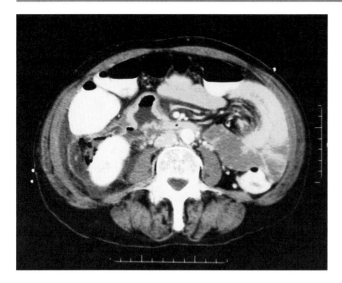

History: A 51-year-old woman presents with right-sided abdominal pain, nausea, and vomiting of brackish dark emesis. She is a long-term user of aspirin and Goody's Powder pain reliever.

1. What should be included in the differential diagnosis of the imaging finding shown in the figure? (Choose all that apply.)
   A. Cholecystitis
   B. Duodenal diverticulitis
   C. Perforated duodenal ulcer
   D. Emphysematous pyelonephritis
   E. Post–endoscopic retrograde cholangiopancreatography (ERCP) and postsphincterotomy

2. Which statement regarding possible causes of duodenal perforation is true?
   A. Duodenal diverticula are most commonly bulbar.
   B. Blunt force trauma usually does not cause duodenal perforation.
   C. Duodenal perforation after ERCP and sphincterotomy is mostly managed surgically.
   D. Peptic ulceration is diagnosed at CT by the presence of circumferential wall thickening.

3. Which of the following conditions is associated with "benign" pneumoretroperitoneum?
   A. Pneumatosis coli cystica
   B. Duodenal diverticulum
   C. Pancreatic pseudocyst
   D. None of the above

4. From where does most of the gas in the bowel come?
   A. Swallowed air
   B. Bacterial fermentation
   C. By-product of food digestion
   D. Product of tissue metabolism

Pneumoretroperitoneum

1. B, C, D, and E

2. B

3. D

4. A

References

Jayaraman MV, Mayo-Smith WW, Movson JS, et al: CT of the duodenum: an overlooked segment gets its due. *Radiographics* 2001;21(Spec No):S147-S160.
Zissin R, Osadchy A, Gayer G, et al: CT of duodenal pathology. *Br J Radiol* 2002;75(889):78-84.

Cross-Reference

Gastrointestinal Imaging: *THE REQUISITES,* 3rd ed, p 98.

Comment

Occasionally, one sees a patient with free intraperitoneal air and no symptoms. Usually the free intraperitoneal air is the result of a burst serosal bleb in patients with the cystic type of pneumatosis coli. However, air in the retroperitoneum is never benign and is always associated with significant underlying causes (see figure). Perhaps the most common cause is a perforated hollow viscus that is located behind the posterior peritoneal layer of the peritoneal cavity (the retroperitoneum), in which lie parts of the duodenum, ascending colon, pancreas, kidney, and adrenal glands.

Besides perforation of peptic ulcer disease, other considerations include perforation secondary to endoscopy or ERCP or trauma. A large pneumomediastinum could also cause some air to percolate through the diaphragmatic hiatus into the retroperitoneum. In cases of significant pneumoretroperitoneum, the air tends to be streaky and linear in nature, following the iliopsoas muscle, perhaps outlining the kidney. There is no Rigler's sign, or air collecting under the diaphragm, or air outlining the falciform ligament, as seen with a pneumoperitoneum. Blunt trauma to the abdomen affecting the retroperitonized portions of the colon and resulting in leakage of air can produce these findings as well. Streaky linear air collections are seen on the plain image of the abdomen shown with this case. However, CT is much more sensitive in the detection of retroperitoneal air, especially small amounts, and is now the standard study.

Notes

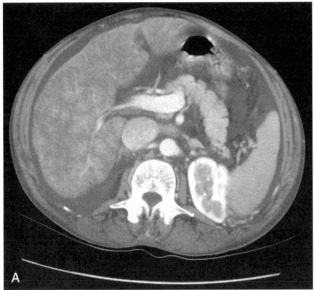

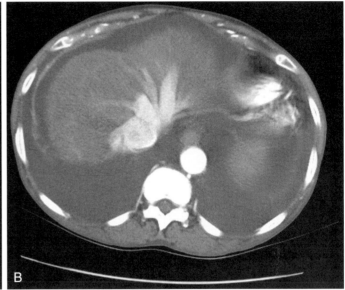

History: A 65-year-old woman presents with abdominal distention.

1. What should be included in the differential diagnosis of the imaging finding shown in Figure A? (Choose all that apply.)
   A. Cirrhosis
   B. Nutmeg liver
   C. Carcinomatosis
   D. Hemochromatosis
   E. Hepatocellular carcinoma

2. What process within the liver gives rise to the appearance of the nutmeg liver?
   A. Chronic systemic venous congestion
   B. Chronic portal venous congestion
   C. Chronic arterial obstruction
   D. Chronic biliary obstruction

3. What is the most common disease resulting in chronic systemic venous congestion?
   A. Left heart failure
   B. Right heart failure
   C. Systemic arterial hypertension
   D. Pulmonary venous congestion

4. Which of the following features suggests Budd-Chiari syndrome instead of systemic venous congestion as the cause of a diffuse mottled nutmeg liver appearance?
   A. Presence of ascites
   B. Biliary duct dilation
   C. Caudate lobe enlargement
   D. Distention of the inferior vena cava

Nutmeg Liver

1. A, B, C, and E

2. A

3. B

4. C

References

Brancatelli G, Vilgrain V, Federle MP, et al: Budd-Chiari syndrome: spectrum of imaging findings. *AJR Am J Roentgenol* 2007;188(2):W168-W176.

Liu WL, Lai CC: Images in emergency medicine: nutmeg liver. *Emerg Med J* 2011:28.

Moulton JS, Miller BL, Dodd GD III, et al: Passive hepatic congestion in heart failure: CT abnormalities. *AJR Am J Roentgenol* 1998;151(5):939-942.

Cross-Reference

Gastrointestinal Imaging: *THE REQUISITES,* 3rd ed, p 183.

Comment

Right-sided heart failure is almost always the basis of a diffuse mottled-appearing, enlarged liver, with distended hepatic veins (see figures). It has been referred to by pathologists as nutmeg liver for more than 100 years and is a very common finding at autopsy. Any chronic preterminal event may result in right-sided heart failure—hence the high incidence seen at autopsy. Nutmeg is a spice, the germ taken from the seed of a tree found in the tropics. The name "nutmeg liver" was used by pathologists to describe sections taken from a chronically passive congested liver, usually caused by right-sided heart failure. The congestion and pigmentation around the central veins of the liver lobules gave it a "nutmeg" appearance to the eyes of early pathologists, who were inclined to give food-related names to disease entities in the early days of histopathology (i.e., "bread and butter pericarditis," "anchovy sauce" liver lesions).

The nutmeg liver would have remained an interesting sidelight of histopathology if not for the advent of CT imaging. When evaluating patients with congestive heart failure, especially right-sided failure, radiologists began to observe that the liver took on a diffuse mottled appearance almost identical to that described by the pathologists. Distention of the hepatic veins and degrees of hepatomegaly were also seen.

The potential problem of the nutmeg liver is that it could conceivably mask some other hepatic disease. The term "nutmeg liver" is now part of the lexicon of radiology and hepatic imaging.

Notes

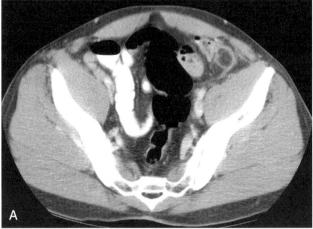
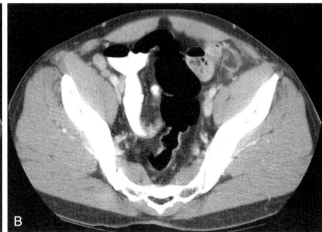

History: A 39-year-old man presents with left lower quadrant pain of 4 days' duration.

1. What should be included in the differential diagnosis of the imaging finding shown in Figure A? (Choose all that apply.)
   A. Diverticulitis
   B. Colonic lipoma
   C. Omental infarction
   D. Epiploic appendagitis
   E. Mesenteric panniculitis

2. What is the etiology of epiploic appendagitis?
   A. Occlusion of the lumen of the appendage with debris
   B. Bacterial contamination of the epiploic appendage
   C. Torsion of the epiploic appendage
   D. Localized perforation

3. The lesion of epiploic appendagitis is described as an oval pericolonic lesion surrounded by inflammatory stranding. What is the density of this oval lesion?
   A. Fat
   B. Gas
   C. Water
   D. Calcium

4. What is the treatment for epiploic appendagitis?
   A. Conservative management
   B. Colonoscopy
   C. Laparotomy
   D. Antibiotics

Epiploic Appendagitis

1. A, D, and E

2. C

3. A

4. A

References

Almeida AT, Melao L, Viamonte B, et al: Epiploic appendagitis: an entity frequently unknown to clinicians—diagnostic imaging, pitfalls, and look-alikes. *AJR Am J Roentgenol* 2009;193(5):1243-1251.

Singh AK, Gervais DA, Hahn PF, et al: Acute epiploic appendagitis and its mimics. *Radiographics* 2005;25(6):1521-1534.

Cross-Reference

Gastrointestinal Imaging: *THE REQUISITES,* 3rd ed, p 319.

Comment

Acute epiploic appendagitis is an unusual self-limiting inflammatory process involving the epiploic appendages of the colon. It is thought to be due to torsion of the appendage pedicle, which results in vascular occlusion, thrombus, and inflammation. The epiploic appendages are fatty extensions arising from the two rows of taeniae coli, which form the well-known haustral pattern of the colon. The taeniae are covered by peritoneum and are found anywhere along the length of the colon.

Before laparoscopy and CT, the condition went undiagnosed and the patient recovered, or it was mistaken for some other intraabdominal disease, and the patient underwent laparotomy. Multidetector CT is excellent not only for revealing the condition but also for excluding other causes of abdominal pain that might require immediate intervention. The treatment is conservative with spontaneous resolution in virtually all patients.

CT shows the inflamed appendage, as in this case, apart from the bowel wall and without inflammatory changes of the bowel wall (see figures). Follow-up CT scans may show involution with some scar tissue in the pericolonic fat. Tiny calcifications or focal fatty scarring in the fat around the pericolic regions may be indicative of prior epiploic appendagitis.

Notes

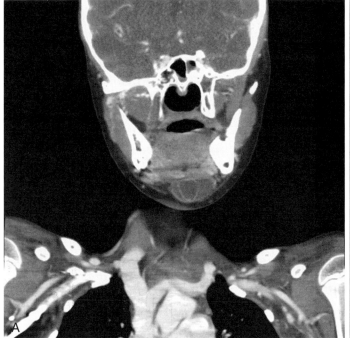
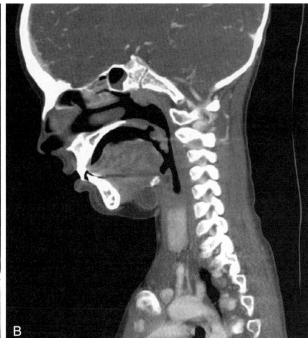

History: An infant presents with a palpable lump under her chin.

1. What should be included in the differential diagnosis of the imaging finding shown in Figure A? (Choose all that apply.)
   A. Thyroglossal duct cyst
   B. Branchial cleft cyst
   C. Sebaceous cyst
   D. Dermoid cyst
   E. Laryngocele

2. What is the most common presentation of a thyroglossal duct cyst?
   A. Dysphagia
   B. Asymptomatic
   C. Palpable mass
   D. Hypothyroidism

3. What is the most common complication of a thyroglossal duct cyst?
   A. Carcinoma
   B. Infection
   C. Fistula
   D. Stridor

4. What is the definitive treatment of a thyroglossal duct cyst?
   A. Surgery
   B. Do nothing
   C. Sclerotherapy
   D. Fine needle aspiration

CASE 167

Thyroglossal Cyst

1. A, B, C, and D

2. B

3. B

4. A

References

Ahuja AT, Wong KT, King AD, et al: Imaging for thyroglossal duct cyst: the bare essentials. *Clin Radiol* 2005;60(2):141-148.

Reede DL, Bergeron RT, Som PM: CT of thyroglossal duct cysts. *Radiology* 1985;157(1):121-125.

Cross-Reference

Gastrointestinal Imaging: *THE REQUISITES,* 3rd ed, p 10.

Comment

A thyroglossal cyst is a cystic structure formed in a persistent thyroglossal duct. This duct usually involutes early in embryonic life (8 to 9 weeks) but may retain some patency in a small percentage of the population, leading to cyst formation at the base of the tongue, often in the midline and occasionally touching the hyoid bone. Most patients are female and asymptomatic.

Occasionally, the cyst may cause a globus sensation or "dysphagia." Barium swallow is usually normal. CT shows the mass at the base of the tongue, usually midline, but not always (see figures). It rarely exceeds 3 cm in size. Complications include infection, in which case the patient presents with painful swallowing (the cyst moves with the tongue) and a painful lump in the neck in a sublingual location. Rarely, an association of thyroglossal cyst with medullary carcinoma of the thyroid gland has been reported.

Other cystic structures in the neck or upper mediastinum to be considered are foregut cysts such as bronchogenic cysts, duplication cysts, neurogenic cysts, and thymic cysts. Many of these conditions produce no symptoms and are often incidental findings. However, as the individual ages, some of these cystic structures may become symptomatic.

Notes

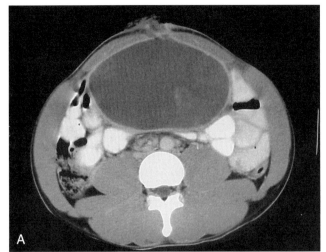

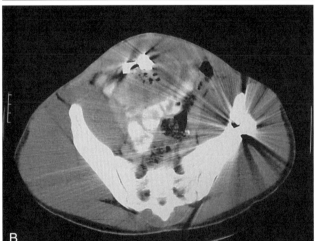

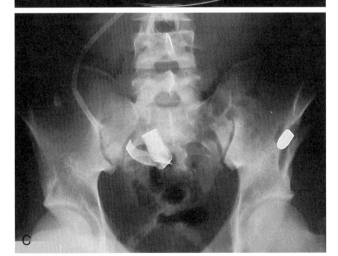

History: A 24-year-old man presents with fever and abdominal pain and distention.

1. What should be included in the differential diagnosis of the imaging finding shown in Figure A? (Choose all that apply.)
   A. Abscess
   B. Mucocele
   C. Hematoma
   D. Stromal tumor
   E. Urinary retention

2. What is the cause for the high-density focus within this abnormality shown in figure 2? (*Hint:* The plain radiograph shown in Figure C may be helpful.)
   A. Calcification
   B. Surgical sponge
   C. Gunshot remnant
   D. Contrast enhancement

3. Why is it radiopaque?
   A. Calcification
   B. Metallic strip
   C. Impregnated material
   D. Contrast enhancement

4. What treatment may be performed by the radiologist?
   A. Angiography and embolization
   B. Percutaneous aspiration
   C. Percutaneous drainage
   D. Sclerotherapy

Gossypiboma (Retained Surgical Sponge and Abscess)

1. A, B, C, and E

2. B

3. C

4. C

References

Hunter TB, Taljanovic MS: Medical devices of the abdomen and pelvis. *Radiographics* 2005;25(2):503-523.

Low VH, Killius JS: Animal, vegetable, or mineral: a collection of abdominal and alimentary foreign bodies. *Appl Radiol* 2000;29:23-30.

Sahin-Akyar G, Yagci C, Aytac S: Pseudotumour due to surgical sponge: gossypiboma. *Australas Radiol* 1997;41(3):288-291.

Cross-Reference

Gastrointestinal Imaging: THE REQUISITES, 3rd ed, p 318.

Comment

This CT scan shows an abnormal collection of mainly fluid and traces of gas within the anterior abdomen consistent with an abscess (see figures). Of greater importance, however, is the presence of a ribbonlike density within the abscess, which is indicative of some type of foreign object within the abdominal cavity (see figures). It can be seen distinctly on the plain image of the abdomen (see figures). This constellation of findings along with a history of prior abdominal surgery raises the likelihood of an iatrogenic cause (i.e., the introduction of some object into the peritoneal cavity during a surgical procedure). This object could be a surgical sponge or towel or perhaps a surgical needle that was dropped into the peritoneal cavity.

This complication is rare, considering the number of procedures performed daily. A retained surgical sponge (also known as a gossypiboma) can sometimes be difficult to diagnose. On plain film, motion artifact can make the radiopaque ribbon all but disappear. An intraoperative image obtained because of the possibility of a retained sponge must be obtained during complete suspended respiration. Motion artifact has been known to make the radiopaque ribbon virtually disappear. The radiopaque ribbon is placed in surgical sponges so that they can be identified on radiographs of the abdomen.

Intraoperative radiographs are obtained if the sponge count taken during surgery is incorrect. Radiography usually detects most sponges that are lost within the abdominal cavity. However, because of incorrect counting, the surgeon often may be unaware that a sponge has been lost within the abdominal cavity. Some of these objects produce no symptoms and are retained within the abdominal cavity until they are later discovered incidentally during a radiologic examination. Others may serve as a nidus for infection, leading to the development of an abscess, as in this patient. Surgery is the primary treatment when complications, such as abscess formation, occur as a result of a retained foreign object. However, in some instances, the abscess can be drained percutaneously if the patient is too ill for immediate surgery.

Notes

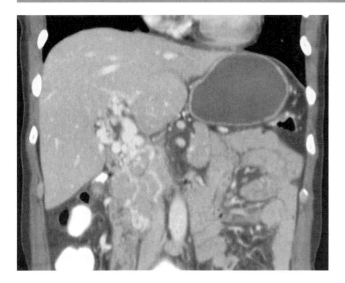

History: A 69-year-old man presents with hematemesis.

1. What should be included in the differential diagnosis of the imaging finding shown in the figure? (Choose all that apply.)
   A. Cavernous transformation of the portal vein
   B. Hepatoportal arteriovenous malformation
   C. Hemangioma of the portal vein
   D. Aneurysm of the portal vein
   E. Agenesis of the portal vein

2. What is the most common cause of portal vein thrombosis in adults?
   A. Cirrhosis
   B. Portal sepsis
   C. Hypercoagulability
   D. Abdominal surgery

3. What is the specific feature of portal venous obstruction that results in cavernous transformation?
   A. Etiology
   B. Malignant
   C. Chronicity
   D. Total obstruction

4. What radiologic intervention has been associated with this condition?
   A. Transjugular intrahepatic portosystemic shunting
   B. Percutaneous transhepatic cholangiography
   C. Transfemoral hepatic arteriography
   D. Transjugular liver biopsy

Cavernous Transformation of the Portal Vein

1. A, B, C, and E

2. A

3. C

4. A

References

Gallego C, Velasco M, Marcuello P, et al: Congenital and acquired anomalies of the portal venous system. *Radiographics* 2002;22(1):141-159.

Tublin ME, Dodd GD III, Baron RL: Benign and malignant portal vein thrombosis: differentiation by CT characteristics. *AJR Am J Roentgenol* 1997;168(3):719-723.

Cross-Reference

Gastrointestinal Imaging: *THE REQUISITES,* 3rd ed, p 185.

Comment

Cavernous transformation of the portal venous system is defined as the formation of numerous serpiginous, wormlike venous channels between the liver and spleen as a result of chronic portal vein occlusion. This condition is usually due to portal vein thrombosis. The occlusive process is usually not acute, and some time is required to allow formation of prominent venous collateralization.

Not all cases of portal vein thrombosis result in cavernous transformation. It has been reported in cases of chronic portal hypertension secondary to fibrosing liver disease, chronic pancreatitis, pancreatic carcinoma, hepatocellular carcinoma, perinatal omphalitis in newborns, pregnancy, hemolytic anemias such as thalassemia, hypercoagulable diseases, and systemic sepsis. It can also progress to such conditions as esophageal varices and gastric varices and gastrointestinal bleeding. The diagnosis of both portal vein thrombosis and cavernous transformation can usually be made using Doppler ultrasound. CT can also show these changes and show the underlying cause in some instances (see the figure).

Notes

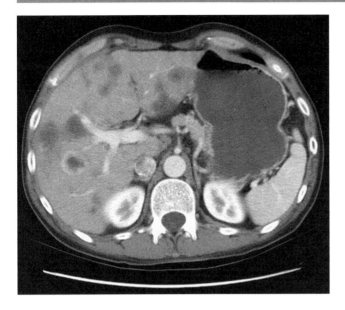

History: A 40-year-old woman presents with right upper quadrant pain and weight loss.

1. What should be included in the differential diagnosis of the imaging finding shown in the figure? (Choose all that apply.)
   A. Metastases
   B. Hamartomas
   C. Hemangiomas
   D. Telangiectasias
   E. Hemangioendotheliomas

2. What is the most common tumor of the liver of vascular origin?
   A. Hemangioma
   B. Angiosarcoma
   C. Lymphangiomatosis
   D. Hemangioendothelioma

3. Which of the following describes the prognosis of hepatic epithelioid hemangioendothelioma (EHE)?
   A. Intermediate between benign and malignant
   B. Benign until transformation to hepatoma
   C. Similar to angiosarcoma
   D. Similar to hemangioma

4. What is the most common site of EHE?
   A. Soft tissues
   B. Bone
   C. Liver
   D. Lung

Epithelioid Hemangioendothelioma

1. A, C, and E

2. A

3. A

4. A

References

Lyburn ID, Torreggiani WC, Harris AC, et al: Hepatic epithelioid hemangioendothelioma: sonographic, CT, and MR imaging appearances. *AJR Am J
Roentgenol* 2003;180(5):1359-1364.

Makhlouf HR, Ishak KG, Goodman ZD: Epithelioid hemangioendothelioma of the liver: a clinicopathologic study of 137 cases. *Cancer* 1999;85(3):
562-582.

Miller WJ, Dodd III GD, Federle MP, et al: Epithelioid hemangioendothelioma of the liver: imaging findings with pathologic correlation. *AJR Am J
Roentgenol* 1992;159(1):53-57.

Cross-Reference

Gastrointestinal Imaging: *THE REQUISITES,* 3rd ed, p 205.

Comment

The hepatic lesions are of soft tissue density, and some have a
well-defined "halo" around them (see figure). This appearance
should not dissuade the radiologist from considering metastatic disease as the first thing to be excluded. However, no
primary disease was present in this patient, and biopsy of the
liver lesions revealed the multinodular lesions of the liver to be
EHE. This is a rare condition mostly seen in soft tissues and
bone. Involvement of the liver resembles metastatic disease.
Although metastatic lesions can have an enhancing halo, EHE
seems to have a more prominent halo sign; however, this does
not apply in all hepatic lesions as seen on the transaxial image
of the liver.

In a setting in which a primary lesion is not evident, and
well-defined peripheral enhancement that is brighter than
usual is present (and is not the "puddling" effect seen with
benign hemangiomas), EHE is a consideration. The tumor is
an unusual vascular lesion characterized by epithelioid endo-
thelial cells. It has been described in adults of all ages. The
tumor has the histologic features of a low-grade malignancy.
In 2002, the World Health Organization defined "hemangioendothelioma" as a definitive, locally aggressive malignant
tumor that rarely metastasizes.

In the liver, EHE is seen as multiple, indolent, slow-growing
progressive lesions, which on CT may show a bright, well-
defined halo effect. It is extremely rare to see spread of the
tumor beyond the liver.

Notes

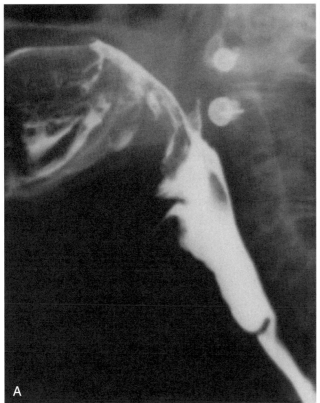
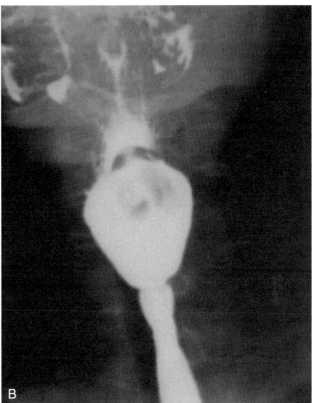

History: A 71-year-old woman presents with dysphagia.

1. What should be included in the differential diagnosis of the imaging finding shown in Figure A? (Choose all that apply.)
   A. Radiation
   B. Congenital
   C. Schatzki ring
   D. Cricopharyngeal spasm
   E. Graft-versus-host disease

2. Where in the esophagus are strictures most commonly seen?
   A. Distal
   B. Diffuse
   C. Proximal
   D. Midsegment

3. In what syndrome are cervical esophageal webs associated with iron deficiency anemia?
   A. Killian-Jamieson
   B. Plummer-Vinson
   C. Zollinger-Ellison
   D. Ivor-Lewis

4. What is the treatment for cervical esophageal webs?
   A. Corticosteroids
   B. Endoscopy
   C. Antibiotics
   D. Surgery

Esophageal Web

1. A, B, and E

2. A

3. B

4. B

References

Luedtke P, Levine MS, Rubesin SE, et al: Radiologic diagnosis of benign esophageal strictures: a pattern approach. *Radiographics* 2003;23(4):897-909.

Smith MS: Diagnosis and management of esophageal rings and webs. *Gastroenterol Hepatol (NY)* 2010;6(11):701-704.

Cross-Reference

Gastrointestinal Imaging: *THE REQUISITES,* 3rd ed, p 32.

Comment

Images from a barium esophagogram show a well-defined web or ring stricture in the proximal esophagus (see figures). These proximal webs are common. If the web is small or noncircumferential, the patient may be asymptomatic. However, if the lumen is sufficiently compromised, such that a 13-mm barium tablet would be held up by the web, the patient is likely to complain of dysphagia. These webs are seen accompanied by iron deficiency anemia in Plummer-Vinson syndrome (also known as Paterson-Kelly syndrome in the United Kingdom). The condition is sometimes referred to as sideropenic dysphagia.

The exact cause of this condition is unclear. Some authors doubt the validity of the association or the syndrome altogether. Plummer-Vinson syndrome has been speculated to be an autoimmune phenomenon, but no conclusive evidence has been offered to prove this hypothesis. The condition was first described and named in the early 20th century, when the incidence was thought to be common. It is now seen rarely, possibly because fewer barium esophagograms are being done, and endoscopy may not see the web or may push by it (and effect a cure), or, alternatively, Plummer-Vinson syndrome may be a nonentity.

Authors who have described the condition have mostly described an esophageal web seen in the cervical esophagus during a barium esophagogram. It has been said to be found predominantly in white women with a predisposition for increased risk of squamous cell carcinoma of the esophagus. However, this risk factor is also disputed. For the radiologist, it is important to rule out strictures related to other conditions, such as skin lesions, epidermolysis bullosa, and pemphigus, and strictures related to gastroesophageal reflux.

Notes

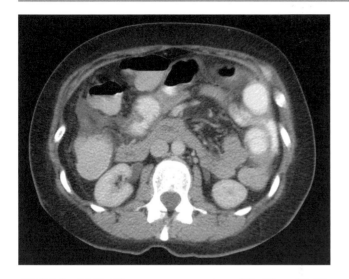

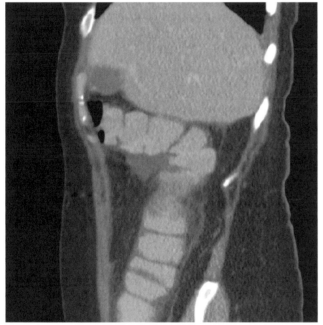

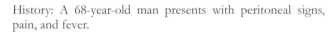

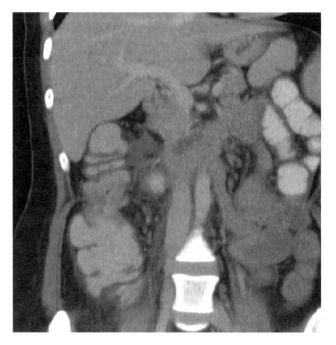

History: A 68-year-old man presents with peritoneal signs, pain, and fever.

1. What should be included in the differential diagnosis of the imaging finding shown in the figures? (Choose all that apply.)
   A. Trauma
   B. Diverticulitis
   C. Colon cancer
   D. Angiodysplasia
   E. Crohn's disease

2. Which of the following statements regarding perforated colon carcinoma is *false*?
   A. Perforation is a serious, often fatal complication of colonic carcinoma.
   B. Perforation is an uncommon complication of primary colonic carcinoma.

C. Perforation of a primary colonic carcinoma is later associated with a higher local recurrence rate.
   D. Most patients with perforation of a primary colonic carcinoma go on to develop peritoneal carcinomatosis.

3. What mode of disease spread occurs with the greatest increased incidence in patients with colon cancer presenting with perforation?
   A. Peritoneal carcinomatosis
   B. Hepatic metastases
   C. Lymphatic spread
   D. Skeletal deposits

4. All of the following are potential causes of a pericolonic fluid collection *except:*
   A. Villous adenoma
   B. Diverticular disease
   C. Colon adenocarcinoma
   D. Ischemic bowel disease

Perforated Colon Carcinoma

1. A, B, C, and E

2. D

3. A

4. A

References

Kriwanek S, Armbruster C, Dittrich K, et al: Perforated colorectal cancer. *Dis Colon Rectum* 1996;39(12):1409-1414.

Cheynel N, Cortet M, Lepage C, et al: Incidence, patterns of failure, and prognosis of perforated colorectal cancers in a well-defined population. *Dis Colon Rectum* 2009;52(3):406-411.

Cross-Reference

Gastrointestinal Imaging: *THE REQUISITES,* 3rd ed, p 302.

Comment

The CT images show inflammatory changes around the colon forming a pericolic abscess (see figures). Although the usual presenting symptoms of obstruction and bleeding (occult or frank bleeding) account for most colonic malignant lesions, perforation is the presentation in a small but significant number of cases (1% to 2%). In most cases, such as in the case presented here, the perforation site is at the site of the tumor. However, perforation proximal to the tumor can be seen in about 30% of these patients. Perforation distal to the tumor is extremely rare. Secondary perforation after radiation treatment has been reported but is also rare.

Perforation linked to colonic carcinoma occurs slightly more frequently on the right side. In such a scenario, the question of a perforated carcinoma is always an issue and must be excluded before considering right-sided diverticulitis. However, when the perforation is left sided and especially in the sigmoid colon, it can mimic diverticulitis almost perfectly.

Notes

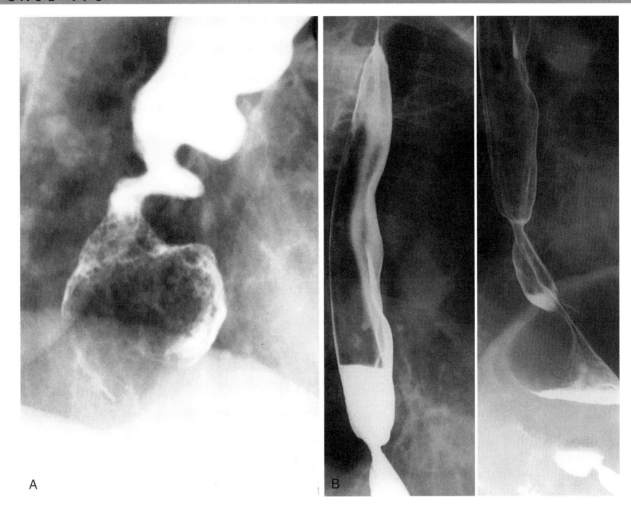

A

B

History: A 63-year-old woman presents with sudden onset of dysphagia; she cannot tolerate pills, fluids, or her own saliva.

1. What should be included in the differential diagnosis of the imaging finding shown in Figure A? (Choose all that apply.)
   A. Intraluminal foreign body
   B. Mucosal polypoid mass
   C. Submucosal mass lesion
   D. Serosal involvement
   E. Extrinsic mass impression

2. What is the most common predisposing factor for esophageal foreign body obstruction?
   A. Child
   B. Elderly
   C. Stricture
   D. Nonaccidental

3. What therapeutic option should a radiologist perform first on discovery of an impacted food bolus in the distal esophagus?
   A. Snare retrieval
   B. Effervescent agent
   C. Parenteral antispasmodic
   D. Proteolytic enzyme via nasogastric tube

4. What is the treatment?
   A. Nothing; peristalsis eventually breaks up the bolus
   B. Interventional radiology
   C. Endoscopy
   D. Surgery

Food Impaction in Esophagus Secondary to Stricture

1. A and B

2. C

3. C

4. C

References

Ginsberg GG: Management of ingested foreign objects and food bolus impactions. *Gastrointest Endosc* 1995;41(1):33-38.

Low VH, Killius JS: Animal, vegetable, or mineral: a collection of abdominal and alimentary foreign bodies. *Appl Radiol* 2000;29:23-30.

Cross-Reference

Gastrointestinal Imaging: *THE REQUISITES,* 3rd ed, p 37.

Comment

Esophageal food impaction is common. In virtually in every case, there is some underlying disease; this is usually in the form of a mild area of narrowing or stricture that is located in the distal esophagus, associated with chronic reflux disease (see figures). It can often turn out to be the symptomatic form of the esophageal "B" ring, referred to as Schatzki ring. This condition is sometimes referred to as the "steakhouse syndrome," suggesting that the patient has swallowed a large, inadequately chewed solid bolus of food. The reasons for this can vary depending on the patient. Mild intoxication has often been implicated, such as in the "café coronary," in which the bolus becomes stuck in the cervical esophagus or the esophagopharyngeal junction, occluding or compressing the airway. In such cases, the more dramatic Heimlich maneuver is called for to prevent asphyxiation.

The capacity for the human gastroesophageal junction to stretch to accommodate a large bolus of food is high. The esophagus may be anatomically divided into the tubular and vestibular esophagus. The vestibule is a short segment of natural widening of the esophagus just above the gastroesophageal junction and should not be confused with a small hiatal hernia. No gastric folds are present in this natural widening, and it is more prominent in some patients than in others. Because of this vestibule, even a large bolus can usually pass the gastroesophageal junction safely.

When a solid bolus becomes impacted near the gastroesophageal junction, the radiologist should appreciate the extremely high probability that some underlying narrowing is present. If the narrowing is mild, it can easily be missed at endoscopy. In follow-up studies, a barium tablet (12.5 mm) should be used; the tablet is often hung up in the narrowed area and subsequently washed down with warm water. The radiologist should explain to the patient that the barium tablet is not a medication.

Notes

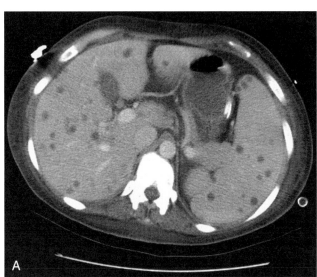

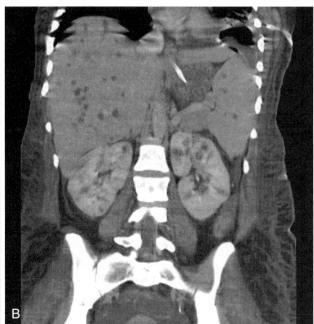

History: A 47-year-old man presents with fever.

1. What should be included in the differential diagnosis of the imaging finding shown in Figure A? (Choose all that apply.)
   A. Metastases
   B. Microabscesses
   C. Polycystic disease
   D. *Echinococcus multilocularis*
   E. Multifocal cholangiocarcinoma

2. What is the most important predisposing factor to the development of hepatic microabscesses?
   A. Travel to endemic areas
   B. Immunosuppression
   C. Portal sepsis
   D. Cirrhosis

3. What is the most common causative organism of hepatic microabscesses?
   A. *Candida*
   B. Tuberculosis
   C. *Escherichia coli*
   D. *Echinococcus granulosus*

4. Which of the following statements regarding liver infection is true?
   A. The liver is the most common site of amebic infection.
   B. On CT, the presence of calcified septa is pathognomonic of schistosomiasis.
   C. Hydatid liver abscesses are most commonly due to *E. multilocularis*.
   D. Acute miliary tuberculosis of the liver is characterized on CT by multiple tiny, dense nodules.

Microabscesses of the Liver and Spleen

1. A, B, and C

2. B

3. A

4. B

References

Moore NJ, Leef JL, Pang Y: Systemic candidiasis. *Radiographics* 2003;23(5): 1287-1290.

Mortele KJ, Segatto E, Ros PR: The infected liver: radiologic-pathologic correlation. *Radiographics* 2004;24(4):937-955.

Cross-Reference

Gastrointestinal Imaging: THE REQUISITES, 3rd ed, p 216.

Comment

Multiple low-density lesions throughout the liver or spleen may be the result of metastasis, which is the most common cause. However, when there are numerous tiny low-density areas occurring diffusely, the possibility of microabscesses must be seriously considered (see figures). The lesions almost always occur in the setting of some type of immunosuppression (e.g., patients with AIDS, transplant recipients, patients with leukemia, and patients with cancer undergoing chemotherapy). Patients receiving steroid therapy are another subgroup to be considered. The microabscesses develop as a result of systemic sepsis with a microorganism, usually fungal. However, many patients may have no irregular findings on blood cultures.

Candida albicans is the organism that most commonly produces this type of appearance. It is believed that this organism often resides in an immunosuppressed patient, and when the immune status of the patient decreases to a certain threshold, a systemic infection occurs. Other organisms that have been implicated include *Cryptococcus* and *Aspergillus* species. Rarely, this radiologic appearance can be attributed to some type of bacterial infection.

On ultrasound, these abscesses have a bright central echogenic focus with a surrounding hypoechoic band and "bull's eye" lesion. Hepatic or splenic enlargement may be present. CT often reveals multiple low-density areas in the liver or spleen that often do not exceed 1 cm in diameter. Sometimes there is a central area of high density. Major differential considerations include metastases, and lymphoma may have a similar appearance.

Notes

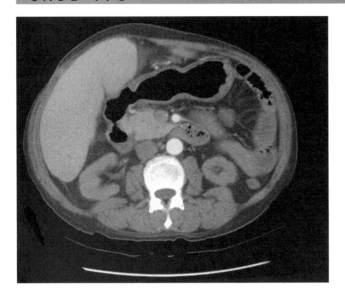

History: A 57-year-old man presents with dyspepsia.

1. What should be included in the differential diagnosis
   of the imaging finding shown in the figure? (Choose all
   that apply.)
   A. Gastritis
   B. Carcinoma
   C. Gastric ulcer
   D. Stromal tumor
   E. Ménétrier's disease

2. If on a barium examination the stomach does not change
   shape, what might you call this condition?
   A. Hallux rigidus
   B. Linitis plastica
   C. Carmen's sign
   D. Gastric incisura

3. What is the most common metastatic malignancy
   that could cause a linitis plastica appearance?
   A. Lymphoma
   B. Breast carcinoma
   C. Malignant melanoma
   D. Hepatocellular carcinoma

4. What is the most common benign etiology for the linitis
   plastica appearance?
   A. Caustic ingestion
   B. Eosinophilic gastritis
   C. Granulomatous gastritis
   D. *Helicobacter pylori* infection

Uremic Gastritis

1. A and B

2. B

3. B

4. A

References

Ba-Ssalamah A, Prokop M, Uffmann M, et al: Dedicated multidetector CT of the stomach: spectrum of diseases. *Radiographics* 2003;23(3):625-644.

Rubesin SE, Levine MS, Laufer I: Double-contrast upper gastrointestinal radiography: a pattern approach for diseases of the stomach. *Radiology* 2008;246(1):33-48.

Cross-Reference

Gastrointestinal Imaging: *THE REQUISITES,* 3rd ed, p 70.

Comment

The usual cause of an atrophic, rigid nonpliant stomach is generally primary or metastatic malignancy. It cannot be totally excluded here, but the lack of a mass makes it much less likely (see figure). Other conditions that diffusely involve the stomach and result in a ridged "linitis-like" picture must be considered. In this case, the patient was a sickle cell patient with chronic renal failure. In such patients, chronic severe gastritis is common. Many also have chronic duodenitis, such as this patient. Uremic gastritis is mostly seen in patients on long-term dialysis. There is also thought to be a higher incidence of peptic ulcer disease in such patients.

A correlation between elevated serum creatinine levels and serum gastrin levels seems to exist, although it is unclear that this is an instigating factor involved with uremic gastritis. Increased urea in the blood may affect the gastric mucosa directly. Endoscopically, uremic gastritis has been described as atrophy and hemorrhagic erosive gastritis. Involvement of *H. pylori* as a causative effect in uremic gastritis has also been considered and found to occur with about the same frequency as in other patients with peptic ulcer disease. Whatever the cause, there seems to be little doubt that patients on long-term dialysis have a higher level of chronic gastritis, duodenitis, and peptic ulceration and erosions and are more predisposed to gastrointestinal bleeding than the normal population.

Notes

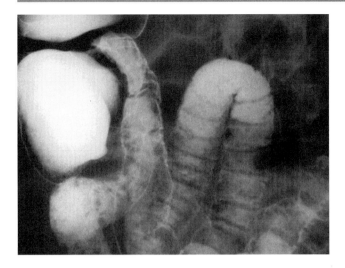

History: A 22-year-old man presents with diarrhea.

1. What should be included in the differential diagnosis
   of the imaging finding shown in the figure? (Choose all
   that apply.)
   A. Lymphoma
   B. Mastocytosis
   C. Villous adenoma
   D. Lymphoid hyperplasia
   E. Familial adenomatous polyposis

2. What disease is considered to be most commonly
   associated with nodular lymphoid hyperplasia?
   A. Hypogammaglobulinemia
   B. Viral infection
   C. Tuberculosis
   D. Giardiasis

3. With what complication is lymphoid hyperplasia associated
   in the pediatric age group?
   A. Mesenteric adenitis
   B. Immunodeficiency
   C. Intussusception
   D. Malabsorption

4. What are normal lymphoid aggregates in the ileum called?
   A. Heberden's nodes
   B. Peyer's patches
   C. Meissner's plexus
   D. Singer's nodes

Lymphoid Hyperplasia of the Terminal Ileum

1. D and E

2. B

3. C

4. B

References

Levine MS, Rubesin SE, Laufer I: Pattern approach for diseases of mesenteric small bowel on barium studies. *Radiology* 2008;249(2):445-460.

Mukhopadhyay S, Harbol T, Floyd FD, et al: Polypoid nodular hyperplasia of the terminal ileum. *Arch Pathol Lab Med* 2004;128(10):1186-1187.

Cross-Reference

Gastrointestinal Imaging: *THE REQUISITES,* 3rd ed, p 127.

Comment

The condition of lymphoid hyperplasia is often a normal finding in children. It is thought by some authors that lymphoid hyperplasia might act as a nidus for childhood idiopathic ileocolic intussusception. The pattern has also been described in patients with immunodeficiency, giardiasis infestation, *Yersinia* infections of the small bowel (usually the terminal ileum), Whipple's disease, and Waldenström's macroglobulinemia. Some investigators believe there is an association of lymphoid hyperplasia of the terminal ileum with the development of Crohn's disease in the distal small bowel. These nodules can range in size from 2 to 5 mm and usually involve the distal small bowel (see figure). Crossover into the colon is unusual, although colonic lymphoid hyperplasia is a known entity. In most cases, these nodules are regarded as a reactive hyperplasia secondary to bowel response to a viral infectious or inflammatory process that is generally self-limiting and eventually disappears.

It is thought that in some cases nodular lymphoid hyperplasia may be a presenting sign of small bowel multifocal lymphoma. Another unusual association that has been reported is lactose intolerance. In some instances in adults, the condition has been pronounced and symptomatic with weight loss, diarrhea, and abdominal pain to the point at which resection of the terminal ileum was undertaken with varying results.

Notes

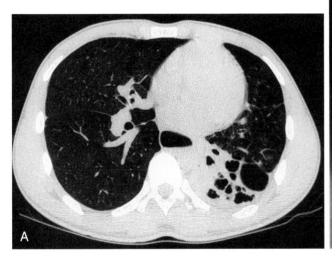

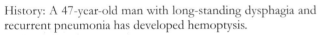

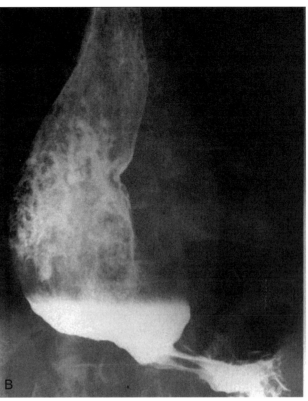

History: A 47-year-old man with long-standing dysphagia and recurrent pneumonia has developed hemoptysis.

1. What should be included in the differential diagnosis of the imaging finding shown in Figure A? (Choose all that apply.)
   A. Achalasia
   B. Scleroderma
   C. Chagas' disease
   D. Esophageal spasm
   E. Gastroesophageal junction cancer

2. What is the underlying pathophysiologic defect in achalasia?
   A. Vagal denervation
   B. Muscularis fibrosis
   C. Anticholinergic effect
   D. Ganglion cell deficiency

3. Which of the following conditions is associated with the highest risk of developing esophageal carcinoma?
   A. Tylosis
   B. Achalasia
   C. Barrett's disease
   D. Head and neck cancers

4. Which of the following statements regarding conditions predisposing to esophageal cancer is true?
   A. In achalasia, cancer develops as a result of chronic stasis.
   B. Carcinoma developing in a lye stricture has a more dismal prognosis.
   C. The Northern Asia cluster of esophageal carcinoma is due to Epstein-Barr virus.
   D. In the United States, the main risk factor for esophageal cancer is chronic gastroesophageal reflux.

Esophageal Carcinoma Developing in Achalasia

1. A, B, C, and E

2. D

3. A

4. A

References

Leeuwenburgh I, Scholten P, Alderliesten J, et al: Long-term esophageal cancer risk in patients with primary achalasia: a prospective study. *Am J Gastroenterol* 2010;105(10):2144-2149.

Pohl D, Tutuian R: Achalasia: an overview of diagnosis and treatment. *J Gastrointest Liver Dis* 2007;16(3):297-303.

Cross-Reference

Gastrointestinal Imaging: *THE REQUISITES,* 3rd ed, p 21.

Comment

Achalasia is a common but poorly understood disorder of esophageal motility, producing lifelong dysfunction. It is a neurogenic disorder marked by a decrease or absence of ganglion cells in the esophagus. Abnormalities also have been found in the vagal trunks and nuclei. The underlying etiology for this loss of innervation is uncertain. The result is decreasing esophageal peristalsis and failure of the lower esophageal sphincter to relax. Achalasia occurs almost equally among men and women. Onset is typically in early adulthood, and later onset should raise suspicions of carcinoma, which may mimic the condition (secondary achalasia). With longstanding achalasia, the esophagus becomes markedly dilated, and food is retained in it (see figures). Scleroderma, peptic strictures, and intramural spread of carcinoma at the gastroesophageal junction may produce a similar appearance.

An unusual complication of this condition is the development of esophageal carcinoma secondary to chronic stasis. This complication is said to affect approximately 5% of patients with achalasia, although there are many who believe the incidence to be much less. Some authors do not classify cancer as a complication of this condition and consider the prevalence of cancer in patients with achalasia no higher than in the general population. Achalasia is usually present 20 or more years before carcinoma is found. Typically, squamous cell carcinoma is present, but adenocarcinoma also has been reported.

Other conditions that have a proven association with an increased incidence of esophageal squamous carcinoma include lye strictures, head and neck tumors, celiac disease, Plummer-Vinson syndrome (Paterson-Kelly syndrome), radiation exposure, palmar and plantar hyperkeratosis, and skin conditions such as epidermolysis bullosa.

Notes

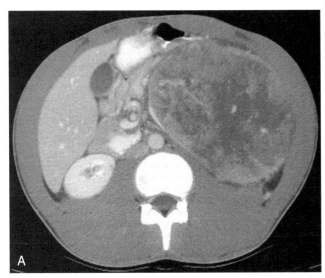

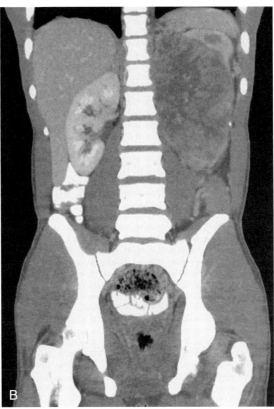

History: A 19-year-old man presents with weight loss and abdominal distention.

1. What should be included in the differential diagnosis of the imaging finding shown in Figure A? (Choose all that apply.)
   A. Renal tumor
   B. Jejunal tumor
   C. Psoas abscess
   D. Retroperitoneal tumor
   E. Pancreatic pseudocyst

2. Which of the following statements regarding Wilms' tumor is true?
   A. Almost all Wilms' tumors are solitary lesions.
   B. Age at presentation is most commonly 5 to 10 years.
   C. The tumor is typically well defined, surrounded by a pseudocapsule.
   D. Children with associated congenital abnormalities usually present later.

3. Which of the following statements regarding renal cell carcinoma (RCC) is true?
   A. Tumor calcification usually forms a thin peripheral rim.
   B. Most patients present with hematuria, flank pain, and a palpable abdominal mass.
   C. Multifocal RCCs are most commonly associated with acquired cystic disease of dialysis.
   D. On contrast-enhanced CT scan, RCCs are most conspicuous on nephrographic phase imaging.

4. Which of the following statements regarding renal tumors is *false*?
   A. Transitional cell carcinomas are most conspicuous on the corticomedullary phase of a contrast-enhanced CT scan.
   B. Lymphoma involving the kidney most commonly occurs as multiple low-attenuation lesions.
   C. Metastatic disease to the kidneys is the most common renal malignancy.
   D. Oncocytomas are the most commonly excised benign solid renal tumor.

Recurrent Wilms' Tumor

1. A, B, and D

2. C

3. D

4. A

References

Dyer R, DiSantis DJ, McClennan BL: Simplified imaging approach for evaluation of the solid renal mass in adults. *Radiology* 2008;247(2):331-343.

Lowe LH, Isuani BH, Heller RM, et al: Pediatric renal masses: Wilms' tumor and beyond. *Radiographics* 2000;20(6):1585-1603.

Cross-Reference

Gastrointestinal Imaging: *THE REQUISITES,* 3rd ed, p 59.

Comment

Wilms' tumor is a solid tumor arising from the kidney that is seen in children and infants. It is the fifth most common cancer in children. It is diagnosed and treated in childhood. Wilms' tumor is currently a treatable and curable condition. Almost 90% of patients survive 5 years after diagnosis as opposed to the poor prognosis of 25 years ago. In this case, the patient had Wilms' tumor of early childhood that was successfully treated. Almost 15 years later, the tumor has recurred, as these tumors are known to do (2% to 3% after nephrectomy) with a much reduced survival rate (20% to 40%).

This tumor falls into the category of large extrinsic masses affecting the bowel (see figures). In the left upper quadrant, splenomegaly, pancreatic pseudocysts, pancreatic masses, subphrenic processes or processes relating to the proximal jejunum, and splenic flexure of the colon would be considerations. In a young patient with a large abdominal mass, the question of recurrent childhood tumor would be raised. Such recurrence is unusual but does occur. Most of the extrinsic processes mentioned compress or displace the adjacent bowel. Rarely, there may be contiguous invasion. In this case, the stomach can be seen sandwiched between the diaphragm and the tumorous mass without local invasion.

Notes

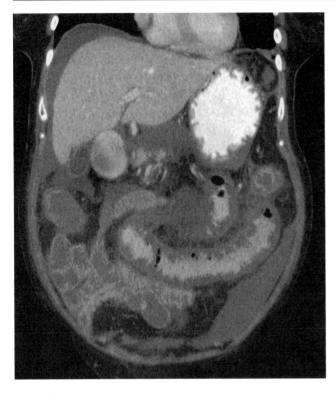

History: A 54-year-old woman referred from the infectious diseases clinic presents with severe abdominal pain and diarrhea.

1. What should be included in the differential diagnosis of the imaging finding shown in the figure? (Choose all that apply.)
   A. Pseudomembranous disease
   B. Infectious disease
   C. Ischemic disease
   D. Carcinoma
   E. Cirrhosis

2. What is the most common organism involved in AIDS-related enteritis?
   A. *Candida*
   B. *Mycobacterium*
   C. Cytomegalovirus (CMV)
   D. *Cryptosporidium parvum*

3. What is the most common cause of symptoms of impaired swallowing (dysphagia and odynophagia) in a patient with AIDS?
   A. CMV ulceration
   B. Mediastinal tuberculosis
   C. *Candida* esophagitis
   D. Kaposi's sarcoma

4. Which of the following diseases occurs in immunocompromised patients after bone marrow transplant but not in patients with AIDS?
   A. Graft-versus-host disease
   B. Opportunistic infections
   C. Kaposi's sarcoma
   D. Lymphoma

Patient with AIDS and Small Bowel Infection

1. B, C, and E

2. D

3. C

4. A

References

Jones B, Wall SD: Gastrointestinal disease in the immunocompromised host. *Radiol Clin North Am* 1992;30(3):555-577.

Lappas JC: Small bowel imaging. *Curr Opin Radiol* 1992;4(3):32-38.

Cross-Reference

Gastrointestinal Imaging: *THE REQUISITES,* 3rd ed, p 342.

Comment

In patients with AIDS, the small bowel is a common site for infection by opportunistic pathogens. The presenting symptoms are almost always abdominal pain and diarrhea. Although cryptosporidiosis appears to be the most common cause, other considerations include *Mycobacterium avium* complex (MAC), CMV infection, giardiasis, microsporidiosis, and histoplasmosis. The organism is usually identified by small bowel aspirates or biopsy. This case was an AIDS-related enteric infection (see figure). Barium studies and CT scans show abnormal small bowel, as in this case, which is nonspecific. In cases of enteric involvement of the small bowel with MAC, barium small bowel studies have described the changes in the small bowel as being similar to changes seen in Whipple's disease. CMV infections are common in the colon and occur less frequently in the esophagus and small bowel of patients with AIDS. Bowel obstructions relating to CMV small bowel infection have been described.

When seen on CT images, the small bowel appears thickened and edematous in most patients. The possibility of small bowel lymphoma (non-Hodgkin's lymphoma is common in patients with AIDS) must always be considered. Obstruction is uncommon. In older patients without AIDS, ischemic changes may have a similar appearance. Other neoplastic lesions described in the small bowel of patients with AIDS include Kaposi's sarcoma.

Notes

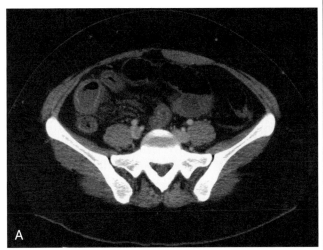

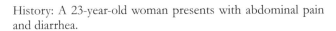

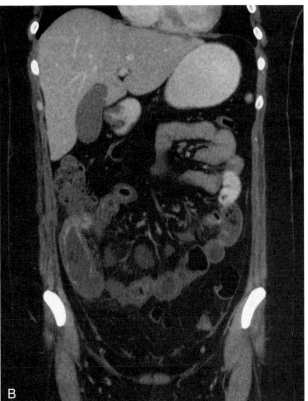

History: A 23-year-old woman presents with abdominal pain and diarrhea.

1. What should be included in the differential diagnosis of the imaging finding shown in Figure A? (Choose all that apply.)
   A. Giardiasis
   B. Celiac disease
   C. Intussusception
   D. Crohn's disease
   E. *Yersinia* enteritis

2. In this case, the thickened ileum has three layers with a middle low-attenuation layer. What is the name of this sign?
   A. String sign
   B. Creeping fat
   C. Fat halo sign
   D. Intramural tract

3. Which of the following statements regarding the CT halo sign is true?
   A. The lucent layer is due to widening of the submucosa.
   B. Intravenous contrast medium is required to render the lucent layer visible.
   C. Halo sign of the colon is most likely due to Crohn's disease.
   D. Halo sign of the terminal ileum is diagnostic of Crohn's disease.

4. Which of the following statements regarding patients with Crohn's disease presenting after age 50 years is true?
   A. Most elderly patients with Crohn's disease are men.
   B. About 10% to 15% of patients with Crohn's disease present after age 50 years.
   C. Crohn's disease in elderly patients more frequently involves the small bowel.
   D. Mortality is higher and response to treatment is poorer in elderly patients with Crohn's disease.

Intramural Fat in Crohn's Disease

1. D and E

2. C

3. A

4. B

References

Ahualli J: The fat halo sign. *Radiology* 2007;242(3):945-946.

Horsthuis K, Bipat S, Bennink RJ, et al: Inflammatory bowel disease diagnosed with US, MR, scintigraphy, and CT: meta-analysis of prospective studies. *Radiology* 2008;247(1):64-79.

Wills JS, Lobis IF, Denstman FJ: Crohn disease: state of the art. *Radiology* 1997;202(3):597-610.

Cross-Reference

Gastrointestinal Imaging: *THE REQUISITES,* 3rd ed, p 294.

Comment

The ring of fat tissue seen in the submucosa of this patient is fast becoming an important CT sign of inflammatory bowel disease (see figures). Generally, the halo sign of submucosal fat is not specific for any particular disease, and it has been described in several inflammatory conditions, including Crohn's disease and ulcerative colitis and some inflammatory processes including radiation enteritis. It also has been described in normal bowel. This is not the creeping fat sign described by pathologists and relating to the gross anatomy of Crohn's disease, in which mesenteric fat around the diseased bowel becomes thickened and rubbery and appears to extend over the inflamed serosal surface similar to "fingers of fat" creeping across the surface of the bowel.

The halo sign (as seen in this case) is seen in gastrointestinal inflammatory conditions as a well-defined ring of submucosal lucency, usually of fat density. This sign has become more noticeable since the advent of high-resolution CT imaging. It has also been described in intestinal lymphangiectasia. Some authors think of the halo sign as nonspecific submucosal edema. It is difficult to measure Hounsfield numbers of the lucent ring.

Subsequent biopsy of this bowel showed this to be Crohn's disease. Edema of the bowel wall usually affects all layers. The halo sign has been described in patients with no evidence of bowel disease. It may be a finding related to obesity in such cases. If one accepts the fact that the halo sign can represent either fat or a ring of edema, other possibilities must be considered, such as ischemic bowel or pseudomembranous colitis. Some authors have deemed the rings of lucency as a double halo sign when edema is seen between the mucosa and submucosa. Generally, a thin single fatty submucosal layer is another manifestation of bowel wall inflammation. In a young patient, such as in this case, with the halo sign involving the terminal ileum, Crohn's disease must be considered first.

Notes

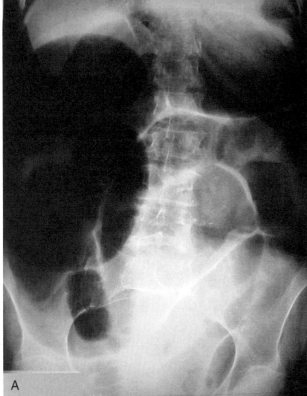

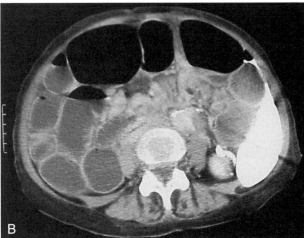

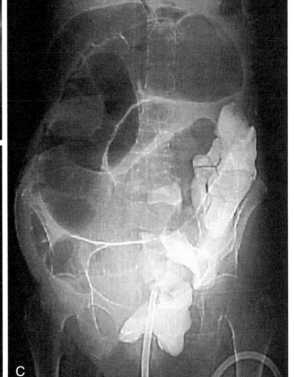

History: An 85-year-old woman presents with abdominal distension.

1. What should be included in the differential diagnosis of the imaging finding shown in Figure A? (Choose all that apply.)
   A. Small bowel paralytic ileus
   B. Large bowel obstruction
   C. Small bowel obstruction
   D. Colonic paralytic ileus
   E. Pneumoperitoneum

2. What is the most common cause of large bowel obstruction?
   A. Tumor
   B. Volvulus
   C. Adhesions
   D. Diverticulitis

3. What is the most common type of colonic volvulus?
   A. Cecal
   B. Rectal
   C. Sigmoid
   D. Transverse

4. What therapeutic option can a radiologist offer this patient?
   A. Nasogastric placement of long small bowel decompression tube
   B. Fluoroscopically guided insertion of rectal decompression tube
   C. Hydrostatic contrast enema reduction
   D. None

Volvulus of the Transverse Colon

1. B and D

2. A

3. C

4. D

References

Newton NA, Reines HD: Transverse colon volvulus: case reports and review. *AJR Am J Roentgenol* 1977;128(1):69-72.

Rahbour G, Ayantunde A, Ullah MR, et al: Transverse colon volvulus in a 15 year old boy and the review of the literature. *World J Emerg Surg* 2010;5: 19-24.

Cross-Reference

Gastrointestinal Imaging: *THE REQUISITES,* 3rd ed, p 310.

Comment

The plain conventional anteroposterior image of this 85-year-old woman, presenting with a distended abdomen and severe pain, shows dilated loops of colon and some small bowel (see figures). The natural history of volvulus and other high-grade colonic obstructions and dilation of the colon can lead to ischemia and perforation. The patient immediately went to surgery where she was found to have a volvulus of the transverse colon.

The most common cause of colonic obstruction is cancer, followed by diverticulitis and volvulus. Most commonly, volvulus is in the sigmoid (80%), but it is also seen in the cecum (15%) and the transverse colon (5%). Predisposing factors are an extra long mesocolon and marked redundancy in the transverse colon. Some authors believe that patients with colonic interposition anterior to the liver (Chilaiditi syndrome), reaching the diaphragm, are at increased risk for volvulus. However, other authors consider the interposition a variant, with no clinical significance. Splenic flexure volvulus, which may be considered a form of transverse volvulus, is the least common type of colonic volvulus. Surgery is the most acceptable form of definitive treatment. The bowel may be complicated by vascular compromise. In such an event, mortality and morbidity rates are high. Simple reduction of all types of colonic volvulus is associated with a high recurrence rate.

Notes

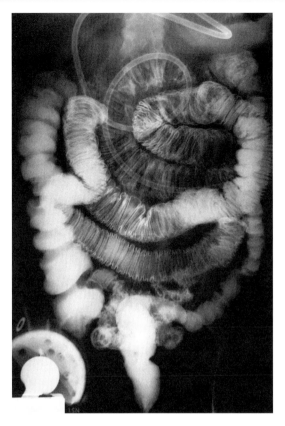

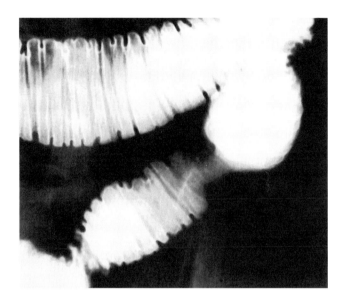

History: A 74-year-old woman presents with intermittent abdominal pain following meals.

1. What should be included in the differential diagnosis of the imaging finding shown in the figures? (Choose all that apply.)
   A. Ischemia
   B. Adhesive band
   C. Ileal dysgenesis
   D. Primary adenocarcinoma
   E. Nonsteroidal anti-inflammatory drugs

2. What is the most common cause of acute mesenteric ischemia?
   A. Superior mesenteric artery thrombosis
   B. Superior mesenteric artery embolism
   C. Mesenteric venous thrombosis
   D. Vasculitis

3. What is the most common CT finding of bowel ischemia?
   A. Bowel wall thickening
   B. Vascular occlusion
   C. Ectopic gas
   D. Dilation

4. Which of the following statements regarding chronic mesenteric ischemia is true?
   A. Chronic mesenteric ischemia is most commonly due to recurrent mesenteric artery emboli.
   B. The typical presentation is postprandial crampy abdominal pain.
   C. MR angiography is the gold standard imaging modality.
   D. Treatment is surgical resection of the ischemic segment of bowel.

C A S E   1 8 2

Small Bowel Ischemic Stricture

1. A, B, D, and E

2. B

3. A

4. B

References

Makanjuola D: Computed tomography compared with small bowel enema in clinically equivocal intestinal obstruction. *Clin Radiol* 1998;53(3):203-208.

Rha SE, Ha HK, Lee SH, et al: CT and MR imaging findings of bowel ischemia from various primary causes. *Radiographics* 2000;20(1):29-42.

Cross-Reference

Gastrointestinal Imaging: *THE REQUISITES,* 3rd ed, p 115.

Comment

This patient presented with an incomplete small bowel obstruction. A barium small bowel examination showed a focal area of narrowing in the ileum (see figures). The fold pattern is distorted but intact without evidence of mucosal destruction, suggesting this is not a malignant obstruction. The possibility of an inflammatory obstruction was considered. The segment of involved ileum was resected, and pathologic examination of the narrowing showed it to be an area of fibrosis and scarring, resulting from prior ischemic disease. These types of small bowel obstructions are uncommon compared with postoperative adhesions causing small bowel obstruction.

Ischemic small bowel obstruction is seen mostly in elderly patients and results from occlusive or low-flow mesenteric arterial disease. However, focal ischemic and resultant fibrotic strictures of the small bowel have been reported in collagen vascular disease and any condition resulting in a vasculitis, such as rheumatoid arthritis, post-transplant cases and trauma cases without perforation, radiation cases, and some malabsorption processes. Ischemic disease of the colon is more likely to result in a residual stricture (40% of cases). Small bowel obstruction is also a well-known complication of neoplasms, such as primary adenocarcinoma and carcinoids, and inflammatory processes such as Crohn's disease.

Notes

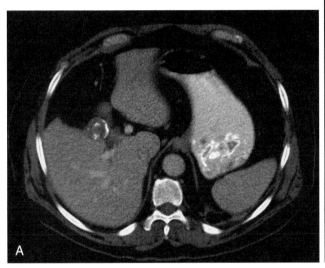

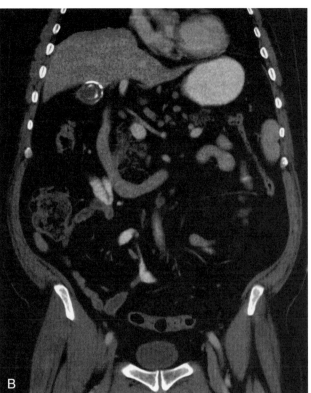

History: A 66-year-old man presents with epigastric pain.

1. What should be included in the differential diagnosis of the imaging finding shown in Figure A? (Choose all that apply.)
   A. Hematoma
   B. Hydatid cyst
   C. Metastatic deposit
   D. Porcelain gallbladder
   E. Focal nodular hyperplasia

2. What serious complication is associated with porcelain gallbladder?
   A. Cholelithiasis
   B. Cholangiocarcinoma
   C. Gallbladder hydrops
   D. Gallbladder adenocarcinoma

3. What is the most common malignancy of the biliary tract?
   A. Klatskin's tumor
   B. Intrahepatic lymphoma
   C. Gallbladder adenocarcinoma
   D. Extrahepatic cholangiocarcinoma

4. What is the prognosis of gallbladder carcinoma?
   A. Tumor behavior is benign.
   B. Mean survival time is about 6 months.
   C. The disease is cured by cholecystectomy.
   D. Disease progresses to gallbladder perforation.

Carcinoma of the Gallbladder

1. A, B, C, and D

2. D

3. C

4. B

References

Furlan A, Ferris V, Hossseinzadeh K, et al: Gallbladder carcinoma update: multimodality imaging evaluation, staging, and treatment options. *AJR Am J Roentgenol* 2008;191(5):1440-1447.

Levy AD, Murakata LA, Rohrmann CA Jr: Gallbladder carcinoma: radiologic-pathologic correlation. *Radiographics* 2001;21(2):295-314.

Cross-Reference

Gastrointestinal Imaging: *THE REQUISITES,* 3rd ed, p 250.

Comment

Although carcinoma of the gallbladder is uncommon, it is the most common malignant biliary disease. It is generally an adenocarcinoma. Patients present with symptoms that are very similar to pancreatic head lesions: jaundice, weight loss, and abdominal pain. The condition of chronic cholecystitis that leads to cystic duct occlusion and (if it does not result in a septic catastrophe) can eventually result in a calcified gallbladder wall—the porcelain gallbladder (see figures). The risk of gallbladder cancer in this setting is high (about 12%). However, other conditions (if not being direct risk factors) are associated with carcinoma of the gallbladder. About 75% of patients with gallbladder cancer have gallstones, especially a high percentage of cholesterol stones.

Owing to the anatomic position of the gallbladder in or around the porta hepatis, the dissemination of the disease to important contiguous structures makes the outlook for survival bleak. CT is not specific but is suggestive. In some cases, a soft tissue–filled gallbladder, still maintaining its gallbladder configuration (the "jam-packed gallbladder") may be seen. In many instances, the finding is an amorphous mass in the porta hepatis with bile duct obstruction. The origin may be pancreatic or biliary. Depending on the clinical presentation, severe gallbladder inflammation would also be a consideration.

Notes

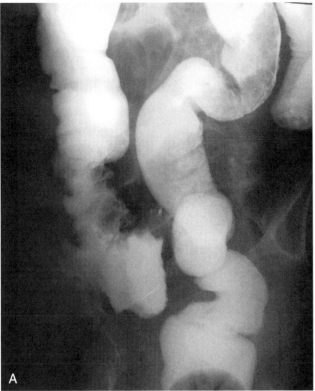

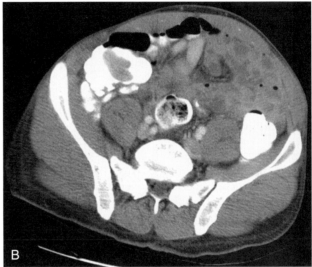

History: An 18-year-old man presents with a right lower quadrant abdominal mass.

1. What should be included in the differential diagnosis of the imaging finding shown in Figure A? (Choose all that apply.)
   A. Carcinoma
   B. Lymphoma
   C. Tuberculosis
   D. Echinococcosis
   E. Crohn's disease

2. What is the most common gastrointestinal tract site of involvement by Burkitt's lymphoma?
   A. Terminal ileum
   B. Pancreas
   C. Stomach
   D. Liver

3. What is the most common site of presentation of Burkitt's lymphoma?
   A. Bone marrow
   B. Ileocecal region
   C. Facial and mandibular
   D. Central nervous system

4. What virus is specifically associated with Burkitt's lymphoma?
   A. HIV
   B. Enteric adenovirus
   C. Epstein-Barr virus
   D. Cytomegalovirus

CASE 184

Burkitt's Lymphoma of the Cecum

1. A, B, C, and E

2. A

3. C

4. C

References

Biko DM, Anupindi SA, Hernandez A, et al: Childhood Burkitt lymphoma: abdominal and pelvic imaging findings. *AJR Am J Roentgenol* 2009;192(5): 1304-1315.

Toma P, Granata C, Rossi A, et al: Multimodality imaging of Hodgkin disease and non-Hodgkin lymphomas in children. *Radiographics* 2007;27(5):1335-1354.

Cross-Reference

Gastrointestinal Imaging: *THE REQUISITES,* 3rd ed, p 282.

Comment

This young patient has a destructive colonic mass in the cecum (see figures). The obvious possibility would be colonic adeno-carcinoma, which is the most common malignant lesion of the colon. Lymphoma is uncommon. However, among the various types of lymphomas seen in the colon is Burkitt's lymphoma, named after the pathologist who first described the relationship of this highly aggressive tumor affecting mostly children in equatorial Africa in areas of endemic malaria. The lesion usually involved the mandible in these children.

Burkitt's lymphoma is one of the most aggressive tumors known, with a doubling rate much greater than the usual adenocarcinoma of the colon. The type found in North America usually manifests as an intra-abdominal process in the distal ileum or proximal colon and can be seen as a mass in the right lower quadrant. It is extremely typical of Burkitt's lymphoma to involve this area, and the diagnosis should be strongly considered in any child who has a painless palpable mass in the region with heme-positive stool. However, in North America, the disease is seen more commonly in young adults.

In the type of lymphoma that Burkitt described in Africa, the jaw and retroperitoneal lymph nodes were frequently involved in children, but this is not typical of the type of Burkitt's lymphoma common in North America. The tumor is usually intra-abdominal and often associated with EBV, similar to some other lymphomas and cancers. A distinctive feature of Burkitt's lymphoma is its rapid doubling time. It grows in an extremely aggressive fashion, involving and displacing bowel loops in the region. It also responds dramatically to chemotherapy. Patients with HIV infection are particularly susceptible to this tumor.

Notes

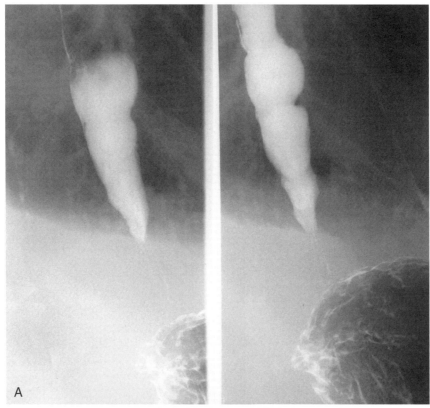

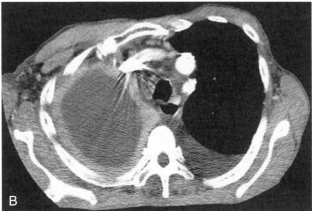

History: A 51-year-old man presents with dysphagia.

1. What should be included in the differential diagnosis of the imaging finding shown in Figure A? (Choose all that apply.)
   A. Achalasia
   B. Presbyesophagus
   C. Esophageal spasm
   D. Paraneoplastic syndrome
   E. Postvagotomy syndrome

2. What is the most common systemic disorder that may be complicated by esophageal motility dysfunction?
   A. Neoplastic disease
   B. Diabetes mellitus
   C. Chagas' disease
   D. Scleroderma

3. What is the most common gastrointestinal (GI) manifestation of paraneoplastic syndrome?
   A. Abdominal distention
   B. Hematochezia
   C. Dysphagia
   D. Diarrhea

4. What is the most common malignancy that gives rise to paraneoplastic syndrome?
   A. Bronchogenic carcinoma
   B. Ovarian carcinoma
   C. Thyroid carcinoma
   D. Gastric carcinoma

Paraneoplastic Syndrome

1. A, D, and E

2. B

3. D

4. A

References

Rutherford GC, Dineen RA, O'Connor A: Imaging in the investigation of paraneoplastic syndromes. *Clin Radiol* 2007;62(11):1021-1035.

Thomas L, Kwok Y, Edelman MJ: Management of paraneoplastic syndromes in lung cancer. *Curr Treat Options Oncol* 2004;5(1):51-62.

Cross-Reference

Gastrointestinal Imaging: *THE REQUISITES,* 3rd ed, p 27.

Comment

In some malignant conditions, secondary (nonmetastatic) systemic effects can be seen accompanying primary malignant disease. The achalasialike appearance of the esophagus, as seen in this case, is an example and is most commonly seen in patients with small cell carcinoma of the lung (see figures). However, paraneoplastic syndromes may encompass much more than the neuromuscular functions of the esophagus. They can affect skin, muscle, joints, kidneys, and endocrine function. Some cases of scleroderma have been determined to be a paraneoplastic syndrome, secondary to a primary lesion elsewhere in the body.

The exact mechanism of paraneoplastic manifestations is not well understood. The tumors may excrete hormones, which affect a specific target organ. There is considerable discussion in the literature of tumor antibodies produced by the body to resist the tumor but that have a secondary effect in the body. The presentation of a patient who has carcinoma of the lung with concomitant achalasialike symptoms and findings is uncommon but is not rare. Other GI manifestations of paraneoplastic syndrome have been reported, including malabsorption in the small bowel (the most common manifestation according to some) and unexplained diarrhea.

GI manifestations of paraneoplastic syndrome are of great interest and the subject of considerable research. It is possible that the problem is much larger than is appreciated at the present time. Although lung tumors have been mostly shown to be involved with paraneoplastic syndromes, more recent work has shown that malignancies from almost every body system have that capability. Imaging may be used to show either the primary lesions or paraneoplastic manifestations. However, most of the paraneoplastic effects have been detected by laboratory studies.

Notes

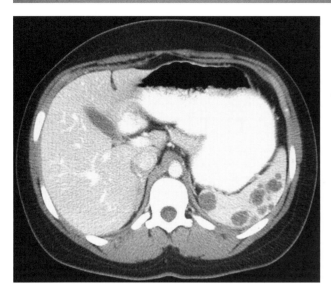

History: A 57-year-old man presents with vague left upper quadrant pain.

1. What should be included in the differential diagnosis of the imaging finding shown in the figure? (Choose all that apply.)
   A. Splenic metastases
   B. Hemangiomas
   C. Myelofibrosis
   D. Abscesses
   E. Cysts

2. What is the most common cause of perfusion defects in the spleen?
   A. Infarcts
   B. Abscesses
   C. Leukemic deposits
   D. Pancreatic pseudocyst

3. What is the most common tumor seen in the spleen?
   A. Lymphoma
   B. Hamartoma
   C. Hemangioma
   D. Angiosarcoma

4. Which of the following statements regarding splenic metastases is true?
   A. Splenic involvement is rare in patients with widespread metastases.
   B. Calcified splenic metastases arise most commonly from an ovarian primary.
   C. The most common primary site of hematogenous metastases is GI tumors.
   D. Involvement of the spleen from an adjacent primary tumor usually results in invasion of the spleen.

Splenic Metastatic Disease

1. A, B, and D

2. A

3. C

4. A

References

Kamaya A, Weinstein S, Desser TS: Multiple lesions of the spleen: differential diagnosis of cystic and solid lesions. *Semin Ultrasound CT MRI* 2006;27(5):389-403.

Sutherland T, Temple F, Hennessy O, et al: Abdomen's forgotten organ: sonography and CT of focal splenic lesions. *J Med Imaging Radiat Oncol* 2010;54(2):120-128.

Cross-Reference

Gastrointestinal Imaging: *THE REQUISITES,* 3rd ed, p 212.

Comment

Marginal perfusion defects in the spleen, often wedge-shaped, are a common finding in the spleen at CT imaging. These defects are almost always old splenic infarcts. Despite the vascularity and the hematogenous "filter" function of the spleen, metastatic disease is rare. Several theories as to why this seemingly unusual situation should be the case have been put forward—ranging from the angle of the splenic artery from its takeoff from the celiac axis to the high concentrations of lymphoid tissue in the spleen. As in this case, the most common primary cancer is lung cancer followed by GI tumors (see figure). Splenic metastatic disease apparently without liver involvement is especially rare, representing less than 5% of cases of reported splenic metastatic disease.

Other differential considerations include congenital and acquired (usually secondary to trauma) splenic cysts. These cysts are almost entirely solitary. Hydatid cyst may also be seen in the spleen as a solitary lesion. Abscesses, which are encountered more frequently in immunocompromised patients, may be single but are usually multiple and often tiny. Hemangiomas, the most common benign tumors of the spleen, can be solitary or multiple. Involvement of the spleen with lymphoma or leukemia usually takes the form of splenomegaly. However, if the spleen is normal in size with multiple defects, these possibilities must also be considered. Pancreatic pseudocysts have been reported as intrasplenic lesions.

Notes

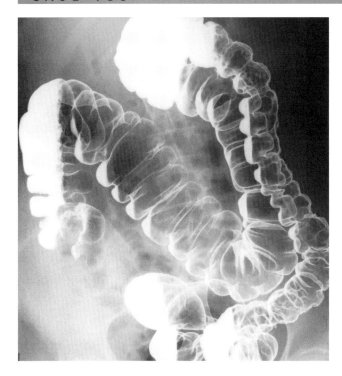
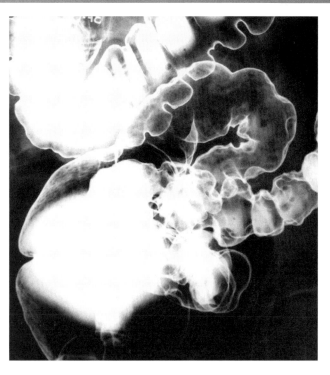

History: A 38-year-old woman presents with bloody diarrhea.

1. What should be included in the differential diagnosis of the imaging finding shown in the figures? (Choose all that apply.)
   A. Inflammatory bowel disease
   B. Polyposis syndrome
   C. Pneumatosis coli
   D. Filiform polyposis
   E. Diverticulosis

2. What is the most common colon polyp?
   A. Adenomatous
   B. Hyperplastic
   C. Hamartoma
   D. Villous

3. This patient has a history of foreign travel including "swimming in the Nile." What diagnostic consideration has the greatest relevance to this history?
   A. Schistosomiasis
   B. Echinococcosis
   C. *Yersinia* colitis
   D. Ascariasis

4. What is the most common clinical manifestation of schistosomal infection?
   A. None
   B. Pruritus
   C. Hematuria
   D. Bloody diarrhea

Schistosomiasis of the Colon

1. A, B, and C

2. B

3. A

4. A

References

Fataar S, Bassiony H, Hamed MS, et al: Radiographic spectrum of rectocolonic calcification from schistosomiasis. *AJR Am J Roentgenol* 1984;141(5):933-936.

Ortaga CD, Ogawa NY, Rocha MS, et al: Helminthic diseases in the abdomen: an epidemiologic and radiologic overview. *Radiographics* 2010;30(1):253-267.

Cross-Reference

Gastrointestinal Imaging: *THE REQUISITES,* 3rd ed, p 290.

Comment

Polypoid processes limited to the distal colon, as in this case, are usually hyperplastic in nature (see figures). Hyperplastic polyps, although the most common colonic polyp, are mostly small (<5 mm) and difficult to image. The polyps shown in this case are larger with a mostly smooth elevated surface (see figures). Some have tiny collections of barium, indicating ulceration. The patient presented with rectal bleeding. Adenomas, which represent about 10% of all colonic polyps, can bleed. However, a cluster of adenomatous polyps limited to the distal colon would be extremely unusual, even in the various polyposis syndromes.

The patient's history of foreign travel and "swimming in the Nile" must be considered in the differential diagnosis. Schistosomiasis is endemic in several places in the world and, until more recently with the return of malaria to the world scene, was the most common infectious (parasitic) disease in the world. Even a single exposure to fresh water in these endemic areas can result in infection, such as in this patient. Humans are the host for this parasitic infection; with world travel becoming commonplace, U.S. physicians and particularly radiologists should be aware of the possibility of tropical diseases, especially new outbreaks of malaria in travelers coming home to the United States.

In schistosomiasis, the organisms are *S. mansoni* and *Schistosoma japonicum*. In fresh water, the tiny worms penetrate the human skin; seek the vascular system of the host; and migrate to the liver, lungs, bladder, and other organs. Bladder involvement is associated with an increased risk of bladder cancer. When in the host organ, in this case, the lower colon (usually *S. mansoni*), the worms infest the venules of the colon wall, and eventually mature eggs are deposited in the wall (hence the polyps) and rupture into the lumen (hence the ulceration on the polyps and bleeding).

Notes

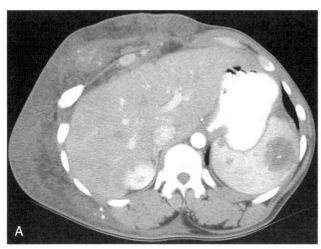

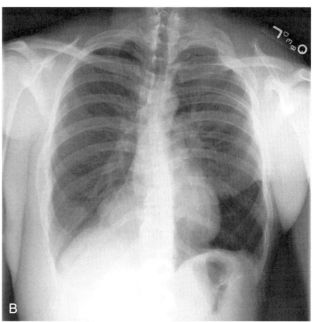

History: A 19-year-old man presents with right costal margin pain and swelling.

1. What should be included in the differential diagnosis of the imaging finding shown in Figure A? (Choose all that apply.)
   A. Infarct
   B. Abscess
   C. Lymphoma
   D. Hemangioma
   E. Lymphangioma

2. Which of the following statements regarding cystic splenic lesions is true?
   A. Most cystic splenic lesions are neoplastic.
   B. Splenic lymphangioma is usually diagnosed in childhood.
   C. Patients with echinococccal cysts develop fever secondary to antigen release.
   D. Post-traumatic cysts are usually less than 5 cm in size, allowing differentiation from congenital cysts, which are larger.

3. What is the most common clinical manifestation of a lymphangioma?
   A. Skin
   B. Cystic hygroma
   C. Mesenteric cyst
   D. Lymphangioleiomyomatosis

4. Which of the following conditions is associated with lymphangiomas?
   A. Osler-Weber-Rendu syndrome
   B. Kasabach-Merritt syndrome
   C. von Hippel-Lindau disease
   D. Fetal alcohol syndrome

Lymphangioma of the Spleen

1. B, C, D, and E

2. B

3. B

4. D

References

Kamaya A, Weinstein S, Desser TS: Multiple lesions of the spleen: differential diagnosis of cystic and solid lesions. *Semin Ultrasound CT MRI* 2006;27(5):389-403.

Warshauer DM, Hall HL: Solitary splenic lesions. *Semin Ultrasound CT MRI* 2006;27(5):370-388.

Cross-Reference

Gastrointestinal Imaging: *THE REQUISITES,* 3rd ed, p 214.

Comment

Lymphangioma is an unusual condition that rarely involves the spleen. The splenic lesions can be solitary or multiple as in this case (see figures). Lymphangioma is a congenital malformation of the lymphatic vessels and system. It can be focal or widespread lymphangiomatosis, as in this case. The lesion is entirely benign with no malignant potential known. Perhaps the most common manifestation in infants is a cystic hygroma, which is thought to represent a form of focal lymphangioma in the neck. Histologically, lymphangiomas are thought to be hamartomas rather than neoplasms.

Splenic involvement can be solitary organ involvement or part of lymphangiomatosis. Bone also can be involved. Deformities of the ribs in this patient are noted (see figures). Lytic expansile lesions of bones in this condition have been called Gorham's disease. However, these bones appear deformed rather than replaced or destroyed. In some cases of splenic lymphangioma, splenectomy has been necessary when the lesion is symptomatic or diagnosis is questionable. The skin thickening seen over this patient's body is a manifestation of lymphangiomatosis, as is the mediastinal and neck involvement. This condition has been classified into three groups: (1) lymphangioma circumscriptum, (2) cavernous lymphangioma (this patient), and (3) cystic lymphangioma (cystic hygroma, which can also be seen in some cases of cavernous lymphangioma).

Notes

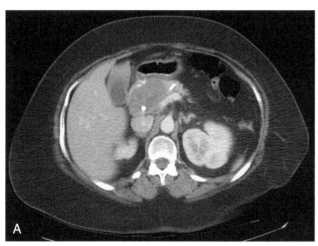

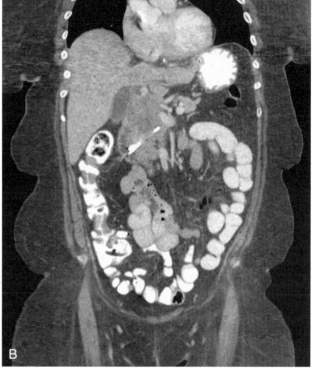

History: A 32-year-old woman presents with mild jaundice.

1. What should be included in the differential diagnosis of the imaging finding shown in Figure A? (Choose all that apply.)
   A. Acute pancreatitis
   B. Pancreatic carcinoma
   C. Pancreatic lymphoma
   D. Pancreatic pseudocyst
   E. Peripancreatic lymphadenopathy

2. Which of the following statements regarding pancreatic lymphoma is *true*?
   A. Pancreatic lymphoma represents less than 1% of pancreatic masses.
   B. The uninvolved part of the pancreas becomes atrophic.
   C. Pancreatic lymphoma is usually due to Hodgkin's disease.
   D. Diffuse lymphomatous infiltration results in high attenuation enlargement.

3. What finding is most suggestive of pancreatic lymphoma instead of carcinoma?
   A. Absence of pancreatic duct dilation
   B. Heterogeneous enhancement
   C. Tumoral calcification
   D. Vascular invasion

4. What is the most common site of lymphomatous involvement of the gastrointestinal tract?
   A. Esophagus
   B. Stomach
   C. Small bowel
   D. Colon

Lymphoma of the Pancreatic Head

1. A, B, C, and E

2. A

3. A

4. B

References

Leite NP, Kased N, Hanna RF, et al: Cross-sectional imaging of extra-nodal involvement in abdominopelvic lymphoproliferative malignancies. *Radiographics* 2007;27(6):1613-1635.

Merkle EM, Bender GN, Brambs HJ: Imaging findings in pancreatic lymphoma: differential aspects. *AJR Am J Roentgenol* 2000;174(3):671-675.

Cross-Reference

Gastrointestinal Imaging: *THE REQUISITES,* 3rd ed, p 169.

Comment

Primary pancreatic head lymphomas are rare; they account for about 0.5% of pancreatic masses. Secondary involvement of the pancreas by a non-Hodgkin's lymphoma resulting from gross peripancreatic lymphadenopathy is more common. However, in cases such as the one shown here (see figures), in which the mass is entirely within the pancreatic substance and there is no evidence of lymphoma elsewhere, pancreatic lymphoma is a possible differential diagnosis. In this case, the lesion was a T-cell lymphoma. Most pancreatic lymphomas are B-cell lymphomas.

Diagnosis usually is confirmed by CT-guided needle aspiration or surgical pathology. Multidetector CT and routine and endoscopic ultrasound have also been useful in the diagnosis of pancreatic head masses. However, none of these imaging modalities can be considered specific. Nevertheless, multidetector CT imaging performed in this case shows a more homogeneous appearance, which might be expected with a hypovascular ductal adenocarcinoma. In addition, the small portion of the distal pancreas included in the images shows no evidence of pancreatic duct obstruction. The biliary duct obstruction that brought the patient to medical attention and resulted in stent placement completely resolved in a few days; this would be highly unlikely for the usual ductal carcinoma of the pancreas. All these observations, although not specific, might suggest alternative diagnostic possibilities. The incidence of lymphoma is increased in patients with AIDS, and the incidence of pancreatic lymphoma may also be increased.

Notes

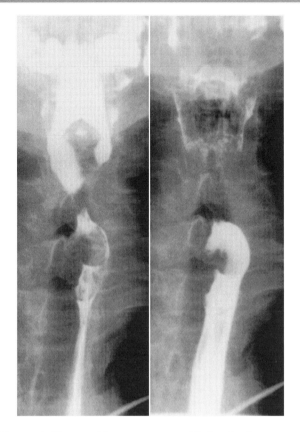

History: A 79-year-old man presents with dysphagia.

1. What should be included in the differential diagnosis of the imaging finding shown in the figure? (Choose all that apply.)
   A. Foreign body
   B. Inflammatory polyp
   C. Fibrovascular polyp
   D. Spindle cell carcinoma
   E. Squamous cell carcinoma

2. What is the most common benign neoplasm of the esophagus?
   A. Leiomyoma (stromal tumor)
   B. Fibrovascular polyp
   C. Papilloma
   D. Adenoma

3. What is the most common clinical presentation of a patient with a fibrovascular polyp of the esophagus?
   A. Dysphagia
   B. Regurgitation
   C. Incidental finding
   D. Acute asphyxiation

4. Which of the following statements regarding fibrovascular polyps of the esophagus is *false*?
   A. These lesions degenerate to malignant sarcomas.
   B. These lesions are usually found in the proximal esophagus.
   C. The lesion may appear of density less than water on CT imaging.
   D. The lesion may appear of high signal intensity on T1-weighted MRI.

Fibrovascular Esophageal Polyp

1. A, C, and E

2. A

3. A

4. A

References

Levine MS, Buck JL, Pantongrag-Brown L, et al: Fibrovascular polyps of the esophagus: clinical, radiographic, and pathologic findings in 16 patients. *AJR Am J Roentgenol* 1996;166(4):781-787.

Rubesin SE, Levine MS: Differential diagnosis of esophageal disease on esophagography. *Appl Radiol* 2001;30:11-21.

Cross-Reference

Gastrointestinal Imaging: THE REQUISITES, 3rd ed, p 10.

Comment

Polyps of the esophagus are unusual; the most common is the benign leiomyoma, or stromal cell tumor. They are usually solitary, but multiple leiomyomatosis of the esophagus has been encountered rarely. Fibrovascular polyps, which are composed of fibrovascular tissue, are also rare. Because of the presence of fatty tissue in some of these tumors, fibrovascular polyps may appear to have low density on CT scan. They have a propensity to develop in the upper portion of the esophagus, as seen in this case (see figure).

Fibrovascular polyps occur particularly in the cervical region of older patients, which is the opposite of most esophageal tumors, occurring typically seen in the middle to distal esophagus. These polyps occur more commonly in men. Because of their soft nature, these tumors can grow quite large before producing symptoms. The cervical location exposes the polyps to repeated peristalsis and dragging by ingested materials that may cause the tumors to become pedunculated or mobile. The most dramatic clinical finding is when the patient states that he or she has regurgitated a mass into the oropharynx and then swallowed it. These tumors may cause bleeding. If large enough, airway obstruction has been reported in these very mobile tumors.

Granular cell tumors are also rare and are believed to originate in Schwann cells. However, only about 10% occur in the gastrointestinal tract, usually the esophagus. Squamous cell papillomas in the esophagus have been reported, more frequently in men. Most are asymptomatic. It is unclear whether papillomas are true neoplasms.

Notes

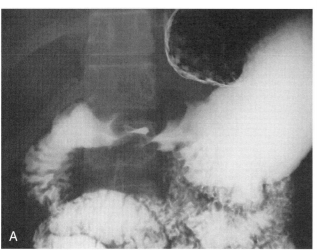

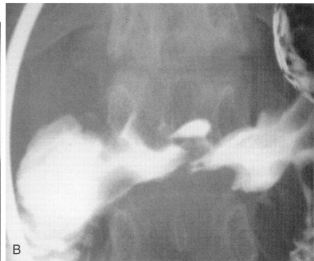

History: A 33-year-old woman presents with epigastric pain and vomiting.

1. What should be included in the differential diagnosis of the imaging finding shown in Figure A? (Choose all that apply.)
   A. Gastric carcinoma
   B. Pseudodiverticulum
   C. Pyloric channel ulcer
   D. Adult pyloric stenosis
   E. Hypertrophic pyloric stenosis

2. What is the eponym for a penetrating ulcer that extends from the distal gastric antrum to the base of the duodenum, paralleling the pyloric channel?
   A. Hampton's line
   B. Marshall's line
   C. Dragsted's ulcer
   D. Cushing's ulcer

3. What is the most common complication of peptic ulceration?
   A. Bleeding
   B. Perforation
   C. Penetration
   D. Obstruction

4. Which of the following radiographic signs would be most useful in diagnosing a lesion seen on a barium upper GI study as a polyp rather than a diverticulum?
   A. Lesion collects barium
   B. Lesion location in the fundus
   C. Filling defect in the barium pool
   D. Bowler hat sign pointing outward

Pyloric Channel Ulcer

1. A, B, C, and D

2. C

3. A

4. C

References

Levine MS: Peptic ulcers. In Gore RM, Levine MS (eds): *Textbook of Gastrointestinal Radiology*, 2nd ed. Philadelphia: Saunders, 2000, pp 514-545.

Thompson G, Stevenson GW, Somers S: Benign gastric ulcer: a reliable radiologic diagnosis. *AJR Am J Roentgenol* 1983;141(2):331-333.

Cross-Reference

Gastrointestinal Imaging: *THE REQUISITES,* 3rd ed, p 97.

Comment

This upper GI double-contrast barium examination clearly shows a persistent collection of barium in the pyloric channel (see figures). Ulcers collect barium because they are essentially holes in the mucosa. An ulcer collects barium in the same manner in which a pothole in the road may collect water. The granulation tissue that forms the base of the ulceration tends to cause the barium to become adherent to the ulcer crater. Diverticula also collect barium in the same manner. Space-occupying lesions such as polyps and masses displace barium, which is called a *filling defect*.

Although this was basic knowledge a decade ago, it seems less basic to current residents. The widespread use of endoscopy and decreased number of upper GI examinations done by radiologists and the great interest in newer modalities seem to have relegated expertise in barium procedures to a small niche in the radiology department of the 21st century. Nevertheless, the examinations are still relevant, and radiologists are still required to have some basic knowledge. Dragsted, who connected hyperacidity to peptic disease (although to some extent this had been done by Beaumont in 1835), was a surgeon whose name is attached to a penetrating ulcer that connects the gastric antrum to the base of the duodenum—the double pyloric channel sign. Dragsted's work was done before Marshall made the connection between *H. pylori* and peptic ulcer disease. Ulcers in the pyloric channel often manifest as gastric outlet obstruction after a chronic history of peptic ulcer disease. The manifestation of gastric outlet obstruction in a patient with no history of peptic ulcer disease is an ominous sign of possible malignancy.

Notes

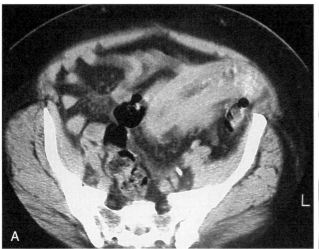

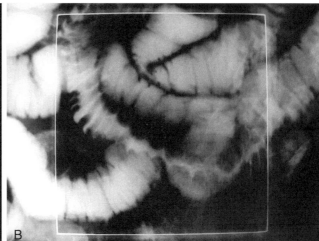

History: A 32-year-old woman presents with lower abdominal pain; a low hematocrit also is discovered.

1. What should be included in the differential diagnosis of the imaging finding shown in Figure A? (Choose all that apply.)
   A. Neoplasia
   B. Intussusception
   C. Intramural hematoma
   D. Meckel's diverticulum
   E. Inflammatory bowel disease

2. What is the most common cause of small bowel hemorrhage?
   A. Trauma
   B. Hemophilia
   C. Anticoagulant therapy
   D. Henoch-Schönlein syndrome

3. What finding on CT is *most* suggestive of small bowel hemorrhage?
   A. Circumferential bowel wall thickening
   B. Intramural hyperdensity
   C. Bowel obstruction
   D. Pneumatosis

4. This patient underwent a barium small bowel study (see figures). In the involved segment, the mucosal folds are thickened but remain straight and parallel. What is this pattern of fold abnormality known as?
   A. Spiculation
   B. Coiled spring
   C. "Stack of coins"
   D. String of beads

Small Bowel Intramural Hemorrhage

1. A, B, C, and E

2. C

3. B

4. C

References

Abbas MA, Collins JM, Olden KW: Spontaneous intramural small-bowel hematoma: imaging findings and outcome. *AJR Am J Roentgenol* 2002;179(6): 1389-1394.

Silva AC, Pimenta M, Guimaraes LS: Small bowel obstruction: what to look for. *Radiographics* 2009;29(2):423-439.

Cross-Reference

Gastrointestinal Imaging: *THE REQUISITES,* 3rd ed, p 120.

Comment

A patient presenting with abdominal pain and CT findings (see figures) such as in this case must raise many diagnostic possibilities in the mind of the radiologist. The fact that this patient is relatively young lessens, but does not exclude, the possibility of ischemic disease and intramural hemorrhage. Hypoperfusion, such as in hypovolemic shocked bowel, would be a consideration. Disease that manifests as an intramural vasculitis, such as Henoch-Schönlein purpura affecting the bowel with intramural bleeding, may also give such a picture. The CT images in this case show thickened small bowel wall and folds.

This patient underwent a barium small bowel study (see figures). In the involved segment, the folds are "stacked" together producing the well-known "stack of coins" or "picket fence" sign. This patient had a severe intramural hemorrhage of the small bowel. Multidetector CT showed no evidence of arterial occlusion of the major mesenteric vessels. The length of involved bowel would make blunt trauma less likely. An infiltrative process, neoplastic or nonneoplastic, is always a possibility. Carcinoid involvement of the bowel might be considered, although the desmoplastic distortion of bowel loops is not present in this case. Metastatic disease would not likely affect such an extended length of bowel. Nonneoplastic diagnostic considerations include intramural edema, intramural bleeding, and less likely possibilities such as lymphangiectasia and amyloid of the bowel. In this case, all findings were the result of mesenteric and intramural small bowel bleeding. A CT scan repeated 3 weeks later showed normal small bowel throughout, which is an almost sure diagnostic sign of bleeding.

Notes

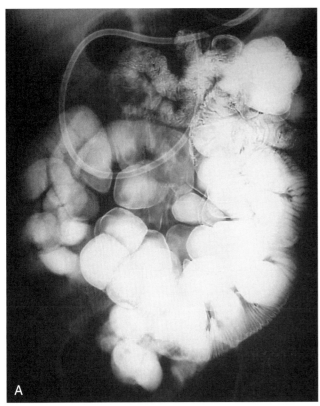

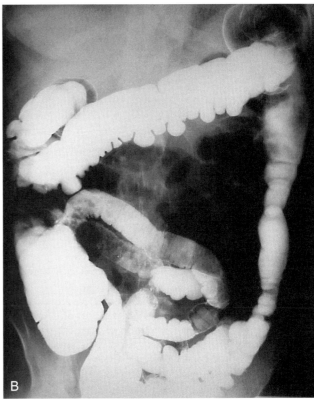

History: A 38-year-old woman presents with diarrhea and abdominal bloating.

1. What should be included in the differential diagnosis of the imaging finding shown in Figure A? (Choose all that apply.)
   A. Scleroderma
   B. Paralytic ileus
   C. Jejunal diverticulosis
   D. Small bowel obstruction
   E. Short small bowel syndrome

2. In scleroderma, what intestinal organ is most commonly involved?
   A. Colon
   B. Stomach
   C. Esophagus
   D. Small bowel

3. What are the underlying pathologic changes seen in the bowel as a result of scleroderma?
   A. Small vessel vasculitis and fibrosis
   B. Bacterial overgrowth
   C. Villous atrophy
   D. Dysmotility

4. What is the term used to describe small bowel that appears dilated with crowding of normal thickness valvulae conniventes?
   A. Hidebound
   B. Obstruction
   C. Jejunization
   D. Thumbprinting

Scleroderma of the Small Bowel and Colon

1. A, B, C, and D

2. C

3. A

4. A

References

Madani G, Katz RD, Haddock JA, et al: The role of radiology in the management of systemic sclerosis. *Clin Radiol* 2008;63(9):959-967.
Pickhardt PJ: The "hide-bound" bowel sign. *Radiology* 1999;213(3):837-838.

Cross-Reference

Gastrointestinal Imaging: THE REQUISITES, 3rd ed, p 113.

Comment

Numerous connective tissue diseases can affect the small bowel and colon. Scleroderma is caused by abnormal deposition of collagen in the skin, adjacent to blood vessels, and in various visceral organs. It may be isolated or may occur as part of CREST syndrome, which includes changes caused by calcinosis, Raynaud's disease, esophageal dysmotility, sclerodactyly, and telangiectasia (CREST). Mixed connective tissue disease is considered a distinct disease that has features of several connective tissue diseases, including systemic lupus erythematosus, scleroderma, polymyositis, and rheumatoid arthritis. In this condition, as in scleroderma, the esophagus is the organ most often involved, with dysmotility being the main feature.

The major abnormality of scleroderma is the abnormal deposition of collagen into various tissues including the bowel. Fibrosis is a major feature of this disease, and although the esophagus is most commonly involved, fibrosis can also be seen in both colon and small bowel. There is also associated small vessel damage, particularly to the intestines, because much of this deposition produces vasculitis-type changes, with resultant long-term ischemia of the bowel. Malabsorption results because of stasis of the bowel contents, bacterial overgrowth, poor absorption of bile salts, and impaired lymphatic drainage. Diarrhea, weight loss, and bloating are symptoms of this condition.

Radiologically, the changes of fibrosis, muscle atrophy, and vasculitis produce dilation of the small bowel, which is often termed *pseudoobstruction*. Pneumatosis is a known finding, especially pneumatosis coli, but its underlying cause is unclear. A pathognomonic change seen in the bowel is crowding of the valvulae, or a "hide-bound" appearance. The fibrosis of the bowel draws the valvulae closer together, producing more valvulae (>5) per inch than normal (see figures). The margins of the intestines also may be flattened. This flattening gives the bowel an accordion-pleated appearance. In the colon, the changes are often a diminished or disordered haustral pattern with wide-mouth diverticula-like deformities (see figures).

Notes

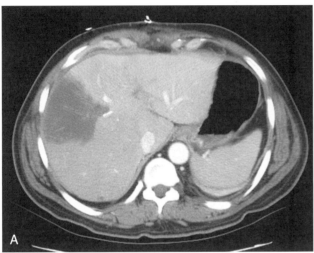

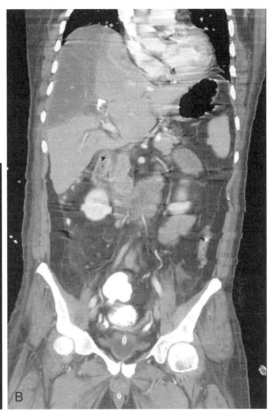

History: A 45-year-old man has abnormal liver function tests.

1. What should be included in the differential diagnosis of the imaging finding shown in Figure A? (Choose all that apply.)
    A. Hepatic artery occlusion
    B. Ischemic hepatitis
    C. Fluid collection
    D. Budd-Chiari syndrome
    E. Metastasis

2. What is the most common cause of hepatic infarction secondary to hepatic artery occlusion?
    A. Liver transplantation
    B. Hypercoagulability
    C. Vasculitis
    D. Infection

3. Which of the following statements regarding the imaging appearances of hepatic infarction is *true*?
    A. The presence of gas is diagnostic of infection.
    B. Infarction may be complicated by formation of bile lakes.
    C. Contrast-enhanced imaging is required to make the diagnosis.
    D. Infarction is characterized by nonenhancement of the affected segment.

4. What is the primary blood supply of the liver?
    A. Portal vein
    B. Hepatic vein
    C. Celiac artery
    D. Hepatic artery

Focal Hepatic Artery Occlusion

1. A, C, and E

2. A

3. B

4. A

References

Lipson JA, Qayyum A, Avrin DE, et al: CT and MRI of hepatic contour abnormalities. *AJR Am J Roentgenol* 2005;184(1):75-81.

Torabi M, Hosseinzaddeh K, Federle MP: CT of nonneoplastic hepatic vascular and perfusion disorders. *Radiographics* 2008;28(7):1967-1982.

Cross-Reference

Gastrointestinal Imaging: *THE REQUISITES,* 3rd ed, p 177.

Comment

The patient in this case developed the wedge-shaped defect after surgery as a result of the hepatic artery vessel being ligated (see figures). The wedge-shaped defect is the hepatic infarction resulting from the interruption of arterial blood to the involved segment. One might think that because the liver has two blood supplies, the portal venous and the hepatic arterial, infarction might be impossible. However, it has been shown that the portal venous system alone cannot protect the liver from possible infarction if there is occlusion of the hepatic artery or its branches. This situation may relate to function. While the portal veins are transporting absorbed content from the gastrointestinal tract to the liver for metabolism, the hepatic artery, rich in oxygen, has the primary function of delivering that oxygen to the hepatocyte.

Most infarcts occur in the right lobe of the liver, which is not surprising because this is the largest part of the liver. The best diagnostic tool at the present time is CT with images obtained in the late arterial phase of scanning. However, even in the portal venous phase, tissue damage still results in the wedge-shaped deformity well described in imaging literature. In the right clinical setting, the diagnosis can be made with confidence. However, the imaging appearance is not specific, especially in patients who present with CT findings similar to infarction but do not have the appropriate clinical history. Other etiologic factors must be considered, such as hepatic abscess, laceration, unusual metastatic lesion, and, in rare cases, lymphoma of the liver. However, with the continued refinement of CT arteriography, the ability to trace the hepatic artery as it swings away from the celiac axis, dividing into its right and left branches in the porta hepatis, has vastly improved.

Notes

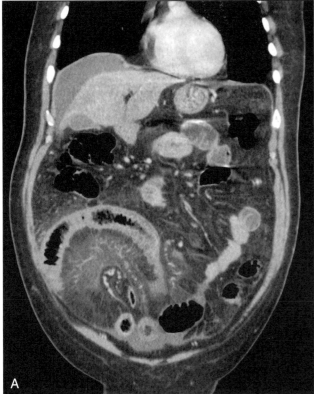 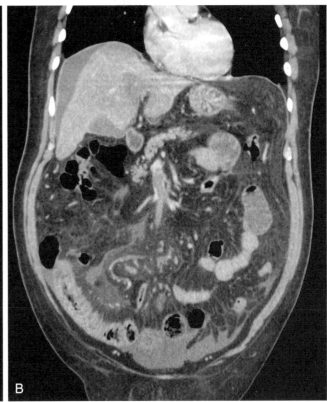

History: A 62-year-old man presents with a 4-day history of nausea and vomiting with a palpable mass in the right iliac fossa.

1. What should be included in the differential diagnosis of the imaging finding shown in Figure A? (Choose all that apply.)
   A. Trauma
   B. Vascular
   C. Neoplastic
   D. Obstruction
   E. Inflammatory

2. What is the most common etiology for superior mesenteric venous occlusion?
   A. Prothrombotic state
   B. Postoperative
   C. Idiopathic
   D. Cirrhosis

3. What is the most specific imaging sign of superior mesenteric venous thrombosis?
   A. Mesenteric stranding
   B. Small bowel pneumatosis
   C. Superior mesenteric vein filling defect
   D. Portal venous cavernous transformation

4. What part of the gastrointestinal tract would you anticipate would be most severely affected by superior mesenteric venous occlusion?
   A. Pharynx and esophagus
   B. Stomach and duodenum
   C. Small bowel and ascending colon
   D. Descending and sigmoid colon

Superior Mesenteric Venous Occlusion

1. A, B, C, and E

2. A

3. C

4. C

References

Bradbury MS, Kavanagh PV, Bechtold RE, et al: Mesenteric venous thrombosis: diagnosis and noninvasive imaging. *Radiographics* 2002;22(3):527-541.
Kumar S, Sarr MG, Kamath PS: Mesenteric venous thrombosis. *N Engl J Med* 2001;345(23):1683-1688.

Cross-Reference

Gastrointestinal Imaging: *THE REQUISITES,* 3rd ed, p 144.

Comment

Mesenteric venous thrombosis is an uncommon form of mesenteric ischemia and infarction. This condition, with a mortality rate of 30% to 40%, is seen in patients with hypercoagulable states, such as intraabdominal sepsis, pregnancy, and polycythemia vera, and in some women taking oral contraceptives. A few cases have been reported in pregnant women who have accidentally taken oral contraceptives. Other wide-ranging causes include blunt trauma and certain malignancies; rarely, it is seen after abdominal surgeries.

The striking findings in this case are the segmental distribution of marked small bowel abnormality (see figures), including congestion in the mesentery, and the filling defect within the lumen of the superior mesenteric vein (see figures). There is also free fluid in the abdomen, which can be expected in this condition. The high mortality rate associated with this condition is most likely due to the prolonged time of seeking medical attention and delayed diagnosis.

Notes

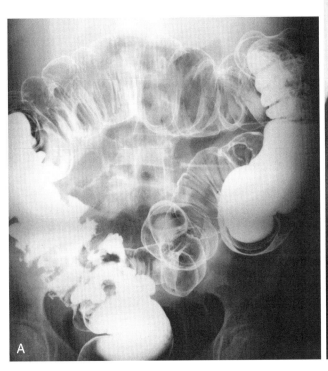

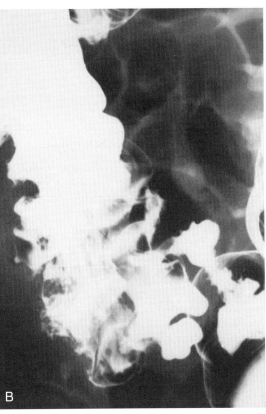

History: A 27-year-old man from Turkey presents with abdominal pain and diarrhea.

1. What should be included in the differential diagnosis of the imaging finding shown in Figure A? (Choose all that apply.)
   A. Tuberculosis
   B. Fecal residue
   C. Crohn's disease
   D. Villous adenoma
   E. Pneumatosis coli

2. This patient had oral aphthous ulcers, skin lesions, uveitis, and genital ulcers. What is your *favored* diagnosis?
   A. Reiter's syndrome
   B. Behçet's disease
   C. Crohn's disease
   D. Syphilis

3. Why is Behçet's disease known as the "silk route" disease?
   A. The geographic distribution
   B. Association with the silk industry
   C. A disease affecting people of Eastern Chinese origin
   D. Disease caused by use of illicit drugs trafficked along this route

4. What is the etiology of Behçet's disease?
   A. Paraneoplastic
   B. Idiopathic
   C. Infection
   D. Allergic

Behçet's Disease of the Colon

1. A, B, C, and D

2. B

3. A

4. B

References

Chung SY, Ha HK, Kim JH, et al: Radiologic findings of Behcet syndrome involving the gastrointestinal tract. *Radiographics* 2001;21(4):911-924.

Iida M, Kobayashi H, Matsumoto T, et al: Intestinal Behcet disease: serial changes at radiography. *Radiology* 1993;188(1):65-69.

Cross-Reference

Gastrointestinal Imaging: *THE REQUISITES,* 3rd ed, p 300.

Comment

Behçet's disease is a rare condition in the West, but is seen with more frequency as people move about the world. It is primarily a condition affecting the population living around the Mediterranean Sea, thought to have been brought back in the Middle Ages along the "silk route" pioneered by Marco Polo in his journey to China. A Turkish physician first described it in the literature in the 1930s, and the disease is known by his name. It affects several organ systems, including the eyes, skin, genitals, joints, and gastrointestinal (GI) system. The colon is almost always the GI organ involved, although cases of esophageal involvement have occurred. The most common site of colonic involvement appears to be the ileocecal region.

Behçet's disease is essentially a vasculitis of unknown origin that leads to inflammation and ulcerative eruptions, often deep and severe, such as in this case (see figures). It may be easily confused with other inflammatory bowel diseases, especially Crohn's disease. Patients usually have other manifestations of Behçet's disease when colonic symptoms are present. Bowel perforations associated with Behçet's disease have been reported. Occasionally, the disease may be seen as an ileocecal inflammatory mass similar to ileocecal phlegmon seen in Crohn's disease.

Notes

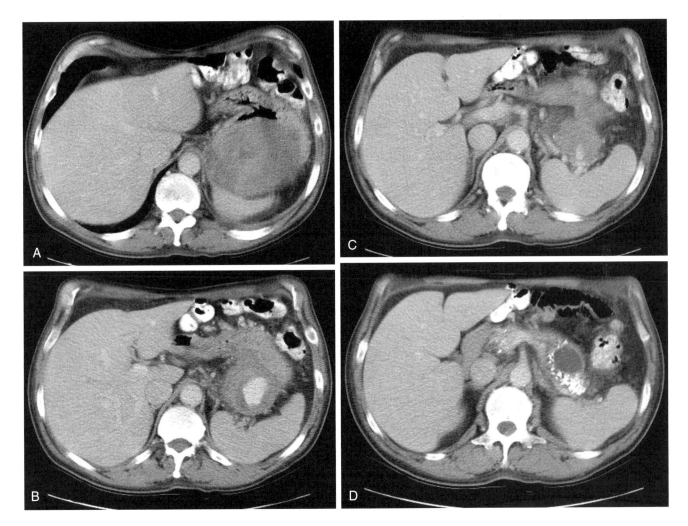

History: A 53-year-old man presents with hematemesis. Upper endoscopy identified an extramucosal mass distorting the gastric greater curvature.

1. What should be included in the differential diagnosis of the imaging finding shown in Figure A? (Choose all that apply.)
   A. Colonic splenic flexure mass
   B. Pancreatic tail mass
   C. Gastric wall mass
   D. Vascular mass
   E. Splenic mass

2. Which of the following statements regarding the differences between splenic artery aneurysms and pseudoaneurysms is *true*?
   A. The aneurysm wall is composed of intima, media, and adventitia; the pseudoaneurysm wall lacks adventitia.
   B. Pseudoaneurysms are usually clinically silent and diagnosed as incidental findings.
   C. Most splenic artery aneurysms occur as a complication of pancreatitis.
   D. Splenic artery pseudoaneurysms are more common than aneurysms.

3. What is the most common site of aneurysm formation in the abdomen?
   A. Iliac arteries
   B. Celiac artery
   C. Splenic artery
   D. Abdominal aorta

4. What is the usual first line of treatment of a splenic artery pseudoaneurysm?
   A. Nothing
   B. Surgery
   C. Endovascular intervention
   D. Percutaneous thrombin injection

Pseudoaneurysm of the Splenic Artery

1. B, C, and D

2. A

3. D

4. C

References

Agrawal GA, Johnson PT, Fishman EK: Splenic artery aneurysms and pseudoaneurysms: clinical distinctions and CT appearances. *Radiographics* 2007;27(4):992-999.

Saad NEA, Saad WEA, Davies MG, et al: Pseudoaneurysms and the role of minimally invasive techniques in their management. *Radiographics* 2005;25(Suppl. 1):S173-S189.

Cross-Reference

Gastrointestinal Imaging: *THE REQUISITES,* 3rd ed, p 161.

Comment

Pseudoaneurysm of vessels in the pancreatic bed associated with chronic pancreatitis is uncommon but can be seen in a small percentage of patients (usually <5%). The most common vascular structure involved is the splenic artery, as in this case (see figures). The gastroduodenal artery is the next most commonly affected vessel. If the abnormality is seen in the region of the head of the pancreas, it is usually the gastroduodenal artery. If it is in the body of the pancreas, it is the splenic artery. Apart from the expected symptoms of chronic pancreatitis, patients often may have other symptoms relative to this vascular abnormality. Cases of gastrointestinal bleeding have been reported if the pseudoaneurysm breaks into the lumen of the gut or pancreatic duct, bile duct, or retroperitoneum itself. A few pancreaticoduodenal artery pseudoaneurysms have also been reported. These findings usually go undiagnosed without the use of CT or Doppler ultrasound.

The differential consideration that has to be excluded is a pancreatic pseudocyst. CT scanning with the use of intravenous contrast material can be definitive in most cases. Blood flow in the pseudoaneurysm can be detected with Doppler ultrasound in most cases. Physical examination is usually not productive, although pulsations detected during physical examination in the pancreatic bed of patients with chronic pancreatitis were diagnostic before widespread imaging; much of this art is lost today. Gastroduodenal artery pseudoaneurysms can occur in settings other than chronic alcoholism. Any condition that can result in pancreatitis can theoretically result in such a complication.

Notes

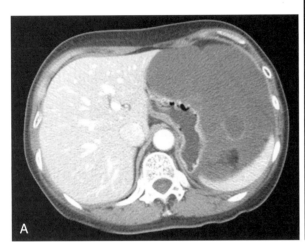

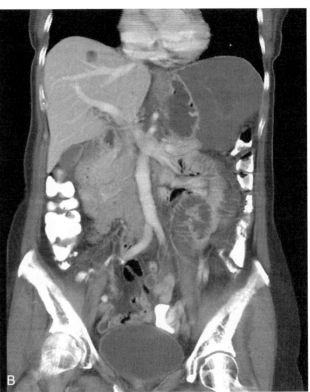

History: A 44-year-old woman presents with abdominal pain.

1. What should be included in the differential diagnosis of the imaging finding shown in Figure A? (Choose all that apply.)
   A. Subphrenic fluid collection
   B. Pancreatic cystic lesion
   C. Gastric cystic mass
   D. Splenic cystic mass
   E. Colon carcinoma

2. Where are gastrointestinal stromal tumors (GISTs) most commonly found?
   A. Small bowel
   B. Esophagus
   C. Stomach
   D. Colon

3. What is the most common imaging morphology of a GIST?
   A. Intraluminal polyp
   B. Predominantly cystic mass
   C. Intramural, submucosal mass
   D. Exophytic, extragastric extension

4. What is the most common cause of a bulky gastric tumor?
   A. Carcinoma
   B. Lymphoma
   C. Metastases
   D. Stromal tumor

Cystic Gastric GIST

1. A, B, C, and D

2. C

3. D

4. A

References

Darnell A, Dalmau E, Pericay C, et al: Gastrointestinal stromal tumors. *Abdom Imaging* 2006;31(4):387-399.

Levy AD, Remotti HE, Thompson WM, et al: Gastrointestinal stromal tumors: radiologic features with pathologic correlation. *Radiographics* 2003;23(2):283-304.

Cross-Reference

Gastrointestinal Imaging: *THE REQUISITES,* 3rd ed, p 77.

Comment

Many GISTs encountered in the bowel and particularly the stomach behave in a benign fashion. They may be ulcerated and bleed if in the wall of the bowel. Most are solid tumors, although some show areas of tumor necrosis and liquefaction and resultant mixed density. The GIST in this case shown on CT is problematic because it does not seem to be "arising" from any particular organ and is almost entirely cystic, with the exception of some foci of density seen on the axial view (see figures). Initially, GISTs were considered mesenchymal or smooth muscle tumors, leiomyomas, or leiomyosarcoma. However, further histologic investigation suggested a surprising lack of smooth muscle elements in the lesion. As a result, the term *gastrointestinal stromal cell tumor* was introduced to denote more correctly the spindle cell and epithelioid elements that compose these tumors.

The tumor can undergo considerable necrosis and manifest as near-cystic lesions in some cases. However, there is also a distinctive morphologic variant of characterized by myxoid content that is well encapsulated, cystic in appearance, mostly seen arising exophytically from the stomach, and mostly seen in women, and such a lesion is shown in this case.

Notes

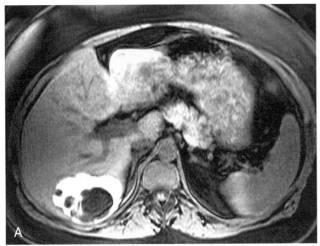
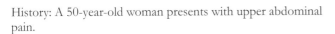
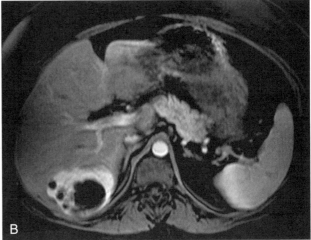

History: A 50-year-old woman presents with upper abdominal pain.

1. What should be included in the differential diagnosis of the imaging finding shown in Figure A? (Choose all that apply.)
   A. Hydatid cyst
   B. Hemangioma
   C. Hepatic abscess
   D. Biliary hamartoma
   E. Biliary cystadenoma

2. Which of the following statements regarding biliary cystadenomas is *true*?
   A. Biliary cystadenomas are more common in women.
   B. The most common presentation is jaundice.
   C. Most progress to cystadenocarcinoma.
   D. The treatment of choice is enucleation of the cyst.

3. Which of the following imaging features is most useful to differentiate a biliary cystic neoplasm from a simple hepatic cyst?
   A. Lesion size
   B. Thick outer wall
   C. Ductal dilation
   D. Lobulated contour

4. What might ultrasound show in a biliary cystadenoma that is not evident in these MRI images and might not be seen with CT?
   A. Septations
   B. Calcification
   C. Mural nodules
   D. Left lobe location

Cystadenoma of the Biliary Ducts

1. A, C, and E

2. A

3. C

4. A

References

Kim JY, Kim SH, Eun HW, et al: Differentiation between biliary cystic neoplasms and simple cysts of the liver: accuracy of CT. *AJR Am J Roentgenol* 2010;195(5):1142-1148.

Korobkin M, Stephens DH, Lee JKT, et al: Biliary cystadenoma and cystadenocarcinoma: CT and sonographic findings. *AJR Am J Roentgenol* 1989;153(3):507-511.

Cross-Reference

Gastrointestinal Imaging: *THE REQUISITES,* 3rd ed, p 203.

Comment

Biliary cystadenomas are rare cystic lesions arising from the bile ducts (see figures). They are most commonly seen in middle-aged women and have some malignant potential. Patients often present with upper abdominal discomfort; rarely, jaundice or mass effect is the presentation. The finding may be incidental most of the time. The lesions are multiloculated and septated, and this is usually more apparent with ultrasound than with CT or MRI.

Because this lesion has malignant potential, and diagnostic imaging is unable to differentiate between a cystadenoma and a cystadenocarcinoma, needle aspiration biopsy or surgical removal is usually required for definitive histologic diagnosis. Both are slow-growing, and both can have similar imaging appearances. The lesions can be of varying sizes, with some 3 to 5 cm and others 30 cm. Alternative diagnostic considerations include hepatic abscess and congenital biliary cysts. The latter are usually multiple, and biliary cystadenomas are usually solitary. In the array of cystic lesions that may be seen in the liver, cystadenomas must be considered relatively rare, accounting for 1% to 5% of all hepatic cystic processes. In some reported cases, symptomatic patients with a cystadenoma were misdiagnosed (i.e., a hydatid cyst). Generally, when a multiloculated septated cyst (usually in the right lobe of the liver) is discovered in a middle-aged woman, biliary cystadenoma or cystadenocarcinoma should be considered in the differential diagnosis.

Notes

Note: Page numbers followed by *f* indicate figures.

C

Killian-Jamieson diverticulum, 275f, 276
Kirkland complex, 61–62
Klatskin's tumor, 70
Kupffer cells, 188

L

Laceration
    liver, 95f, 96
    splenic, 26
Ladd's bands, 316
Laennec's cirrhosis, 112
Laryngeal nerve injury, recurrent, 259
Laxative abuse, 244
Left colon, indolent lesion of, 302
Left pleural effusion, 144
Left-sided colonic cancer obstruction with perforation, 302
Leiomyomas, 67
    benign, 388
    huge myometrial, 318
    uterine, 318
Leiomyosarcomas, 67
Leomyomatosis of esophagus, multiple, 388
LES (lower esophageal sphincter), 10
Lesions
    APUD (amine precursor uptake and decarboxylation), 116
    bull's-eye, 77–78
    of epiploic appendagitis, 337
    intrahepatic cystic, 324
    malignant and benign pelvic, 87
    presacral space, 21
    primary duodenal, 230
    right-sided, 302
    skin conditions and tiny esophageal nodular, 73
Lesions of bones, lytic expansile, 384
Lesions of mesentery, fibrotic, 126
Lesions to stomach
    hematogenous metastatic, 77
    metastatic, 78
Leukemia, 174
Ligament
    spread of gastric carcinoma to colon via gastrocolic, 242
    of Treitz, 288
Linea semilunaris, 104
Linitis plastica of stomach, 93f, 94, 355
"Linitis-like" picture, 356
Lipogenic tumors, 148
Lipomas and small bowel tumors, 16
Lipomatosis or fibrosis, retroperitoneal, 22
Liposarcomas of abdomen, 147f, 148
Liver, 149
    alcoholic cirrhosis of, 202
    cirrhosis of, 112
    focal nodular hyperplasia (FNH) of, 188
    gas in periphery of, 65
    hemangiomas of, 214
    high density in fluid adjacent to, 95
    injuries to spleen and, 142
    iron deposition in, 195, 196
    laceration, 95f, 96
    nutmeg, 336
    portal venous system of, 65
    transplantation, 395
Liver and speen, microabscesses of, 354
Liver disease, cirrhosis and severe, 181
Liver enzymes, abnormalities of, 150
Liver in chest, diaphragmatic rupture with, 258
Liver in young patients, neoplasms of, 262
Liver lesions in children, calcified, 217
Liver trauma, blunt, 96
Lobe enlargement, caudate, 335
Lobular carcinoma, 253
Lower rib fractures and splenic injury in blunt trauma, 25
Lung
    cancer, 152

Lung (Continued)
    distal metastatic disease to, 60
    small cell carcinoma of, 78
    tumors involved with paraneoplastic syndrome, 378
Lymph nodes
    abdominal tuberculosis site, 297
    pericolic, 301
Lymph tissue, pharynx and hypopharynx of, 152
Lymphangioma
    cavernous, 384
    circumscriptum, 384
    cystic, 384
    fetal alcohol syndrome and, 383
    of spleen, 383f, 384
Lymphoid aggregates in ileum, 357–358
Lymphoid follicles, 120
Lymphoid hyperplasia
    benign, 36
    normal finding in children, 358
    of terminal ileum, 357f, 358
Lymphoma, 38, 78. See also Pseudolymphoma
    and adenocarcinomas, gastric malignancies, 264
    Burkitt's, 374
    B-cell, 386
    colon and Burkitt's, 374
    development of, 224
    EBV and Burkitt's, 374
    and esophageal varices, 206
    gastric, 42
    gastrointestinal, 41
    HIV and Burkitt's, 374
    Hodgkin's, 42
    non-Hodgkin's, 42, 364, 386
    of pancreatic head, 385f, 386
    small bowel, 52, 224
        and stomach, 42, 223
    of stomach
        desmoplastic, 94
        primary, 41
    T-cell, 386
Lymphomatous masses, 280
Lymphomatous nodes, foamy, 52
Lynch syndrome, 227
Lytic expansile lesions of bones, 384

M

Macklin's pathway, 32
Macroglobulinemia, Waldenström's, 358
Malabsorption, small bowel, 98
Male patients, hemochromatosis and, 195
Malignancies
    gastric, 19–20
    IBD and, 63
    ulcerated gastric, 62
Malignancies, perivaterian, 156
Malignant lesion of duodenum, primary, 37
Malignant melanoma, 77
Malignant neoplasms, primary gastric, 42
Malignant ulcer of stomach, 19f, 20
Mallory-Weiss
    syndrome, 209
    tear, 210
Malrotation associated with heterotaxy, 287
Marfan's syndrome, 192
Mass effect displacing bowel, 182
Mastocytosis of small bowel, 271f, 272
Mature cystic teratomas, 72
McBurney's point, 6
Mechanical small bowel obstruction, 175
Meckel's diverticulum, 103, 255f, 256
Medulloblastomas, 80
Melanoma, 152, 164
    malignant, 77
    metastasis and gastrointestinal tract, 77